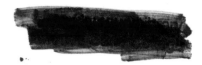

Atlas of
Sleep
Medicine

Atlas of Sleep Medicine

Sudhansu Chokroverty, M.D., F.R.C.P., F.A.C.P.
Professor and Co-Chair of Neurology
Program Director, Clinical Neurophysiology
   and Sleep Medicine
New Jersey Neuroscience Institute at JFK and
   Seton Hall University
Edison, New Jersey

Meeta Bhatt, M.D., Ph.D.
Assistant Professor
Department of Neurology
New York University Medical Center
Director
New York Sleep Institute
New York, New York

Robert J. Thomas, M.D., M.M.Sc.
Instructor in Medicine
Harvard Medical School
Instructor in Medicine, Pulmonary, Critical
   Care and Sleep
Beth Israel Deaconess Medical Center
Boston, Massachusetts

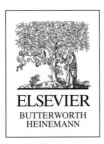

ELSEVIER
BUTTERWORTH
HEINEMANN

ELSEVIER
BUTTERWORTH
HEINEMANN

The Curtis Center
170 S Independence Mall W 300E
Philadelphia, Pennsylvania 19106

ATLAS OF SLEEP MEDICINE
Copyright 2005, Elsevier, Inc. All rights reserved.

Notice

Medicine is an ever-changing field. Standard safety precautions must be followed, but as new research and clinical experience broaden our knowledge, changes in treatment and drug therapy may become necessary or appropriate. Readers are advised to check the most current product information provided by the manufacturer of each drug to be administered to verify the recommended dose, the method and duration of administration, and contraindications. It is the responsibility of the treating physician, relying on experience and knowledge of the patient, to determine dosages and the best treatment for each individual patient. Neither the Publisher nor the author assume any liability for any injury and/or damage to persons or property arising from this publication.

The Publisher

Library of Congress Control Number: 2005921969

ISBN-13: 978-0-7506-7398-3
ISBN-10: 0-7506-7398-2

Acquisitions Editor: *Susan Pioli*
Developmental Editor: *Laurie Anello*
Project Manager: *David Saltzberg*

Printed in the United States of America.

Last digit is the print number: 9 8 7 6 5 4 3

Contents

Contributors

JÉRÔME ARGOD, Ph.D.
Department of Physiology and HP2 Laboratory (Hypoxia Pathophysiology)
Inserm Espri
Joseph Fourier University
Sleep Laboratory
Clinical Physiology
University Hospital
Grenoble, France

ALON Y. AVIDAN, M.D., M.P.H.
Clinical Assistant Professor
Department of Neurology
University of Michigan Medical Center
Director,
Sleep Disorders Clinic
Sleep Disorders Center
Ann Arbor, Michigan

MEETA BHATT, M.D., Ph.D.
Assistant Professor
Department of Neurology
New York University Medical Center
Director
New York Sleep Institute
New York, New York

SUDHANSU CHOKROVERTY, M.D., F.R.C.P., F.A.C.P.
Professor and Co-Chair of Neurology
Clinical Neurophysiology and Sleep Medicine
New Jersey Neuroscience Institute at JFK and
    Seton Hall University
Edison, New Jersey

DEBORAH DALE, M.Sc.
Department of Physiology and HP2 Laboratory (Hypoxia Pathophysiology)
Inserm Espri
Joseph Fourier University
Sleep Laboratory
Clinical Physiology
University Hospital
Grenoble, France

TAMMY GOLDHAMMER, R. EEGT, R. PSG-T, B.S.
Supervisor
Clinical Neurophysiology Section
Department of Neurology
Saint Vincent Catholic Medical Center
New York, New York

TIMOTHY F. HOBAN, M.D.
Clinical Associate Professor
Departments of Pediatrics and Neurology
University of Michigan
Ann Arbor, Michigan

PATRICK LÉVY, M.D., Ph.D.
Professor and Head
Department of Physiology and HP2 Laboratory (Hypoxia Pathophysiology)
Inserm Espri
Joseph Fourier University
Chief
Sleep Laboratory and Department of Clinical Physiology
University Hospital
Grenoble, France

PASQUALE MONTAGNA, M.D.
Professor of Neurology
Department of Neurological Sciences
University of Bologna Medical School
Bologna, Italy

LIBORIO PARRINO, M.D., Ph.D.
University Researcher
Department of Neuroscience
University of Parma
Parma, Italy

JEAN-LOUIS PÉPIN, M.D., Ph.D.
Professor of Clinical Physiology
Physiology Department and HP2 Laboratory (Hypoxia
    Pathophysiology)
Inserm Espri
Joseph Fourier University
Clinical and Research Physician
Sleep Laboratory and Department of Respiratory
    Medicine
University Hospital
Grenoble, France

STEPHEN D. PITTMAN, MSBME, R. PSG-T
Research Technologist
Division of Sleep Medicine
Brigham and Women's Hospital
Boston, Massachusetts

ARIANNA SMERIERI, Ph.D.
Department of Neuroscience and Sleep Disorders
    Center
University of Parma
Parma, Italy

MARIO GIOVANNI TERANZO, M.D.
Professor of Neurology
Department of Neuroscience
University of Parma
Parma, Italy

ROBERT J. THOMAS, M.D., M.M.Sc.
Instructor in Medicine
Harvard Medical School
Instructor in Medicine
Department of Pulmonary, Critical Care and Sleep
Beth Israel Deaconess Medical Center
Boston, Massachusetts

MARCO ZUCCONI, M.D.
Assistant Professor of Neurology
Department of Neurology
Vita-Salute San Raffaele University
Senior Neurologist
Sleep Disorders Center
Hospital San Rafaele
Milan, Italy

Preface

The importance of sleep has been reflected in the writings of Eastern and Western religions and civilization since time immemorial. The history of sleep research has been a history of remarkable progress and remarkable ignorance. In the 1940s and 1950s sleep had been in the forefront of neuroscience. Again in the 1990s there was a resurgence in our understanding of the neurobiology of sleep. Several textbooks of sleep medicine, including a couple of atlases, have been published attesting to such growth. The basic knowledge in the text can be significantly augmented by including a number of illustrations, proving the old adage that a picture is worth a thousand words. Hence the usefulness of an atlas encompassing some textual materials accompanied by appropriate illustrations that emphasize clinical-physiological correlation for the sake of a correct diagnosis and treatment of a sleep disorder. The best way to learn is to take a look at a tracing, identify the deviation from normal, and understand the significance in light of the clinical features. Laboratory techniques, particularly polysomnographic (PSG) study as well as other related procedures, remain the cornerstone for definitive diagnosis of a number of sleep disorders. It must be remembered, however, that these laboratory techniques must be subservient to a careful evaluation of the clinical history and physical examination. Thus, we have tried in this atlas to provide correlation of the clinical features with the physiologic findings as recorded by the PSG and other laboratory techniques. Our objective is to produce a comprehensive and contemporary atlas illustrating numerous examples of PSG and other tracings accompanied by sufficient clinical details so that the reader can formulate a clear view of the big picture.

The *Atlas* is divided into 13 chapters covering the techniques, clinical pattern recognition, continuous and bi- level positive airway pressure titration (CPAP and BIPAP), and PSG changes, and a section on pediatric sleep medicine. Chapter 11, dealing with specialized techniques, includes recently introduced topics of pulse transit time and peripheral arterial tonometry in addition to the recognition and usefulness of the cyclic alternating pattern (CAP), which has great potential for understanding the microstructure of sleep.

The *Atlas* should be useful not only to all sleep specialists in a variety of fields, including neurologists, pulmonologists, cardiologists and other internists, psychiatrists, psychologists, otolaryngologists, and dentists, but also to others who may have an interest in advancing the practical knowledge in sleep medicine, such as the EEG and PSG technologists, fellows, residents, and medical students.

We must express our gratitude to all the contributing authors for their scholarly contributions. We'd like to acknowledge Susan Pioli, Executive Publisher of Global Medicine at Elsevier Science for her professionalism, helpful attitude and patience during all stages of production of the *Atlas*. We wish to thank also Laurie Anello at Elsevier Science and the staff at Graphic World Publishing Services for their efforts in trying to speed up the process of publication. The senior editor would like to acknowledge his indebtedness to his wife, Manisha Chokroverty, M.D., for her unfailing support, love and patience during the long and arduous preparation of this *Atlas*. Finally, all of us would like to thank our patients and the trainees for motivating us to reach the highest level of excellence in patient care and education.

Sudhansu Chokroverty
Robert J. Thomas
Meeta Bhatt

Abbreviations

ABD	abdominal respiratory effort	OSA	obstructive sleep apnea
BiPAP	bilevel positive airway pressure	OSAS	obstructive sleep apnea syndrome
BKUP	backup EMG channel	PLEDS	periodic or pseudoperiodic lateralized epileptiform discharges
CAPN	capnogram		
CHIN	chin EMG	PES	esophageal pressure
CMRR	common mode rejection ratio	PLMD	periodic limb movement disorder
CPAP	continuous positive airway pressure	PLMS	periodic limb movements in sleep
EDS	excessive daytime sleepiness	PSG	polysomnogram
EEG	electroencephalogram	PTT	pulse transit time
EKG	electrocardiogram	RAT	right anterior tibialis surface electromyogram
EMG	electromyogram		
EOG	electrooculogram	REM	rapid eye movement sleep
EPSP	excitatory postsynaptic potentials	NREM	non-rapid eye movement sleep
ESS	Epworth Sleepiness Scale	ROC	right electrooculogram
ETCO2	average end-tidal CO_2	SaO2	hemoglobin oxygen saturation
IPSP	inhibitory postsynaptic potentials	SNOR	snore channel
LAT	left anterior tibialis surface electromyogram	SNORE	snore sensor
LOC	left electrooculogram	SOREM	sleep-onset REM period
MAs	microarousals	SpO2	pulse oximetry
MID	mid-abdominal effort	SSS	Stanford Sleepiness Scale
MSLT	multiple sleep latency test	TIRDA	temporal intermittent rhythmic delta activity
MWT	maintenance of wakefulness test	THOR	thoracic respiratory effort
N/O	nasal and oral airflow	UARES	upper airway resistance episodes
NPRE	nasal pressure transducer	UARS	upper airway resistance syndrome

1

Polysomnographic Recording Technique

SUDHANSU CHOKROVERTY, MEETA BHATT, AND TAMMY GOLDHAMMER

Polysomnography (PSG) is the single most important laboratory technique for assessment of sleep and its disorders. PSG records multiple physiological characteristics simultaneously during sleep at night. These recordings allow assessment of sleep stages and wakefulness, respiration, cardiocirculatory functions, and body movements. Electroencephalography (EEG), electrooculography (EOG), and electromyography (EMG) of the chin muscles are recorded to score sleep staging. Respiratory recording includes measurements of airflow and respiratory effort. PSG also records electrocardiography (EKG), finger oximetry, limb muscle activity, particularly EMG of the tibialis anterior muscles bilaterally, snoring, and body positions. Special techniques, which are not used routinely, include measurements of intraesophageal pressure, esophageal pH, and penile tumescence for assessment of patient with erectile dysfunction. After recording, the data are then analyzed and interpreted by the sleep clinician. A single daytime nap study generally does not record rapid eye movement (REM) sleep, the stage in which most severe apneic episodes and maximum oxygen desaturation are noted. Hence, a daytime study cannot assess the severity of symptoms. There may be false-negative studies as mild cases of sleep apnea may be missed during daytime study. Furthermore, during continuous positive airway pressure (CPAP) titration, an all night sleep study is essential to determine the optimum level of titration pressure during both REM and non-REM (NREM) sleep.

It is important to remember that polysomnographic study is really an extension of the physical examination of the sleeping patient. Before the actual recording an adequate knowledge of patient preparation, laboratory environment, and some technical aspect of the equipment is needed.

PATIENT PREPARATION AND LABORATORY ENVIRONMENT

The technologist performing the study must have basic knowledge about the PSG equipment including the amplifiers, filters, sensitivities, and simple troubleshooting. The technologist should also have an adequate knowledge about the PSG findings of important sleep disorders and must have full clinical information so that he or she may make the necessary protocol adjustments for the most efficient recording. On arrival in the laboratory, the patient should be adequately informed about the entire procedure and should be shown through the laboratory. Ideally, the laboratory should be located in an area that is free from noise and the room temperature should be optimal. The sleeping room in the laboratory should be a comfortable room, similar to the patient's bedroom at home, so that it is easy for the patient to relax and fall asleep. The recording equipment should be in an adjacent room and the patient should be advised about the audiovisual equipment. Some patients might feel comfortable if they are allowed to bring their own pillow as well as their pajamas and a book for reading.

Technical Considerations and Polysomnography Equipment

Equipment for recording PSG contains a series of amplifiers with high- and low-frequency filters and different sensitivity settings. The amplifiers used consist of both alternating current (AC) and direct current (DC) amplifiers. The AC amplifiers are used to record physiological characteristics showing high frequencies such as EEGs, EOGs, EMGs, and EKGs. The AC amplifier contains both high- and low-frequency filters. Using appropriate filters, one may record a specific band within the signal; for example, slow potentials can be attenuated by using low-frequency filters. DC amplifiers have no low-frequency filters and are typically used to record potentials with slow frequency such as the output from the oximeter, the output from the pH meter, CPAP titration pressure changes, and intraesophageal pressure readings. AC or DC amplifiers may be used to record respiratory flow and effort. An understanding of the amplifiers, along with the filters, and sensitivities is important for optimal PSG recording. The PSG equipment uses differential amplifiers, which amplify the difference between the two amplifier inputs. The differential amplifier augments the difference between two electrode inputs, which is an advantage because unwanted extraneous environmental noise, which is likely to be seen at the two electrodes, is subtracted out and therefore cannot contaminate the recording. The ability of the amplifier to suppress an extraneous signal such as noise that is simultaneously present in both electrodes is measured by the common mode rejection ratio (CMRR). Ideally, this ratio must exceed 1000 to 1, but most contemporary PSG amplifiers use a ratio in excess of 10,000 to 1. The currents and voltages generated by the cerebral cortex, eyes, and heart during the PSG recordings are extremely small and through amplification this tiny voltage is transformed into an interpretable record by manipulating the sensitivity switch. Sensitivity is expressed in microvolts per millimeter or millivolts per centimeter. Sensitivity switches should be adjusted to obtain sufficient amplitude for interpretation. Sensitivity and filter settings vary according to the physiological characteristics recorded. (See Table 1–1.)

Following subtraction and amplification of the voltages at the two inputs, the signal is then passed through a series of filters. Two types of filters are used in PSG recordings: a high-pass filter (also known as a low-frequency filter) and a low-pass filter (also known as a high-frequency filter). A high-pass filter allows higher frequencies to pass unchanged while attenuating lower frequencies. A

low-pass filter, in contrast, allows lower frequencies to pass unchanged while attenuating higher frequencies. The other filter, present in most PSG amplifiers, is a 60-hertz notch filter, which attenuates main frequency while attenuating activity of surrounding frequency less extensively. EEG recording is easily contaminated by 60-hertz artifact if the electrode application and impedance are suboptimal. The 60-hertz filter, however, should be used sparingly because some important components in the recording, such as muscle activity and epileptiform spikes, may be attenuated by a notch filter. Most of the time the differential amplifier is sufficient to reject 60-hertz artifacts.

The standard speed for recording traditional PSG is 10 mm/sec, so that each monitor screen or page is a 30-second epoch. A 30-mm/sec recording speed is used for easy identification of epileptiform activities. Analog recording using paper is being replaced in most of the laboratories by digital system recordings (see later).

It is important to have a facility for simultaneous video recording to monitor behavior during sleep. It is advantageous to use two cameras to view the entire body. A low light level camera should be used to obtain good quality video in the dark, and an infrared light source should be available after turning the laboratory lights off. The monitoring station should have remote control that can zoom, tilt, or pan the camera for adequate viewing. The camera should be mounted on the wall across from the head end of the bed. An intercom from a microphone near the patient should be available.

Electroencephalography

It is important for the polysomnographer and the polysomnographic technologist to be familiar with the principles of EEG recording and should have adequate knowledge about normal waking and sleep EEG rhythms in various age groups as well as major patterns of abnormalities that may be encountered during PSG recording (see Section II).

Table 1–1. Filter and sensitivity settings for polysomnographic studies

Characteristics	High-Frequency Filter (Hz)	Time Constant (sec)	Low-Frequency Filter (Hz)	Sensitivity
Electroencephalogram	70 or 35	0.4	0.3	5–7 µV/mm
Electro-oculogram	70 or 35	0.4	0.3	5–7 µV/mm
Electromyogram	90	0.04	5.0	2–3 µV/mm
Electrocardiogram	15	0.12	1.0	1 mV/cm to start; adjust
Airflow and effort	15	1	0.1	5–7 µV/mm; adjust

Electrooculography

EOG records corneoretinal (relative positivity at the cornea and a relative negativity at the retina) potential difference. Any eye movement changes the orientation of the dipole and it is the movement of the dipole that is recorded by the EOG. Gold cup or silver-silver chloride electrodes can be used to monitor the EOG. A typical electrode placement is 1 centimeter superior and lateral to the outer canthus of one eye with a second electrode placed one cm inferior and lateral to the outer canthus of the opposite eye. Both these electrodes are then connected to a single reference electrode, either the same ear or the mastoid process of the temporal bone. Therefore, right outer canthus (ROC) and left outer canthus (LOC) electrodes are referred to as either A1 or A2. In this arrangement, conjugate eye movements produce out-of-phase deflections in the two channels whereas the EEG slow activities contaminating the eye electrodes are in-phase. Both conjugate horizontal and vertical eye movements are detected by this placement scheme. The sensitivity and filter settings for EOG are similar to those used for EEG.

Several varieties of eye movements are recorded during routine PSG: waking eye movements (WEMs), slow eye movements (SEMs), and REMs. During wakefulness both eye blinks and saccadic eye movements produce WEMs. During stage I sleep, SEMs are recorded consistently in the horizontal axis. SEMs generally disappear in the deeper stages of NREM sleep. During REM sleep, characteristic REMs appear which are noted in all directions (horizontal, oblique, and vertical), although they are most prominently seen in the horizontal axis. REMs typically occur in bursts. In addition to finding these three types of eye movements, Santamaria and Chiappa, using a sensitive motion transducer, recorded small, fast, irregular eye movements in about 60 percent of normal subjects in early drowsiness before the appearance of SEMs. They also noted small, fast, rhythmic eye movements generally associated with the traditional SEMs in about 30 percent of normal subjects.

Electromyography Recording During Standard Polysomnography

EMG activities are important physiological characteristics that need to be recorded for sleep staging as well as for diagnosis and classification of a variety of sleep disorders. EMG represents electrical activities of muscle fibers as a result of depolarization of the muscles following transmission of electrical impulses along the nerves and neuromuscular junctions. There is a fundamental tone in the muscle during wakefulness and NREM sleep, but this is markedly diminished or absent in major muscle groups during REM sleep. EMG activities could be tonic, dystonic and phasic (including myoclonic bursts), or rhythmic. A dystonic muscle burst refers to prolonged EMG activities lasting for 500 to 1000 milliseconds or longer. Phasic bursts may include EMG activities phasically related to inspiratory bursts. Myoclonic muscle bursts are also phasic bursts, which are characteristically noted during REM sleep and may be seen as excessive fragmentary myoclonus also during NREM sleep in many sleep disorders. Myoclonic bursts refer to EMG activities lasting for a brief duration of generally 20 to 250 milliseconds, sometimes up to 500 milliseconds. In patients with tremor, EMG may record rhythmic activities.

In a standard PSG recording, EMGs are recorded from mentalis or submental and right and left tibialis anterior muscles. Mental or submental EMG activity is monitored to record axial muscle tone, which is significantly decreased during REM sleep and, therefore, an important physiological characteristic for identifying REM sleep. EMG is recorded using a gold cup or a silver-silver chloride electrode applied to a clean surface using a tape or electrode glue. For chin EMG recordings, at least three EMG electrodes are applied so that in the event of a problem with one of the electrodes the additional electrode can be connected during the recording without disturbing the patient. Generally, the mentalis muscle on one side is connected to the mentalis muscle on the other side, and an additional electrode is placed in the submental muscle. The electrode impedance should be less than 5 K. The high- and low-frequency filter settings for the EMG recordings are different from those used for EEG and EOG, and are listed in Table 1–1. The sensitivity should be at least 20 microvolts per centimeter for mental or submental EMG activity. Additional electrodes may be needed in patients with bruxism (tooth grinding) over the masseter muscles to document associated bursts of EMG activities.

For recording from tibialis anterior muscles surface electrodes are used over tibialis anterior muscles and the distance between the two electrodes is 2 to 2.5 centimeters. Bilateral tibialis anterior EMG is important to record in patients suspected of restless legs syndrome (RLS) because the periodic limb movements in sleep (PLMS), which are noted in 80 percent of such patients, may alternate between the two legs. Ideally, the recording should also include one or two EMG channels from the upper limbs in patients with RLS as occasionally PLMS are noted in the upper limbs. For patients with suspected REM behavior disorder, multiple muscle EMGs from all four limbs are essential as there is often a dissociation of the activities between upper and lower limb muscles in such patients. The upper limb surface electrodes could be placed over extensor digitorum communis muscles with a separation of distance of 2 to 2.5 centimeters. If the upper limbs are not included in the EMG in patients suspected of REM behavior disorder, REM sleep without atonia may be missed in some cases.

Other EMG recordings include intercostal and diaphragmatic EMG to record respiratory muscle activities. The intercostal EMG recorded from the seventh to ninth intercostal space with active electrodes on the anterior axillary line and the reference electrodes on the midaxillary line may also include some diaphragmatic muscle activity in addition to the intercostal activity. The diaphragmatic activities can be recorded by placing surface electrodes over the right or left side of the umbilicus or over the anterior costal margin, but these are contaminated by a mixture of intercostal activity and such noninvasive techniques are unreliable for quantitative assessment of diaphragmatic EMG. The true diaphragmatic activities are typically recorded by intraesophageal recording.

EMG shows progressively decreasing tone from wakefulness through stages I to IV of NREM sleep. In REM sleep, the EMG is markedly diminished or absent. In REM behavior disorder, a characteristic finding is absence of muscle atonia during REM sleep in the EMG recording and the presence of phasic muscle bursts repeatedly during REM sleep.

Electrocardiography

A single channel of EKG is sufficient during PSG recording by placing one electrode over the sternum and the other electrode at a lateral chest location. This recording detects bradytachyarrhythmias or other arrhythmias seen in many patients with obstructive sleep apnea syndrome (OSAS). Gold cup surface electrodes are used to record the EKG and Table 1–1 lists the filter settings and sensitivities for such recording.

RESPIRATORY MONITORING TECHNIQUE

Respiratory monitoring during PSG recording is a very important procedure. In fact, the common reason for referring a patient to a sleep laboratory for PSG is to exclude a diagnosis of sleep apnea-hypopnea syndrome. Therefore, the PSG recording must routinely include methods to monitor airflow and respiratory effort adequately to correctly classify and diagnose sleep-related breathing disorders.

Recording of Respiratory Effort

Respiratory effort can be measured by mercury-filled or piezoelectric strain gauges, inductive plethysmography, impedance pneumography, respiratory magnetometers, and respiratory muscle EMG. Most commonly, piezoelec-

tric strain gauges and inductive plethysmography are used to monitor respiratory effort.

Strain Gauges

Strain gauges are used to record thoracic and abdominal and, thus, respiratory movements. A piezoelectric strain gauge consists of a crystal that emits an electrical signal in response to changes in length or pressure. For all these devices, one belt is placed around the chest and another one is placed around the abdomen, which allows detection of the paradoxical movements indicating upper airway OSAS. Sometimes strain gauges may not be able to differentiate central from obstructive apneas. The other disadvantage of strain gauge includes displacement by body position and body movements interfering with the accuracy of measurements.

Respiratory Inductive Plethysmography

This measures changes in thoracoabdominal cross-sectional areas and the sum of these two compartments is proportional to airflow. Inductance refers to resistance to current flow. Transducers across the chest and abdomen detect changes in the cross-sectional areas of the thorax and abdomen during breathing. Similar to strain gauges, body movements and changes in body positions may displace the transducers, causing inaccuracy in measurements of the respiratory effort.

Impedance Pneumography

This technique may not precisely measure the respiratory pattern and the volume. Furthermore, there may be electrical interference and therefore, this technique is not generally used.

Respiratory Magnetometers

Respiratory magnetometers record the chest and abdominal motions in both the anteroposterior and lateral directions. This was used as a research technique but has not been popular in practical PSG.

Respiratory Muscle Electromyography

Intercostal and diaphragmatic EMG activities may be recorded to measure indirectly effort of breathing by attaching surface electrodes over the intercostal spaces and upper abdomen near the margins of the rectus abdominis muscles. It is really not possible to detect pure uncontaminated intercostal or diaphragmatic muscle activities by these techniques.

MEASUREMENT OF AIRFLOW

Airflow can be measured by thermistors, thermocouples, or nasal cannula–pressure transducers recording nasal pressure. A thermistor or thermocouple device between the nose and mouth is commonly used to monitor airflow to detect changes in temperature (e.g., cool air flows during inspiration and warm air flows during expiration). A thermistor consisting of wires records changes in electrical resistance, and thermocouples consisting of dissimilar metals (e.g., copper and constantan) register changes in voltage that result from temperature variation. Thermistors or thermocouples are not as sensitive as nasal pressure transducers for detecting airflow limitations and, hence, may miss hypopnea. For these reasons, nasal pressure technique to detect airflow should be used routinely during PSG recording. The other problems with thermistors or thermocouples are that they are easily displaced, causing false changes in airflow. Also, certain precautions should be taken while using thermistors and thermocouples. The thermistor or thermocouple temperature must be below body temperature in order to sense the temperature difference between expired and inspired air. Oronasal transducers also must not be in contact with the skin, otherwise the transducer temperature will not be below the body temperature.

Nasal Pressure Monitoring

During inspiration nasal airway pressure decreases and during expiration it increases. This alternate decrement and increment of nasal pressure produces electrical signals, which indirectly register airflow. In nasal pressure monitoring, a nasal cannula is connected to a pressure-sensitive transducer, which measures the pressure difference. Nasal pressure monitoring is more sensitive than thermocouples or thermistors in detecting airflow limitation and hypopnea. If there is airflow limitation and increased upper airway resistance, the nasal pressure monitor will register a plateau indicating a flow limitation. During nasal pressure recording, a DC amplifier or an AC amplifier with a long time constant should be used. One disadvantage is that nasal pressure cannula cannot be used to measure airflow in the mouth breathers and in patients with nasal obstruction.

Pneumotachography

This is an excellent technique to measure quantitatively the tidal volume and direct airflow measurement. However, this requires a sealed face mask, creating patient discomfort and sleep disturbance. Hence, it is not used in most of the laboratories.

Intraesophageal Pressure Monitoring

This is the best technique and, in fact, the gold standard for measuring respiratory effort. However, this is somewhat uncomfortable and invasive, requiring special expertise in acquiring the technique. It requires placing a nasogastric balloon-tipped catheter into the distal esophagus, which is very uncomfortable for the patient. Recently small fluid-filled esophageal catheters became available which are more comfortable and cause less disturbance of sleep. This technique is not used in most laboratories. Nasal pressure monitoring can also detect respiratory flow limitation and increased upper airway resistance. Whether nasal pressure monitoring is as good as esophageal pressure monitoring remains somewhat controversial. Esophageal pressure monitoring registers pleural pressure changes. In normal individuals during wakefulness, the pressure change is less than 5 centimeters of water and in sleep it is between 5 and 10 centimeters of water. Inspiration causes more negative pleural and hence esophageal pressure than expiration. Indications for esophageal pressure monitoring include correct classification of apneas as central or obstructive, detection of increased upper airway resistance, diagnosis of upper airway resistance syndrome, and correct classification of hypopnea as obstructive type.

Expired Carbon Dioxide

Capnography detects the expired carbon dioxide (CO_2) level, which closely approximates intra-alveolar CO_2. Capnography does detect both airflow and the partial pressure of CO_2 in alveoli, which is useful for evaluating OSAS, sleep hypoventilation, and an underlying pulmonary disease. An infrared analyzer over the nose and mouth detects CO_2 in the expired air, which qualitatively measures the airflow. This is the best noninvasive method to detect alveolar hypoventilation. The method is costly and therefore not used in most laboratories, but it should be used in children with suspected OSA.

Oxygen Saturation

The best way to detect arterial O_2 content (PaO_2) is by invasive method using an arterial cannula. This is not viable from the practical standpoint and in any case intermittent sampling of blood through the cannula may not reflect the severity of hypoxemia during a particular disordered breathing event. Therefore noninvasive method by finger pulse oximetry is routinely used to monitor arterial oxygen saturation (SaO_2) or arterial oxyhemoglobin saturation, which reflects the percentage of hemoglobin that is oxygenated. The difference in light absorption between oxyhemoglobin and deoxyhemoglobin determines oxygen saturation. Continuous monitoring of SaO_2 is crucial because it provides important information about the severity of respiratory dysfunction.

ESOPHAGEAL pH

This technique is a specialized procedure and is not used in standard PSG laboratories. Esophageal pH is monitored by asking patients to swallow a pH probe. Recording the output using a DC amplifier detects nocturnal gastro-esophageal reflux disease, which may be mistaken for sleep apnea or nocturnal angina as the patient may wake up choking or have severe chest pain as a result of acid eructation.

BODY POSITION MONITORING

Body position is monitored by placing sensors over one shoulder and using a DC channel. Snoring and apneas are generally worse in the supine position and therefore CPAP titration must include observing patients in the supine position for evaluating optimal pressure for titration.

SNORING

This can be monitored by placing a miniature microphone on the patient's neck. There is no generally accepted standardized technique to record quantitatively the intensity of snoring.

MONITORING OF PENILE TUMESCENCE

This is not used routinely in most of the sleep laboratories. Study of sleep-related penile erections remains limited to those researchers interested in understanding physiology of penile erections and occasionally used in some sleep laboratories to differentiate difficult and confusing cases of organic versus psychogenic impotence, and also for legal purposes to settle compensation claims. Strain gauges are used to measure penile tumescence. In normal adult men, penile tumescence occurs during REM sleep and this persists in psychogenic but not in organic impotence.

Table 1–2 lists the EEG montages and other monitors as recorded routinely for an overnight PSG study in our laboratory.

Figure 1–1 is a representative sample of an overnight PSG recording from our laboratory showing PLMS.

POLYSOMNOGRAPHY DOCUMENTATION

Important information should be clearly documented by the technologist before beginning the recording. This must include the patient's name, age, date of study, identifica-

Table 1–2. Typical overnight polysomnographic montage with continuous positive airway pressure titration used in our laboratory*

Channel Number	Name
1	F3-C3
2	F7-T3
3	T3-T5
4	T5-O1
5	F4-C4
6	F8-T4
7	T4-T6
8	T6-O2
9	C3-A2
10	C4-A1
11	Left electro-oculogram
12	Right electro-oculogram
13	Chin electromyogram (EMG)
14	Left tibialis EMG
15	Right tibialis EMG
16	Oronasal
17	Chest
18	Abdomen
19	Snoring
20	Electrocardiogram
21	Heart rate
22	Position
23	Arterial oxygen saturation
24	Continuous positive airway pressure

*Channels 1–10 record electroencephalogram using the 10–20 International System of electrode placement. Channel 16 records airflow. Channels 17 and 18 record respiratory effort.

tion number, purpose of the recording (before referring the patient to the laboratory for PSG study, sleep clinicians should have performed complete history and physical examination formulating a provisional diagnosis), and the name of the technician. Also "lights out" and "lights on" must be clearly marked, and a detailed description of any unusual behavior or motor events should be clearly indicated.

EQUIPMENT CALIBRATION

It is important to calibrate the PSG equipment and also to perform physiologic calibration prior to beginning testing in order to ensure that all amplifiers are functioning adequately. All-channel calibration followed by individual channel calibration is the first step. A known signal is sent through all the amplifiers, which are set to the same low- and high-frequency filter settings and sensitivities, thus testing proper functioning of all amplifiers. Appropriate filter settings and sensitivities are then set for each channel recording the various physiological characteristics, documenting individual channel calibration.

Montage: SLEEP   High Cut: 15 Hz   Low Cut: 1.00 Hz   Sensitivity: 7 µV/mm   Speed: 30 s/page

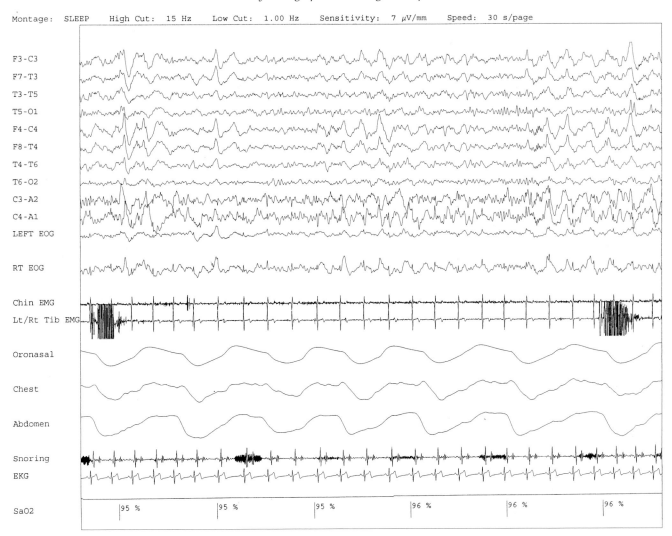

FIGURE 1–1. *A 30-second epoch of a representative sample of an overnight PSG recording from our laboratory showing PLMS. The sample is taken in stage II NREM sleep as shown by the presence of sleep spindles best defined in C3- and C4-derived EEG channels. Few slow waves of sleep are recorded on the EOC channels. Two PLMS are recorded in the Lt./Rt. Tib. EMG channel. The EKG artifact is noted to contaminate the chin EMG, Lt./Rt. Tib. EMG, and snoring channels. The in-phase deflections of respiratory channels are noted. A snore artifact is also recorded on the snoring channel. EEG, Top 10 channels; Lt. and Rt. EOG, left and right electrooculograms; chin EMG, electromyography of chin; Lt./Rt. Tib. EMG, left and right tibialis anterior electromyography; oronasal thermistor; chest and abdomen effort channels; snore monitor; EKG, electrocardiography; SaO2, oxygen saturation by finger oximetry.*

Physiologic Calibration

This is performed after application of the electrodes and other monitors to document proper functioning of these devices. Table 1–3 lists the instructions given for physiologic calibrations. On completion of all calibration procedures, the lights are turned out in the room and the patient is asked to lie down and try to sleep. Throughout the recording, the technologist should watch for any artifacts and make appropriate adjustments to obtain a good quality, relatively artifact-free recording for proper scoring and interpretation of the PSG.

ENDING THE TEST

When the patient is awakened in the morning (either spontaneously or at a set time), equipment and physiologic calibrations should be performed again to ensure that the equipment and all the devices have been continuously functioning properly throughout the night. The patient is then asked to fill out a post-study questionnaire, which includes estimation of time to fall asleep, total sleep time, number of awakenings, and the quality of sleep. For the safety of the patient, it is important to inquire about the

Table 1–3. Instructions for physiologic calibrations

Open eyes and look straight for 30 secs
Close eyes for 30 secs
Look left, right, up, and down
Blink eyes five times
Clench teeth
Inhale and exhale
Hold breath for 10 secs
Extend right hand and then left hand
Dorsiflex right foot and then left foot

mode of transportation that will be used by the patient before leaving the sleep laboratory.

SCORING OF AROUSALS

When EEG shows waking activities for 15 seconds or longer in a 30-second epoch, the scoring stage is *wakefulness*. Arousals are transient phenomena causing fragmentation of sleep and lasting less than 15 seconds. The American Academy of Sleep Medicine (AASM) established a task force to develop preliminary scoring rules for arousal. According to these preliminary rules, an EEG arousal is an abrupt shift in EEG frequency that may include alpha, theta, or beta activities but no spindle or delta waves (Figure 1–2) lasting for 3 to 14 seconds. The subject must be asleep for at least 10 continuous seconds before an arousal can be scored. Similarly, a minimum of 10 continuous seconds of intervening sleep is needed to score a second arousal. Arousals during REM sleep are scored only when accompanied by concurrent increase in submental EMG amplitude. It should be noted that in NREM sleep, arousals may occur without an increase in submental EMG amplitudes. Therefore, based only on submental EMG amplitude augmentation, an arousal cannot be scored. Delta waves, K complexes, and artifacts are not counted as arousals unless they are accompanied by frequency shifts. An arousal index is defined as the number of arousals per hour of sleep and an index above 10 can be considered abnormal.

SCORING OF PERIODIC LIMB MOVEMENTS IN SLEEP

PLMS are counted from the right and left tibialis anterior EMG recordings. The scoring criteria for PLMS can be summarized as follows: the movements must occur as part of four consecutive movements; the duration of each

EMG burst should be 0.5 to 5 seconds; the interval between bursts should be 4 to 90 seconds; the amplitude of the EMG bursts, although variable, should be more than 25 percent of the EMG bursts recorded during the presleep calibration recording. PLMS (Figures 1–3 through 1–5) may or may not be associated with arousals and they should be scored separately. To score PLMS associated with arousal, the arousal must occur within 3 seconds of onset of PLMS. PLMS is expressed as an index consisting of number of PLMS per hour of sleep. To be of pathological significance, the PLMS index should be 5 or more. Leg movements may be noted occurring periodically associated with resumption of breathing following recurrent episodes of apneas or hypopneas. These respiratory-related leg movements should not be counted as PLMS. PLMS are generally seen during NREM sleep but they can occur rarely during REM sleep. In patients with RLS, however, PLMS may also occur during wakefulness (Figure 1–6) when they are termed periodic limb movements in wakefulness (PLMW).

INDICATIONS FOR POLYSOMNOGRAPHY

The guidelines proposed by the AASM for performing overnight in-house attended PSG include the following:

- PSG is routinely indicated for the diagnosis of sleep-related breathing disorders.
- PSG is indicated for CPAP titration in patients with sleep-related breathing disorders.
- PSG is indicated in patients to evaluate for the presence of OSAS before undergoing laser-assisted uvulopalatopharyngoplasty (LAUP).
- PSG is indicated for assessment of therapeutic benefits after dental appliance treatment or after surgical treatment with moderately severe OSAS, including in patients whose symptoms reappear despite an initial good response.
- If the patient has lost or gained substantial weight, a follow-up PSG is indicated for assessment of treatment when the clinical response is insufficient or when symptoms reappear despite a good initial response to treatment with CPAP.
- An overnight PSG followed by a multiple sleep latency test is routinely indicated in patients suspected to have narcolepsy.
- PSG is indicated in patients with parasomnias that are unusual or atypical or behaviors that are violent or injurious to the patient or others. In uncomplicated and typical parasomnias, however, PSG is not routinely indicated.

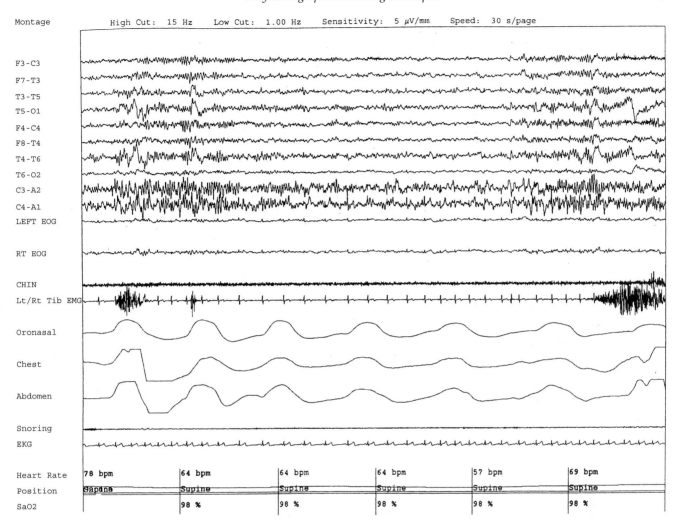

Montage   High Cut: 15 Hz   Low Cut: 1.00 Hz   Sensitivity: 5 µV/mm   Speed: 30 s/page

FIGURE 1–2. *PSG recording shows two brief periods of arousals in the left and right segments of the recording, each lasting about 6 to 7 seconds. Note 9- to 10-hertz alpha activities during arousals in the EEG channels and muscle bursts in the tibialis EMG. Also note movement artifacts in O1 and T6 electrodes. There is more than a 10-second segment of sleep between two arousals. EEG, Top 10 channels; Lt. and Rt. EOG, left and right electrooculograms; chin electromyography, Lt./Rt. Tib. EMG, left and right tibialis anterior electromyography; oronasal airflow, chest respiratory effort; abdomen respiratory effort; snoring; EKG, electrocardiography; SaO2, oxygen saturation by finger oxymetry. (From Chokroverty S. An overview of normal sleep. In Sleep and Movement Disorders, Figure 3–7. Philadelphia: Butterworth Heinemann, 2003, with permission.)*

- PSG is indicated in patients suspected of nocturnal seizures.
- PSG is not routinely performed to diagnose RLS but overnight PSG is indicated for patients with suspected PLMS.
- In patients with insomnia, PSG may be indicated if the response to a comprehensive behavioral or pharmacological treatment program for the management of insomnia is unsatisfactory. If, however, there is a strong suspicion of an associated sleep-related breathing disorder or associated PLMS in patients with insomnia, an overnight PSG is indicated.

There is some controversy regarding the diagnosis of periodic limb movement disorder (PLMD) causing sleep fragmentation, arousals, and excessive daytime sleepiness. PLMS have been noted in a number of sleep disorders as well as in normal individuals, particularly in patients over 60 to 65. Although the specificity of PLMS is not defined, at least 80 percent of patients with RLS show PLMS on PSG recordings. Therefore, to document PLMS in RLS, PSG may be indicated. However, the diagnosis of RLS is a clinical one and has been based on international study group criteria. PLMS are not part of these criteria nor is a sleep disturbance part of the minimal or essential criteria

Montage: SLEEP   High Cut: 35 Hz   Low Cut: 1.00 Hz   Sensitivity: 7 μV/mm   Speed: 120 s/page

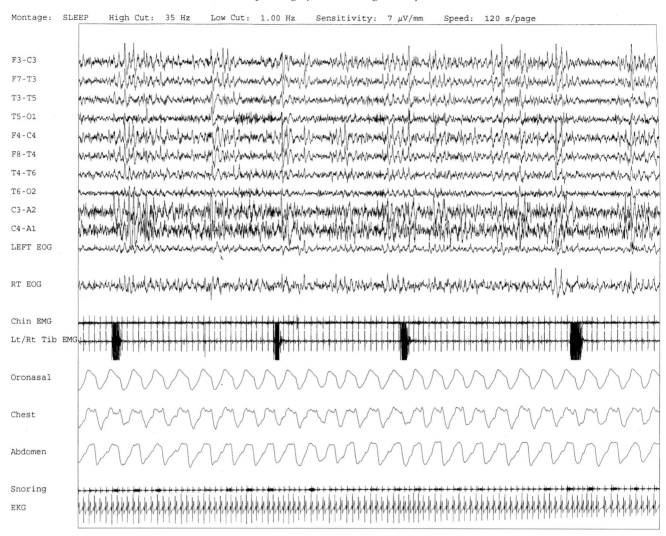

FIGURE 1–3. *A 120-second excerpt in stage II NREM sleep from an overnight PSG recording in a 29-year-old man with complaint of snoring since adolescence recently getting worse. He denies sensation of choking or difficulty breathing at night or excessive sleepiness in the daytime. Overnight PSG study did not show any evidence of sleep apnea, but showed an excessive number of periodic limb movements in sleep (PLMS) with a moderately increased periodic limb movement index of 28 and four sequential bursts of PLMS. The PLMS are not preceded by respiratory events or followed by electroencephalographic arousals. The montage used is the same as in Figure 1–1 without oxymetry display.*

for the diagnosis of RLS. PSG indications, therefore, for RLS-PLMS remain somewhat dubious and contentious. Some investigators do not believe in the existence of PLMD as a separate sleep disorder causing sleep dysfunction and excessive daytime somnolence (ESD). The indications for pure PLMS or PLMD currently remain undetermined and further investigations including outcome studies are needed to document that PLMS or PLMD may cause sleep disturbance and EDS.

Recently the German Sleep Society gathered a group of experts and developed consensus criteria for performing overnight PSG study in patients with RLS and these have

been recently published. These indications, however, have not been accepted generally outside the German Sleep Society at the present time.

VIDEO-POLYSOMNOGRAPHY RECORDING AND INDICATIONS

Video-PSG, which combines PSG with multiple EEG channels and simultaneous video recording, can help assess abnormal movements and behavior occurring during sleep. Such recordings can differentiate parasomnias from noc-

Montage: RLS Study   High Cut: 70 Hz   Low Cut: 0.53 Hz   Sensitivity: 10 μV/mm   Speed: 120 s/page

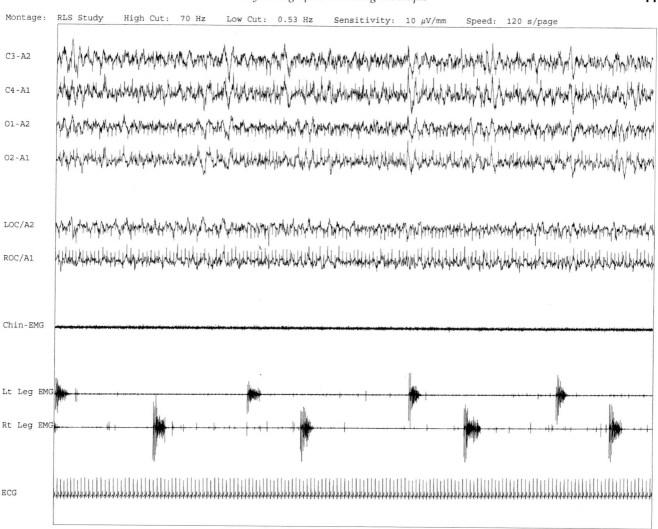

FIGURE 1–4. *A 33-year-old man with history of loud snoring for many years, frequent awakenings at night, and occasional gasping for breath in sleep. Additionally he complains of uncomfortable sensation in the legs at sleep onset with relief on movement or massage for the last 2 years. Clinical suspicion of mild upper airway obstructive sleep apnea and restless legs syndrome was raised. A 120-second excerpt from stage IV NREM sleep showing the presence of alternating limb movements on the left and right leg electromyography (EMG) channels. The limb movements occur at a frequency of approximately two per minute, each lasting about 3.9 to 6.7 seconds with alternation of sides, which has been well described. However, alternating leg muscle activation (ALMA) in sleep has been described recently and future studies may throw further light on the subject. Incidentally an electrocardiographic (EKG) artifact is noted superimposed on the electroencephalography (EEG) and oculogram channels. A modified montage shows the following: EEG, Top 4 channels; LOC/A2, left outer canthus referred to right ear electrode; ROC/A1, right outer canthus referred to left ear electrode; chin EMG, electromyography of chin; Lt. Leg EMG, left leg electromyography; Rt. Leg EMG, right leg electromyography; EKG, electrocardiography.*

turnal seizures, psychogenic dissociative disorders, and other diurnal movement disorders persisting during sleep at night. Clear documentation of abnormal motor manifestations, unusual and complex behaviors, characteristic EEG features of seizures, and other abnormal movements is possible. The video recording can include multiplexed analog signals captured on a tape, but many commercially available systems include digital video directly synchroniz-

ing and time-locking the abnormal behavior to the PSG signals. Depending on the availability of the channels and the electrode inputs in the equipment, multiple channels of EEGs (e.g., for a suspected nocturnal seizure disorder) and EMGs to include additional muscles (e.g., to record from forearm flexor and extensor muscles, masseter, and other muscles for patients with suspected REM behavior disorder [RBD] and bruxism) are recommended.

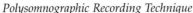

Montage: SLEEP   High Cut: 15 Hz   Low Cut: 1.00 Hz   Sensitivity: 7 μV/mm   Speed: 30 s/page

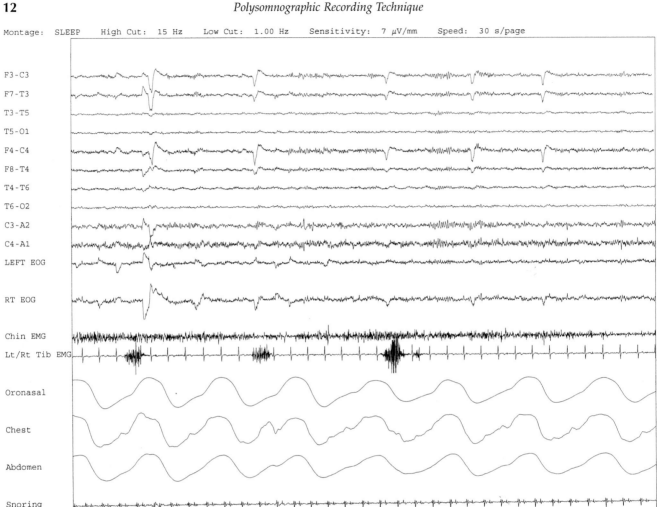

FIGURE 1–5. *A 30-second excerpt from an overnight PSG in 44-year-old man with complaints of unusual electrical sensation in the legs followed by twitching and jerking in the legs and frequent awakenings at night. He also reports occasional similar involvement in the arms. There is no accompanying history of urge to move or relief on movement. Three sequential bursts of periodic limb movements in waking (PLMW) are seen on tibialis anterior electromyography channel. Blink artifacts recur in the frontal and anterior temporal electrodes bilaterally. PLMW have been described in periodic limb movement disorder (PLMD) and restless legs syndrome (RLS). PLMW have the same definition as PLMS except the duration may be longer (0.5 to 10 seconds). EEG, Top 10 channels; left and right EOG, electrooculograms; electromyography of chin; Lt./Rt. Tib EMG, left/right tibialis anterior electromyography; oronasal thermistor; chest and abdomen effort channels; snore monitor; EKG, electrocardiography.*

COMPUTERIZED POLYSOMNOGRAPHY

The advantages of computerized PSG include easy data acquisition, display, and storage. It is easy to review the record on-line (i.e., the ability to look back at early tracing during progression of recording). The other advantages include the ability to manipulate large quantity of data for review and storage for permanent record keeping. It is easy to click on a particular event of interest or a particular sleep stage to simultaneously display all the physiologic data. It is also easy to perform review using a variety of filter settings, sensitivities, monitor speeds, and reformatted montages (i.e., new montages may be created retrospectively from the electrode derivations used during actual recording). In a particular segment with a question of a potentially epileptiform event (e.g., spikes, sharp waves, spike and waves, and sharp and slow waves), the standard PSG speed of 10 millimeters per second can be quickly changed to the usual EEG speed of 30 millimeters per second for recognizing the evolving pattern of activation for a correct

Montage: SLEEP   High Cut: 15 Hz   Low Cut: 1.00 Hz   Sensitivity: 7 μV/mm   Speed: 120 s/page

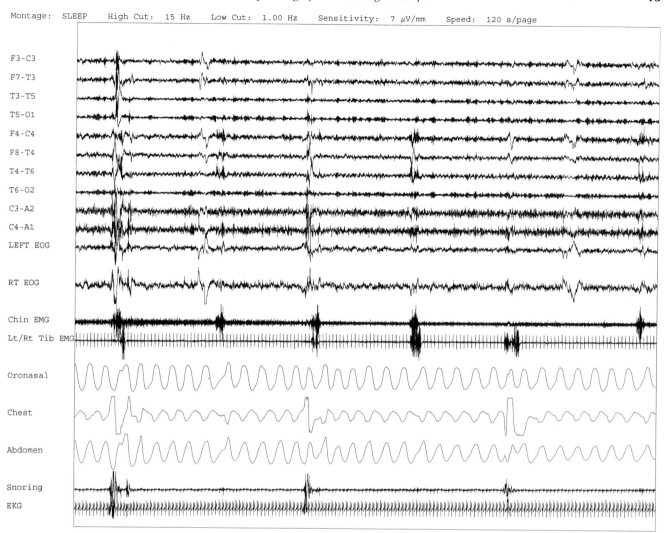

FIGURE 1–6. *A 120-second excerpt from an overnight PSG recording is from the same subject as in Figure 1–5. It shows the presence of periodic limb movements in waking not only on tibialis anterior electromyography channel but also on some occasions both simultaneously and independently on the chin electromyography recording. Montage used is the same as in Figure 1–5.*

diagnosis. These capabilities help identify an abnormal EEG pattern and distinguish artifacts from true cerebral events.

Computerized PSG recording replaces paper and makes PSG paperless, thus making it easy to store the data and conserve space. Computerized PSG makes it easy to document all events during recording digitally and makes it easy to edit and report. The computerized PSG can store the raw data on relatively inexpensive CD-ROM or other suitable media, making it easy to keep a database and access raw data. European data format (EDF) is the most common format for exchange of digital PSGs between different laboratories in different countries.

There are certain minimal requirements for digital PSG. The sampling rate for EEG, EOG, and EMG should

ideally be 200 hertz. A 12-bit analog-digital conversion is a suggested minimum acceptable for the digital amplitude resolution. It is important to have scroll-back mode without interrupting data acquisition so that a particular change during recording can be compared with the previous signals. The computer screen must be of sufficient size and have high resolution.

Simultaneous video monitoring during PSG recording is essential to obtain patient's behavior and motor manifestations, particularly in patients with parasomnias and nocturnal seizures. Recently introduced digital video incorporated into the computerized PSG system is an important advance over the traditional videotape recording. Digital video recordings, however, use a lot of space on the hard disk and one way to handle this problem is to save only small segments of digital video. The latest digital versatile disk (DVD) may solve the storage problems in the future.

COMPUTER-ASSISTED SLEEP SCORING

Manual scoring of sleep using Rechtschaffen-Kales (R-K) technique and scoring of other physiological characteristics (e.g., breathing events, arousals, PLMS) are labor intensive and time consuming, show wide interrater variability, and can be very difficult to score abnormal records. In spite of the fact that R-K system remains the gold standard for scoring sleep, there are severe limitations to R-K scoring system. In the original recommendation, only one central EEG derivation (C3-A2 or C4-Al) was suggested. It was also suggested that epoch-by-epoch scoring be undertaken, and this method of scoring misses short stage changes and many short periods of wakefulness after sleep onset. The R-K system is meant for normal adult sleep patterns. In abnormal sleep with repeated stage and state changes, scoring results do not reflect the real sleep architecture. The R-K system is based on the assumption that the signals are stationary, which is not true from a physiological standpoint. Another serious deficiency in the R-K system is that the amplitude and frequency criteria for delta waves are arbitrarily determined and no justification is given for the use of those criteria. Amplitude criteria are easy to apply in young adults but in the elderly subjects the amplitude of the delta waves decreases and hence the amount of slow-wave sleep will decrease in old age because many of the these delta waves do not reach 75 microvolts of amplitude criteria. One suggestion has been to ignore amplitude criteria in the elderly PSG recording but this has not been generally accepted.

The minimum duration of 0.5 second for sleep spindles and K-complexes is also arbitrary and no justification was given in the original rules of the R-K system. Also, R-K rules do not take into consideration spindle intensity and sleep microstructure. REM sleep scoring in this system implies certain complicated rules. The beginning and ending of REM sleep are often difficult to score. In sleep apnea with repeated arousals, it is difficult to estimate the correct percentage of wakefulness and a particular sleep stage. In the R-K system, sleep scoring is fallacious in patients with OSAS and parasomnias including RBD, narcolepsy, and seizure disorder. The interrater agreement in the R-K system is around 90 percent, which is not quite satisfactory. The R-K sleep manual also does not address scoring and recording of arousals, sleep-disordered breathing events, snoring, sleep-related penile erections, leg muscle activities, or EKG events.

In order to overcome the limitations and fallacies of the R-K system and to reduce the time needed for scoring, automatic computer-assisted scoring techniques have been proposed and are commercially available. The proposed sleep scoring techniques have included period/amplitude analysis, EEG spectral analysis based on fast Fourier transform (FFT), the hybrid system concept combining analog and digital techniques, pattern recognition, the interval histogram method, the bayesian approach, an expert system approach, the neural network model, adaptive sleep stage scoring, and segmentation and self-organization to cluster the different PSG patterns. Some of the latter methods are still evolving, but none of the techniques have received wide popularity because of serious limitations in obtaining an acceptable scoring and because of lack of standardization, validation, and precision in the methods. Some of the problems in computer-assisted scoring include artifact recognition, differentiating stage I NREM sleep from REM sleep, discriminating different sleep stages, inability to differentiate eye movements from high-amplitude delta waves, and failure to detect upper airway resistance. Attempts have also been made to develop computer methods to identify obstructive, central and mixed apneas, and hypopneas as well as arousals and PLMS, but the methods remain ambiguous, imprecise, and variable, resulting in lack of universal acceptance at this time.

Computerized scoring has no real gold standard to compare the data. Another disadvantage of computer scoring is that there is no standardized procedure for scoring of various physiological characteristics. Furthermore, for comparison between visual and computerized scoring, sampling remains a problem. R-K manual scoring still remains today the gold standard in clinical practice.

ARTIFACTS DURING POLYSOMNOGRAPHY RECORDING

The extraneous electrical activities not recorded from the regions of interest (e.g., the brain, muscles, eyes, and heart) generate artifacts in the PSG recording. These extraneous electrical activities may obscure the biological signals of interest and, therefore, recognition and correction of these artifacts is an important task for the PSG technologist. The artifacts can be divided into three categories: physiologic, environmental, and instrumental.

Physiologic Artifacts

These include myogenic potentials, artifacts resulting from movements of the head, eyes, tongue, mouth, and other body parts, sweating, pulse and EKG artifacts, as well as rhythmic tremorogenic artifacts. Potentials originating from the scalp muscles may obscure the EEG activities and may simulate beta rhythms, and obscure

Montage: PSG limbs-PFLOW   High Cut: 70 Hz   Low Cut: 0.53 Hz   Sensitivity: 7 μV/mm   Speed: 30 s/page

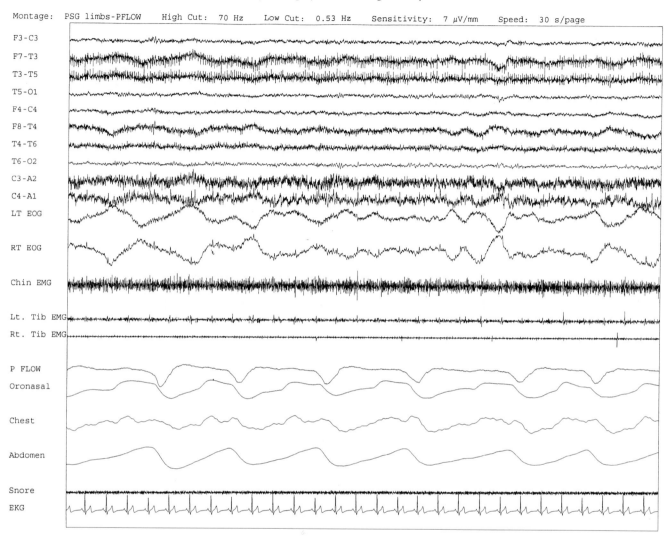

FIGURE 1–7. *A 30-second excerpt of PSG recording shows spike-like potentials of varying amplitude and frequency denoting muscle activity not only on the chin electromyography channel but also in all electroencephalography (EEG) channels, particularly prominent in T3, T4, A2 and A1 electrode derivations. EEG, Top 10 channels; Lt. and Rt. EOG, left and right electrooculograms; electromyography of chin; Lt. and Rt. Tib. EMG, left and right tibialis anterior electromyography; P. Flow, peak flow; oronasal thermistor; chest and abdomen effort channels; snore monitor; EKG, electrocardiography.*

low-amplitude cerebral activities. Figure 1–7 documents muscle activities during PSG recordings. Movements of the head, eyes, tongue, mouth, and other body parts will produce movement artifacts (Figure 1–8) and sometimes resemble slow waves in the EEG or may obscure the EEG activities, causing difficulty in scoring the different sleep stages. The rhythmic movements sometimes generated by rhythmic movements of the head, tongue, and legs as well as rhythmic movements generated by tremor in a patient may produce apparent slow waves, thus causing difficulty in scoring the slow-wave sleep. Sweating may cause excessive baseline swaying, producing a very slow-frequency wave lasting for 1 to 3 seconds, which is noticed promi-

nently in the frontal electrodes (Figures 1–9 and 1–10). The electrical potentials result from salt content of the sweat glands. Eye movement artifacts can be confused with actual cerebral activities (Figure 1–11). Pulse artifact occurs when the electrode is placed over the scalp arteries. Slow waves are generated by electrode movement caused by the pulsations. Temporal relation of these waves to the EKG recording helps identify such extracerebral activity. EKG artifacts can contaminate the EEG recordings, particularly in patients who are obese with short neck (Figure 1–12). Tongue movements may produce characteristic glossokinetic potentials that obscure the EEG activities.

Text continued on p. 25

Montage: PSG limbs-PFLOW   High Cut: 70 Hz   Low Cut: 0.53 Hz   Sensitivity: 15 µV/mm   Speed: 30 s/page

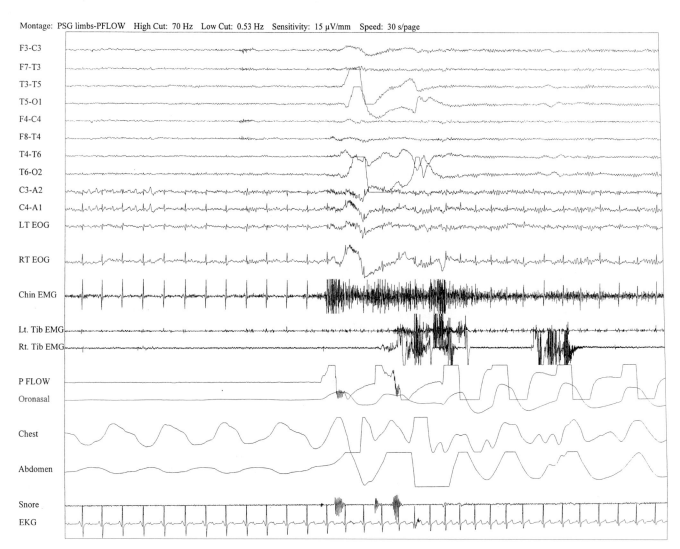

FIGURE 1–8. A: *A 30-second excerpt from overnight PSG recording shows body movement artifact following an obstructive apnea as demonstrated by variable, high-voltage, asymmetrical and asynchronous slow activity on electroencephalography (EEG) channels and increased electromyography activity on chin and tibialis anterior electrode channels. EEG, Top 10 channels; Lt. and Rt. EOG, left and right electrooculograms; electromyography of chin; Lt. and Rt. Tib. EMG, left and right tibialis anterior electromyography; P. Flow, peak flow; oronasal thermistor; chest and abdomen effort channels; snore monitor; EKG, electrocardiography.*

Montage: SLEEP   High Cut: 70 Hz   Low Cut: 1.00 Hz   Sensitivity: 7 μV/mm   Speed: 30 s/page

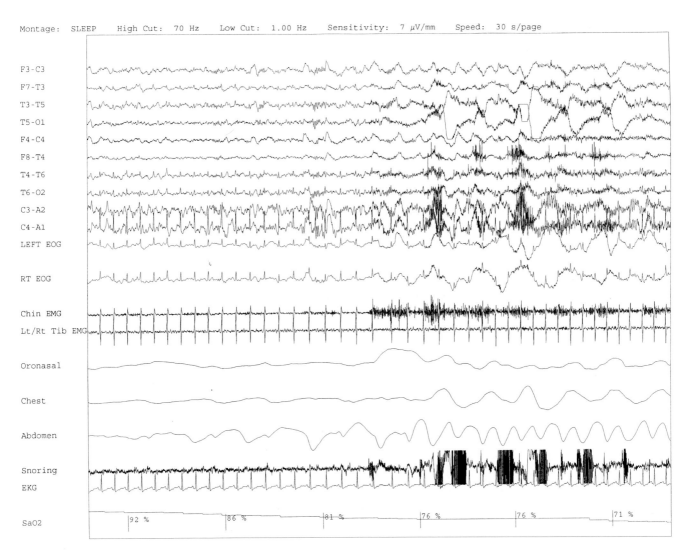

FIGURE 1–8, cont'd B: *A 64-year-old man was referred for evaluation of upper airway obstructive sleep apnea syndrome. The abdomen effort channel in the PSG recording reveals a double-peaked waveform in the post-apnea recovery breaths. This may be related to the clinical finding of a large protuberant abdomen with a ventral midline hernia. EEG, Top 10 channels; Lt. and Rt. EOG, left and right electrooculograms; electromyography of chin; Lt./Rt. Tib. EMG, left and right tibialis anterior electromyography; oronasal thermistor; chest and abdomen effort channels; snore monitor; EKG, electrocardiography; SaO₂, oxygen saturation by finger oxymetry.*

Montage: PSG limbs-PFLOW   High Cut: 70 Hz   Low Cut: 0.53 Hz   Sensitivity: 10 µV/mm   Speed: 30 s/page

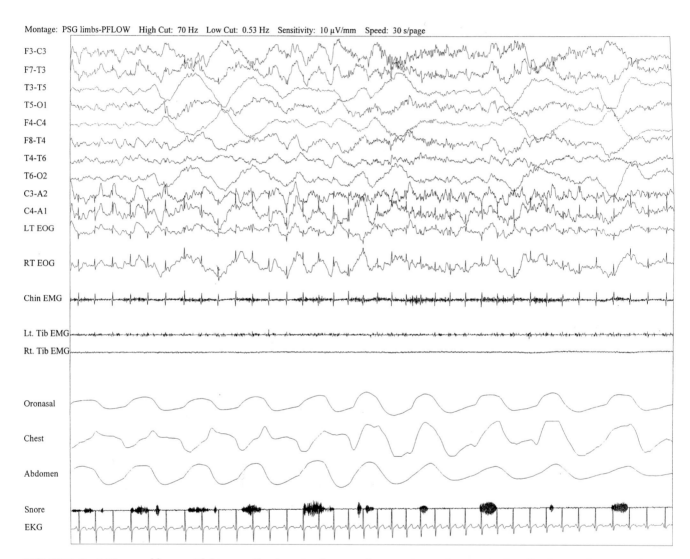

FIGURE 1–9. *A 58-year-old man with history of loud snoring for several years, witnessed apneas in sleep for the past 5 years, and excessive daytime sleepiness. Overnight PSG showed severe obstructive sleep apnea with an apnea-hypopnea index of 75.6. A 30-second excerpt from the study shows the presence of sweat artifact characterized by chaotic, asynchronous, high-voltage slow activity in delta range, randomly distributed over all the EEG channels and electrooculogram electrodes. Sweating occurs commonly in NREM sleep and may need to be differentiated from focal or diffuse slow activity of cerebral origin. EEG, Top 10 channels; Lt. and Rt. EOG, left and right electrooculograms; electromyography of chin; Lt. and Rt. Tib. EMG, left and right tibialis anterior electromyography; oronasal thermistor; chest and abdomen effort channels; snore monitor; EKG, electrocardiography.*

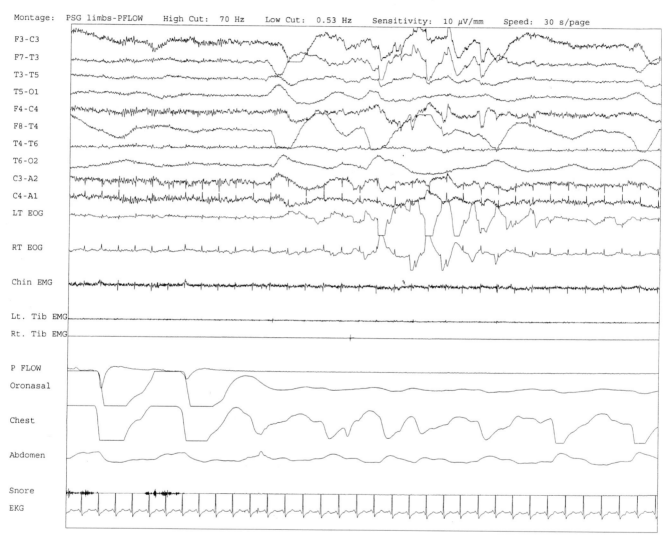

Montage: PSG limbs-PFLOW   High Cut: 70 Hz   Low Cut: 0.53 Hz   Sensitivity: 10 µV/mm   Speed: 30 s/page

FIGURE 1–10. *Overnight PSG shows evidence of severe upper airway obstructive sleep apnea with an apnea-hypopnea index of 51.3 in a 71-year-old man with history of snoring, difficulty breathing in sleep, and excessive daytime sleepiness despite uvulopalatoplasty performed 2 years ago for treatment of obstructive sleep apnea. Medical history is significant for hypertension. Additionally, the PSG shows the presence of sweating recurrently and exclusively during REM sleep while being conspicuously absent during non-REM sleep. This is an atypical finding, raising the suggestion of REM sleep dysregulation. This figure shows a 30-second excerpt in REM sleep taken from overnight PSG recording showing sweat artifact as described for Figure 1–9 and upper airway obstructive apnea. EEG, Top 10 channels;, Lt. and Rt. EOG, left and right electrooculograms; electromyography of chin; Lt. and Rt. Tib. EMG, left and right tibialis anterior electromyography; P. flow, peak flow; oronasal thermistor; chest and abdomen effort channels; snore monitor; EKG, electrocardiography.*

Montage: MSLT-NEW   High Cut: 70 Hz   Low Cut: 0.53 Hz   Sensitivity: 7 μV/mm   Speed: 30 s/page

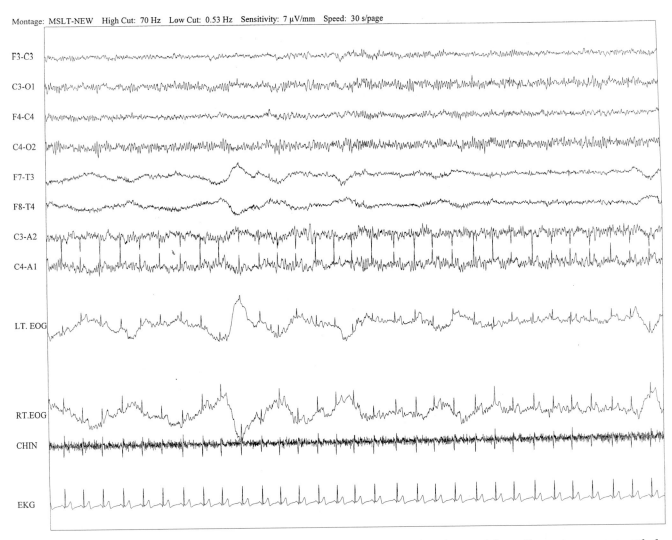

FIGURE 1–11. A: *A 30-second excerpt from a multiple sleep latency test showing the presence of slow rolling eye movements with the onset of stage I non-REM sleep. The slow rolling eye movements are not only recorded on the left and right electrooculogram channels but are also noted on the anterior temporal electroencephalography (EEG) electrode recordings. This can be confused with focal or diffuse slow activity of cerebral origin. EEG, Top eight channels; Lt. and Rt. EOG, left and right electrooculograms; electromyography of chin; EKG, electrocardiography.*

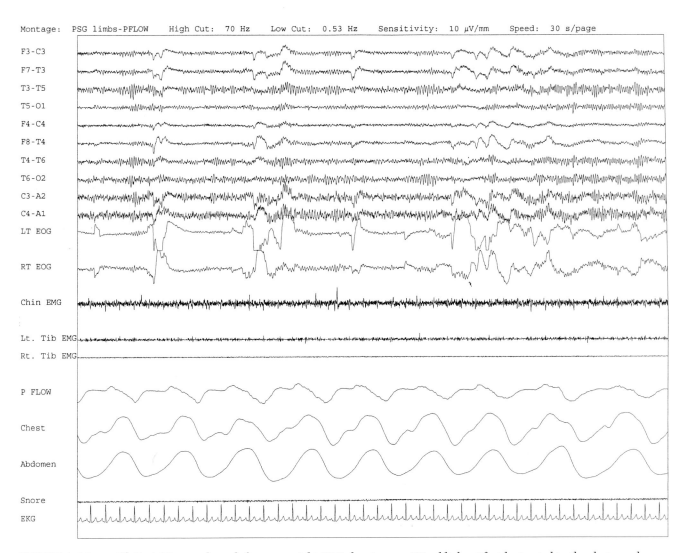

Montage: PSG limbs-PFLOW   High Cut: 70 Hz   Low Cut: 0.53 Hz   Sensitivity: 10 μV/mm   Speed: 30 s/page

FIGURE 1–11, cont'd B: *A 30-second epoch from overnight PSG showing repetitive blink artifact best noted in the electrooculogram channels and on the frontal and anterior temporal EEG electrode recordings. This can be misinterpreted for abnormal cerebral activity. EEG, Top 10 channels; Lt. and Rt. EOG, left and right electrooculograms; electromyography of chin; Lt. and Rt. Tib. EMG, left and right tibialis anterior electromyography; P. flow, peak flow; chest and abdomen effort channels; snore monitor; EKG, electrocardiography.*

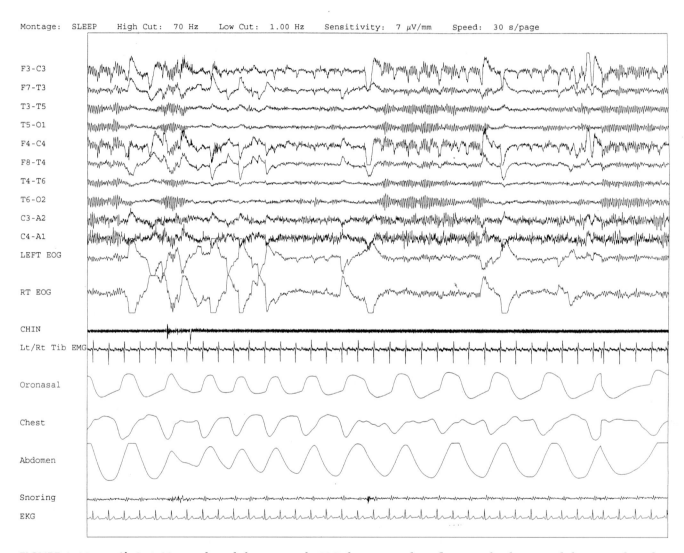

Montage: SLEEP   High Cut: 70 Hz   Low Cut: 1.00 Hz   Sensitivity: 7 µV/mm   Speed: 30 s/page

FIGURE 1–11, cont'd C: *A 30-second epoch from overnight PSG showing rapid eye flutter artifact best recorded in F3 and F4 electrode recordings during the latter half of the epoch. A blink artifact is noted in the initial part of the recording and is best seen on the electrooculogram channels. Well-formed alpha rhythm is noted in the background on all EEG channels when eyes are closed.*

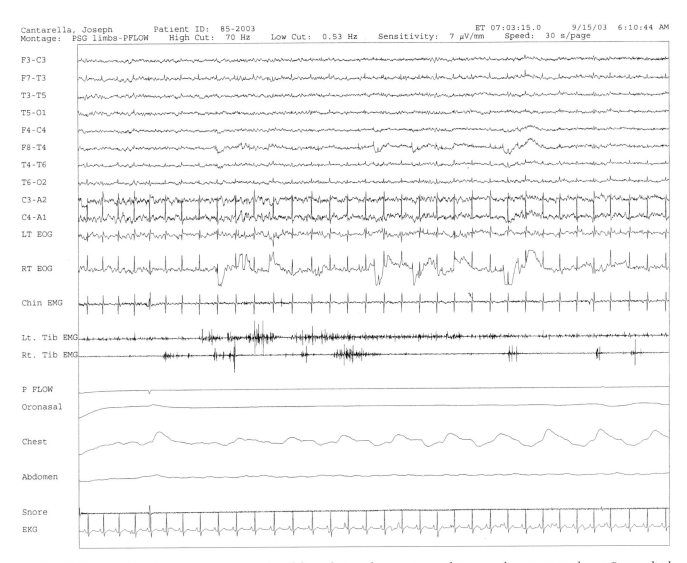

Cantarella, Joseph   Patient ID: 85-2003   ET 07:03:15.0   9/15/03 6:10:44 AM
Montage: PSG limbs-PFLOW   High Cut: 70 Hz   Low Cut: 0.53 Hz   Sensitivity: 7 μV/mm   Speed: 30 s/page

FIGURE 1–11, cont'd D: *A 50-year-old man is referred for exclusion of upper airway obstructive sleep apnea syndrome. Past medical history is significant for an artificial left eye and limited vision in the right eye secondary to severe uveitis. A 30-second excerpt in REM sleep from overnight PSG shows the presence of unilateral eye movement artifact in right electrooculogram and anterior temporal EEG electrodes but not in the corresponding channels on the left side. Myoclonic bursts of electromyographic activity are recorded in the tibialis electromyography channels and a mixed apnea is recorded on the oronasal thermistor and effort channels. A superimposed electrocardiography artifact is also noted. EEG, Top 10 channels; Lt. and Rt. EOG, left and right electrooculograms; electromyography of chin; Lt. and Rt. Tib. EMG, left and right tibialis anterior electromyography; P. flow, peak flow; oronasal thermistor; chest and abdomen effort channels; snore monitor; EKG, electrocardiography.*

Montage: SLEEP   High Cut: 70 Hz   Low Cut: 1.00 Hz   Sensitivity: 5 μV/mm   Speed: 30 s/page

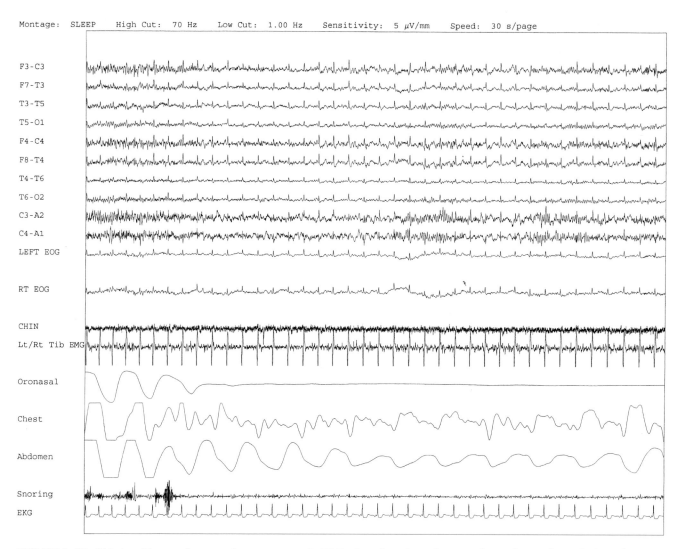

FIGURE 1–12. *This is a 30-second excerpt from an overnight PSG selected to show electrocardiography artifact, which is characterized by its morphology, rhythm, and synchrony with electrocardiographic recording. It is seen throughout the epoch on electroencephalography, electrooculography, and tibialis electromyography channels. Incidentally an obstructive apnea is seen in the airflow and effort channels. EEG, Top 10 channels; Lt. and Rt. EOG, left and right electrooculograms; electromyography of chin; Lt./Rt. Tib. EMG, left and right tibialis anterior electromyography; oronasal thermistor; chest and abdomen effort channels; snore monitor; EKG, electrocardiography.*

Environmental Sources of Electrical Signals

These may simulate electrocerebral activity or obscure EEG activities. The 60-hertz (or 50-hertz) signals from telephone or pager systems can result in artifacts. Electrostatic artifacts result from movements of the subject in the environment. Sixty-hertz electromagnetic radiation from AC current in power lines may contaminate the recording (Figure 1–13). The main frequency is 50 hertz in many other countries. The 60-hertz artifact may be mistaken for myogenic artifact in the slow paper speed of 10 millimeters per second commonly used for PSG recording. The PSG technician should identify this problem and locate the source of this artifact and try to eliminate the artifact. Most important is keeping the impedance below 5 K.

Instrumental Artifacts

These arise from faulty electrodes, electrode wires, switches, and the polygraph machine itself. Electrode "pops" may produce transient sharp waves or slow waves

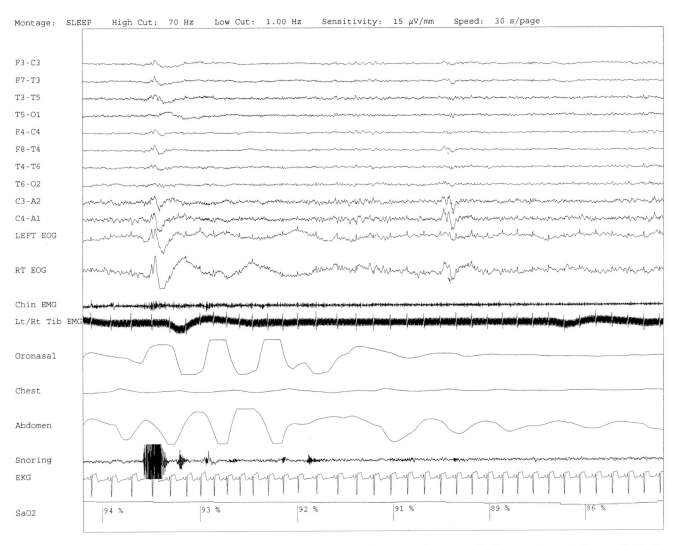

FIGURE 1–13. A: *A 30-second excerpt from an overnight PSG recording shows a uniform monorhythmic artifact at 60 hertz on left/right tibialis electromyography channel, which is further superimposed by an electrocardiography artifact. The 60-Hz artifact is due to electrical interference from power lines and equipment occurring at a frequency of 60 hertz in North America (but at 50 hertz in many other countries). Maximum interference is seen in the presence of poor electrode contact. Incidentally an obstructive apnea is noted in the airflow and respiratory effort channels. EEG, Top 10 channels; Lt. and Rt. EOG, left and right electrooculograms; electromyography of chin; Lt./Rt. Tib. EMG, left and right tibialis anterior electromyography; oronasal thermistor; chest and abdomen effort channels; snore monitor; EKG, electrocardiography; SaO2, oxygen saturation.*

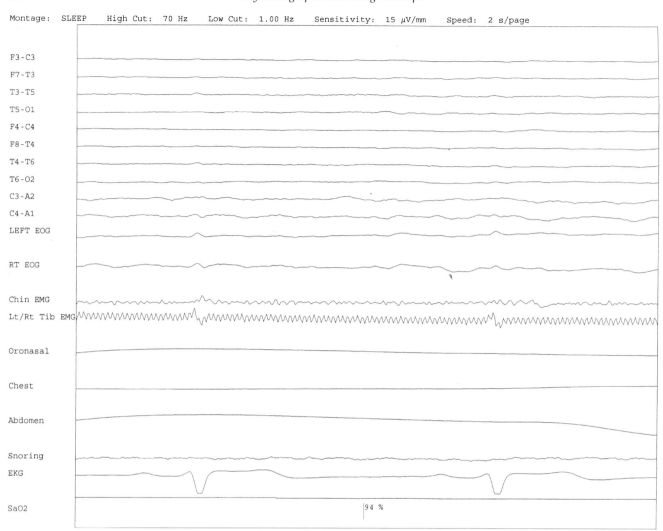

Montage: SLEEP   High Cut: 70 Hz   Low Cut: 1.00 Hz   Sensitivity: 15 μV/mm   Speed: 2 s/page

FIGURE 1–13, cont'd B: *The 60-hertz artifact described in* **A** *is shown at a paper speed of 2 seconds per epoch.*

limited to one electrode (see Figure 1–14 and Figure 2–13). These artifacts are very common and result from faulty electrode placement of insufficient electrode gel causing abrupt changes in impedance. The electrode should be reset and gel applied. If the artifact persists, then electrodes need to be changed. Other sources of artifacts are the electrode wires, the cables, and the switches. In the PSG machine, random fluctuations of charges result in some instrumental noise artifacts. If the sensitivity is greater than 2 microvolts per millimeter, which is not generally used in PSG recordings, then these instrument artifacts may interfere with the recording. Loose contacts in switches or wires may also cause sudden changes in voltage or loss of signal.

PSG artifacts must be eliminated or reduced to a minimum for proper identification of the EEG, EMG, and other bioelectrical potentials for correct staging of the sleep and for diagnosis and classification of sleep disorders. Identification of all these artifacts is best made at the time of the recording by the skilled PSG technologist. Particular attention should be paid to the electrodes, electrode gel application, and impedance. Preparation of the patient and electrode application is fundamental for recording a good quality PSG.

PITFALLS OF POLYSOMNOGRAPHY

PSG is the single most important laboratory test for assessment of sleep disorders, particularly in patients presenting with excessive daytime somnolence. However, PSG has considerable limitations. First, there is no standardized

Montage: SLEEP   High Cut: 70 Hz   Low Cut: 1.00 Hz   Sensitivity: 15 μV/mm   Speed: 30 s/page

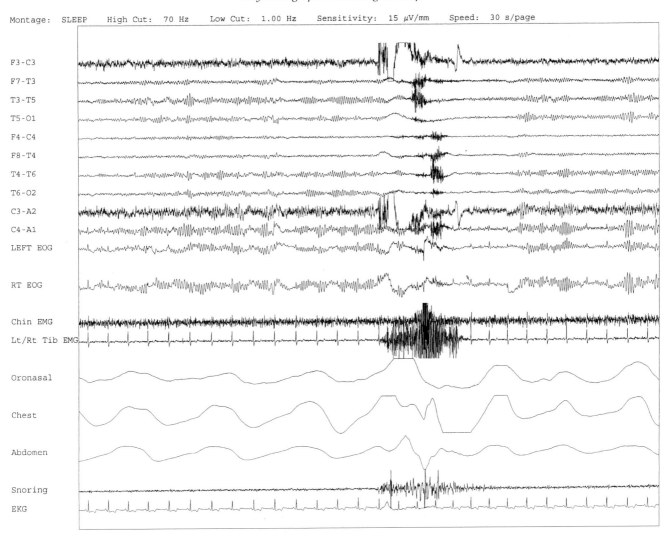

FIGURE 1–14. *A 30-second excerpt from an overnight PSG recording shows the presence of a C3 electrode pop artifact. Near the middle of the epoch it is accentuated by a movement artifact simultaneously recorded on the chin electromyography, left and right tibialis anterior electromyography, and snoring channel. EEG, Top 10 channels; Lt. and Rt. EOG, left and right electrooculograms; electromyography of chin; Lt./Rt. Tib. EMG, left and right tibialis anterior electromyography; oronasal thermistor; chest and abdomen effort channels; snore monitor; EKG, electrocardiography.*

uniform protocol used in all sleep laboratories, and this may make the comparison of the data from one laboratory to another somewhat misleading. The most serious limitation is that the overnight in-laboratory PSG is labor intensive, time consuming, and expensive. A single night's PSG may miss the diagnosis of mild OSAS, PLMS, parasomnias, or nocturnal seizures. PSG data and the patient's clinical findings may not be concordant. Standard PSG study cannot diagnose upper airway resistance syndrome definitively. PSG cannot determine etiology of apnea-hypopnea syndrome. PSG is not helpful in the diagnosis of insomnia, the most common sleep disorder in the general population. PSG is not useful in the diagnosis or treatment of circadian

rhythm sleep disorders. PSG data may be confounded by the first night effects (e.g., increased wakefulness and stage I NREM sleep and decreased slow-wave and REM sleep). Standard PSG does not measure $PaCO_2$ and thus may miss hypoventilation, which is an early abnormality (particularly REM-related hypoventilation) in neuromuscular disorders. Standard PSG does not adequately measure cardiac function (one channel of EKG is inadequate), which may affect the prognosis of OSAS. Furthermore, cardiorespiratory sleep studies, which do not include EEG, may produce false negative findings in mild to moderate OSAS patients. Standard PSG does not include autonomic monitoring, which may be important for assessment of autonomic arousal as well as for assessing autonomic changes which are intense during sleep. Finally, lack of a standardized definition of hypopnea remains a serious limitation to the diagnosis and outcome studies of patients with sleep apnea-hypopnea syndrome.

BIBLIOGRAPHY

1. Keenan S. Polysomnographic technique: An overview. In: Chokroverty S, ed. *Sleep Disorders Medicine: Basic Science, Technical Considerations, and Clinical Aspects*, 2nd Ed. Boston: Butterworth-Heinemann, 1999:151–174.

2. Chokroverty S. Polysomnography and related procedures. In: Hallett M, ed. *Movement Disorders. Handbook of Clinical Neurophysiology*, Vol. 1, Amsterdam: Elsevier, 2003:139–151.

3. Broughton RJ. Polysomnography: Principles and applications in sleep and arousal disorders. In: Niedermeyer E, Lopes Da Silva, eds. *Electroencephalography: Basic Principles, Clinical Science, and Related Fields*, 4th Ed. Philadelphia: Lippincott, Williams and Wilkins, 1999:858–895.

2

Electroencephalography for the Sleep Specialists

SUDHANSU CHOKROVERTY, MEETA BHATT, AND TAMMY GOLDHAMMER

Electroencephalography (EEG) records the difference in electrical potentials between two electrode sites over the scalp. The EEG recorded over the scalp results from extracerebral current flow due to the summated excitatory postsynaptic potentials (EPSP) and inhibitory postsynaptic potentials (IPSP). Rhythmic oscillations of the thalamocortical neuronal projections cause synchronous synaptic EPSP and IPSP over the areas of the cortex. The scalp EEG recording voltages are attenuated and reflect about one tenth of the voltage recorded over the cortical surface.

The electrical signals are transmitted by the electrodes and conducting gel through the electrode wires, which are attached between the electrodes and the jack box of the polysomnography (PSG) equipment. Different types of electrodes are available but for recording EEG activities, the best electrodes to use are the gold cup electrodes with holes in the center and the silver-silver chloride electrodes. Silver-silver chloride electrodes need repeated chloriding for proper maintenance. Electrode paste or conducting gel is used to secure the electrodes. Positive and negative chargers are generated between the scalp and recording electrode as a result of ionic dissociation. The electrode-electrolyte interface is the most critical link in the PSG machine, as most of the artifacts originate at this site and careful preparation is therefore very important. The impedance in a pair of electrodes should be measured by an impedance meter and should not be greater than 5000 (5K) ohms. High impedance impairs the ability of the electrical signal to reach the amplifier and interferes with the capacity of the amplifier to eliminate environmental noise, thus increasing the artifacts. All electrode wires terminate in a pin, which is plugged into the electrode box, called a

jack. All the wires from the head are gathered into a ponytail in the back of the head and then secured by tying them together. A wrap around the scalp secures the electrodes and the wires. The arrangement is therefore as follows: electrodes from the surface of the scalp are connected by electrode wires into the jacks, which are numbered, and then the wires from the jack box are connected through a shielded conductor cable to the electrode montage selector containing rows of switches in pairs corresponding to the inputs of the amplifier.

The placement of the electrodes is determined by the 10-20 electrode placement system which is recommended by the International Federation of Societies for EEG and Clinical Neurophysiology, and was published by Jasper in 1958. The 10-20 system is based on definable anatomical landmarks (Figure 2–1). The system consists of letters denoting the parts of the brain underneath the area of the scalp and numbers denoting specific location. The odd numbers refer to the left side and the even numbers refer to the right side. In the original Rechtschaffen-Kales (R-K) scoring technique, only one channel (C3-A2 or C4-Al) was recommended. One channel may be sufficient to record the background waking activities as well as vertex sharp waves, K complexes, and sleep spindles. However, most of the laboratories use at least four channels (C3-A2, C4-Al, O1-A1, O2-A2) to clearly document the onset of sleep. Some laboratories use eight to ten channels of EEG (see Figure 1–1) to cover the parasagittal and the temporal areas of the brain to record possible focal or diffuse EEG abnormalities as well as for recording epileptiform activities. The technician should be familiar with the measurement technique for placement of the electrodes according to the 10-20 international system. Important

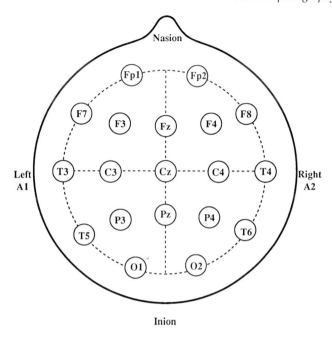

Standard international 10-20 electrode placement (superior view)

FIGURE 2–1. *(From Keenan S. Polysomnographic technique: An overview. In Chokroverty S, ed. Sleep Disorders Medicine. Boston: Butterworth-Heinemann, 1999, with permission.)*

landmarks for measuring include the inion, the nasion, and the right and left preauricular points. The distance from the nasion to inion along the midline through the vertex should be measured. FPz in the midline is 10 percent above the nasion of the total distance between the inion and nasion. The electrodes marked FP_1 and FP_2 are located laterally 10 percent above the nasion of the total distance between the inion and nasion measured along the temporal regions through the preauricular points. Oz denotes an electrode placed at a distance of 10 percent above the inion of the total distance between the nasion and inion. T3 and T4 electrodes are placed in a location 10 percent above the preauricular points of a total distance between the two preauricular points. The rest of the electrodes are located at a distance of 20 percent measured from inion to nasion anteroposteriorly or laterally through the ears as well as transversely between the ears. The montage refers to an arrangement of two electrodes (derivations). Both bipolar montage (connection of the electrodes between two relatively active sites over the scalp) and referential montage (connection of the electrodes

between an active and relatively inactive site, e.g., A1, A2, Cz, Pz) are recommended.

NORMAL WAKING AND SLEEP ELECTROENCEPHALOGRAPHY RHYTHMS IN ADULTS

The dominant rhythm in adults during wakefulness is the alpha rhythm, which consists of 8 to 13 hertz and is distributed synchronously and symmetrically over the parieto-occipital regions (Figure 2–2). The frequency of the rhythm between the two hemispheres should not vary by more than 1 hertz and the amplitude should not vary by more than 50 percent. The alpha rhythm is best seen during quiet wakefulness with eyes closed and is significantly attenuated by eye opening or mental concentration. A small percentage of normal adults show no alpha rhythm and their EEG is characterized by the dominant rhythm of low-amplitude EEG in the beta frequencies (greater than 13 hertz) with amplitude varying between 10 and 25 microvolts (Figure 2–3). In most adults, the beta rhythms are seen predominately in the frontal and central regions intermixed with the posterior alpha rhythms.

There are characteristic changes in the background EEG rhythms as an individual goes into non–rapid eye movement (NREM) sleep consisting of four stages and REM sleep consisting of tonic and phasic stages. The various characteristics during different sleep stages are described under the section of sleep scoring technique (Chapter 3).

EEG in elderly subjects shows a progressive slowing of the alpha frequency during wakefulness and diminution of alpha blocking and photic driving responses. Focal temporal slow waves, particularly in the left temporal region, often called *benign temporal delta transients* (Figure 2–4) of the elderly, are seen in many apparently normal elderly individuals and are sometimes associated with sharp transients. Transient bursts of anteriorly dominant rhythmic delta waves may also be seen in some elderly subjects in the early stage of sleep. Other changes in older adults consist of sleep fragmentation with frequent awakenings, including early morning awakening and multiple sleep stage shifts. Another important finding in the sleep EEG of older adults is the reduction of amplitude of the delta waves and therefore, according to R-K scoring technique, they do not meet the amplitude criteria and slow-wave sleep is thought to be reduced in these subjects.

Text continued on p. 36

Montage: 2 DBL BANANA   High Cut: 70 Hz   Low Cut: 1.00 Hz   Sensitivity: 10 μV/mm   Speed: 10 s/page

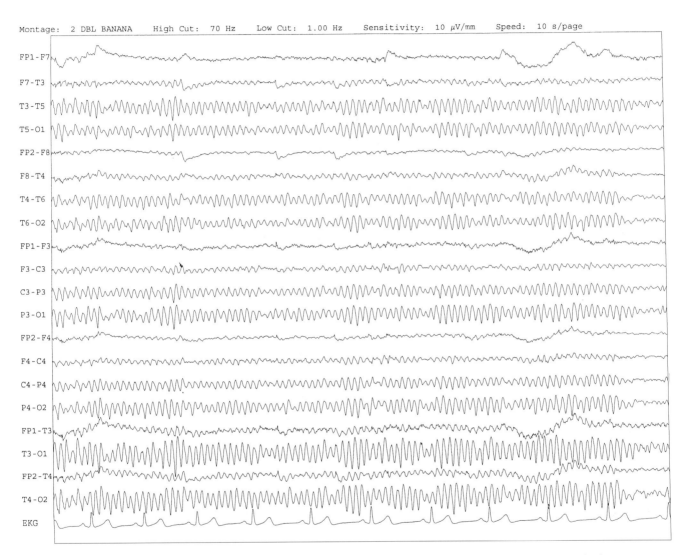

FIGURE 2–2. A: *Normal awake EEG pattern characterized by symmetrical, sinusoidal posterior dominant alpha rhythm at 11 to 12 hertz, 82 to 105 microvolts in a 40-year-old woman at a conventional EEG paper speed of 10 seconds per page. Eye movement artifact is noted in channels linked to frontal FP1 and FP2 electrodes.*

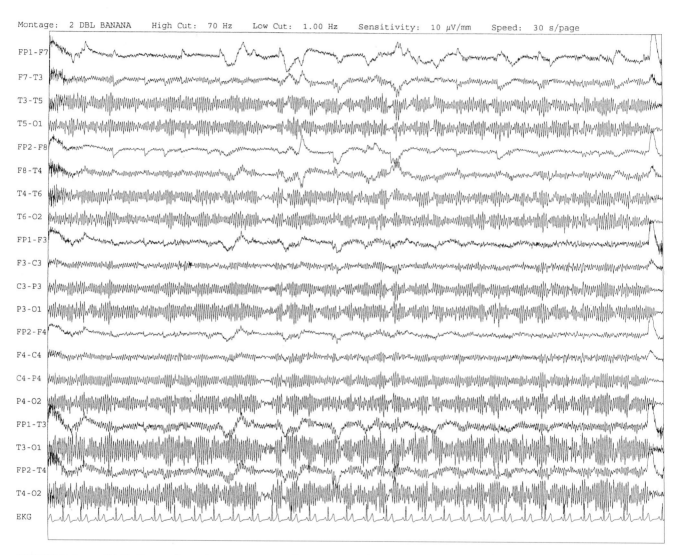

Montage: 2 DBL BANANA   High Cut: 70 Hz   Low Cut: 1.00 Hz   Sensitivity: 10 μV/mm   Speed: 30 s/page

FP1-F7
F7-T3
T3-T5
T5-O1
FP2-F8
F8-T4
T4-T6
T6-O2
FP1-F3
F3-C3
C3-P3
P3-O1
FP2-F4
F4-C4
C4-P4
P4-O2
FP1-T3
T3-O1
FP2-T4
T4-O2
EKG

FIGURE 2–2, cont'd B: *Same subject data as in* **A** *viewed at a 30-second epoch.*

Montage: 2 DBL BANANA   High Cut: 70 Hz   Low Cut: 1.00 Hz   Sensitivity: 5 μV/mm   Speed: 10 s/page

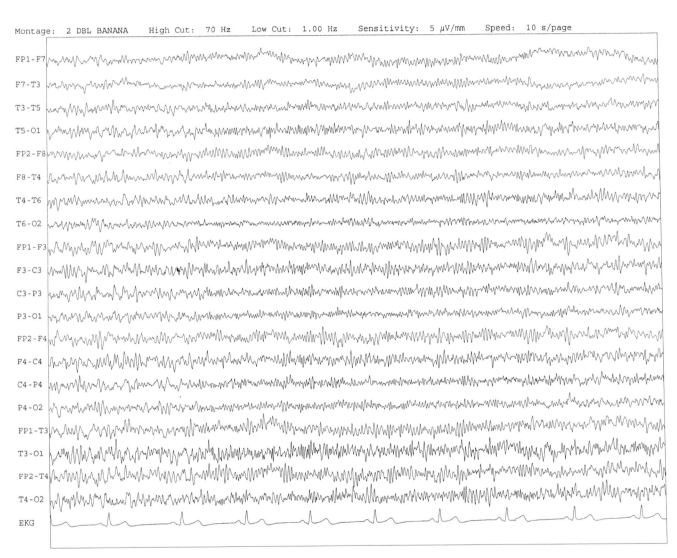

FIGURE 2–3. A: *Normal awake EEG pattern characterized by diffuse low-voltage beta rhythm in a 23-year-old man at a conventional EEG paper speed of 10 seconds per page.*

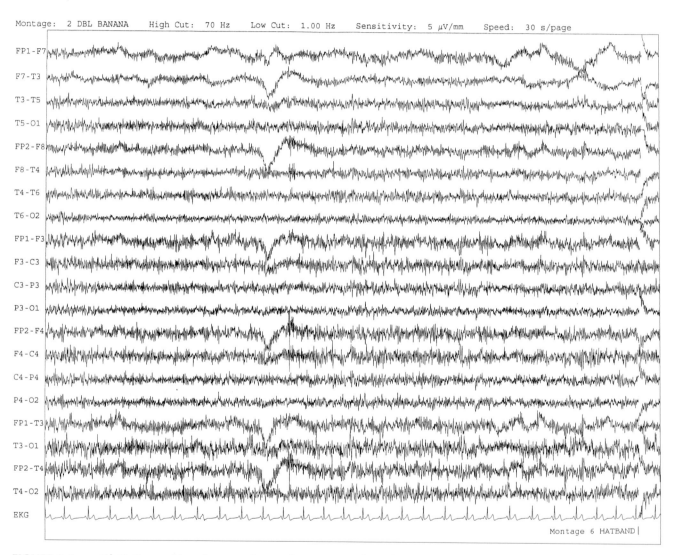

FIGURE 2–3, cont'd ***B:*** *Same subject data as in* **A** *viewed at a 30-second epoch.*

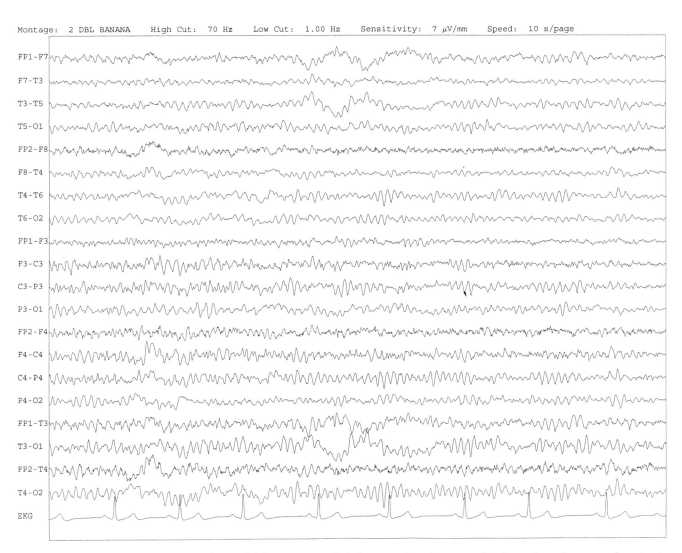

FIGURE 2–4. A: *EEG shows transient burst of delta activity in the left temporal, and occasionally also in the right temporal, region in a 94-year-old woman with history of syncope.*

Montage: 2 DBL BANANA   High Cut: 70 Hz   Low Cut: 1.00 Hz   Sensitivity: 7 µV/mm   Speed: 30 s/page

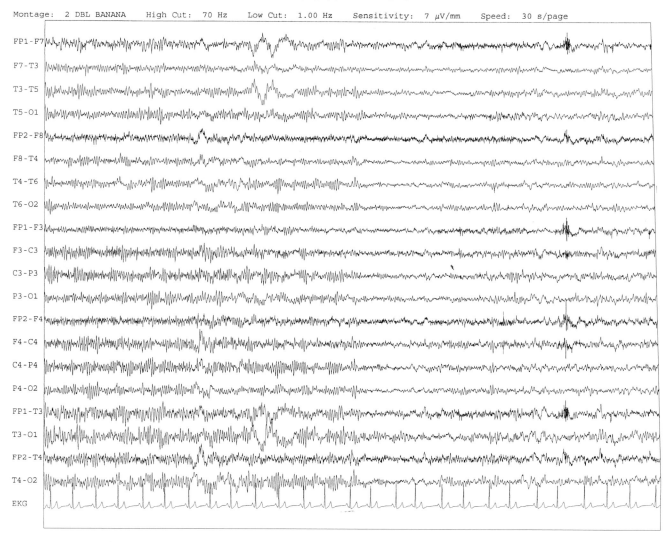

FIGURE 2–4, cont'd *B:* *Same subject data as in* **A** *viewed at a 30-second epoch.*

ABNORMAL EEG PATTERNS

The abnormal pattern may consist of focal or diffuse slow waves and epileptiform discharges. The importance of multiple channel EEG recordings is to document those focal (Figure 2–5) or diffuse (Figure 2–6) slow waves and epileptiform discharges. Many patients are referred to the PSG laboratory for a possible diagnosis of nocturnal seizures. The standard recommended EEG recordings of one to two channels or even four channels of recordings miss most of the epileptiform discharges during all-night recording. Therefore, in patients suspected of nocturnal seizures, PSG study should include multiple channels of EEG covering temporal and parasagittal regions and simultaneous video recording (video-PSG study) for correlation of the electrical activities with the actual behavior of the patients. In computerized PSG

recordings (digital PSG recordings), which are currently performed in most laboratories, it is easy to change the recording speed from the standard 10 millimeters per second of the usual sleep recording to 30 millimeters per second of the standard EEG recording for proper identification of the epileptiform discharges. Full complement of electrodes and special electrode placements (e.g., Tl and T2 electrodes) should be used.

RECOGNITION OF EPILEPTIFORM PATTERNS IN THE POLYSOMNOGRAPHIC TRACING

First, it should be remembered that epilepsy is a clinical diagnosis; therefore history must be obtained from patients, relatives, witnesses, or medical personnel if a patient

Text continued on p. 42

Montage: 2 DBL BANANAeyes   High Cut: 70 Hz   Low Cut: 1.00 Hz   Sensitivity: 10 µV/mm   Speed: 10 s/page

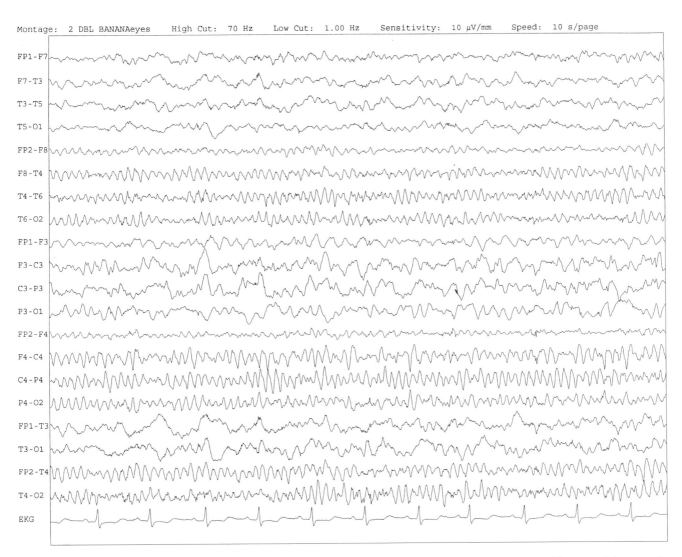

FIGURE 2–5. A: *EEG shows focal slowing at 3 to 6 hertz over the left temporoparietal region in an 85-year-old man with history of a stroke. Normal alpha rhythm at 10 to 11 hertz is noted on the right side.*

Montage: 2 DBL BANANA   High Cut: 70 Hz   Low Cut: 1.00 Hz   Sensitivity: 7 μV/mm   Speed: 30 s/page

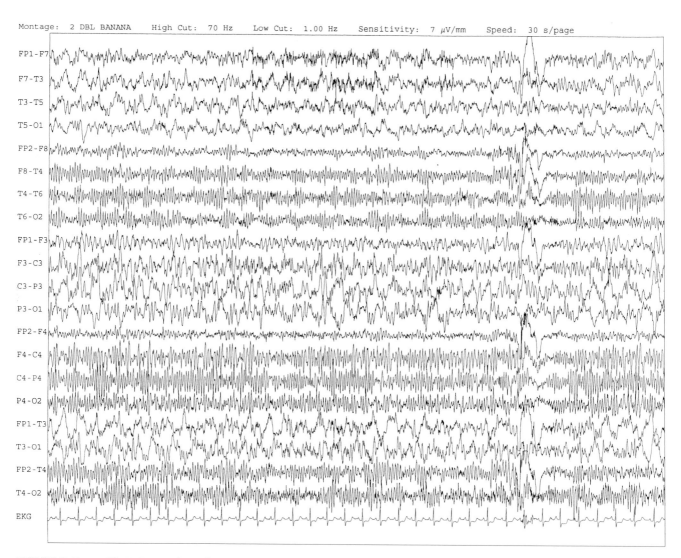

FIGURE 2–5, cont'd *B: Same subject data as in* **A** *viewed at a 30-second epoch.*

Montage: 2 DBL BANANA   High Cut: 70 Hz   Low Cut: 1.00 Hz   Sensitivity: 7 µV/mm   Speed: 10 s/page

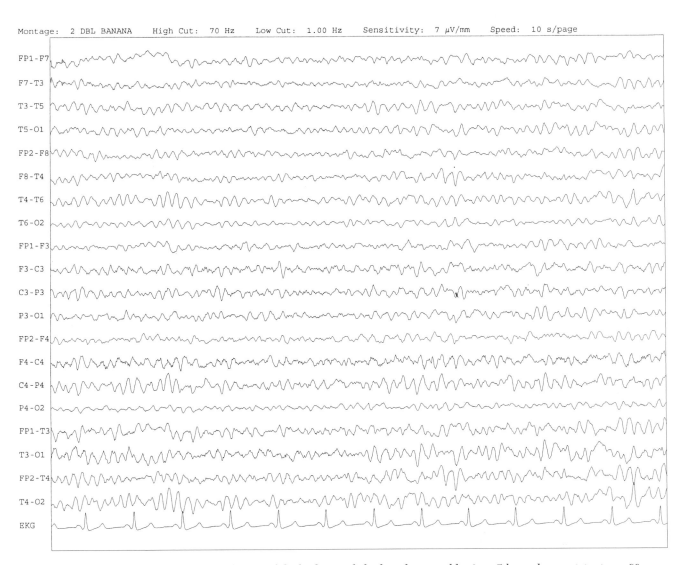

FIGURE 2–6. A: *EEG shows mild diffuse slowing of the background rhythm, dominated by 6- to 7-hertz theta activity in an 80-year-old woman with history of hypertension, diabetes mellitus, and bacteremia.*

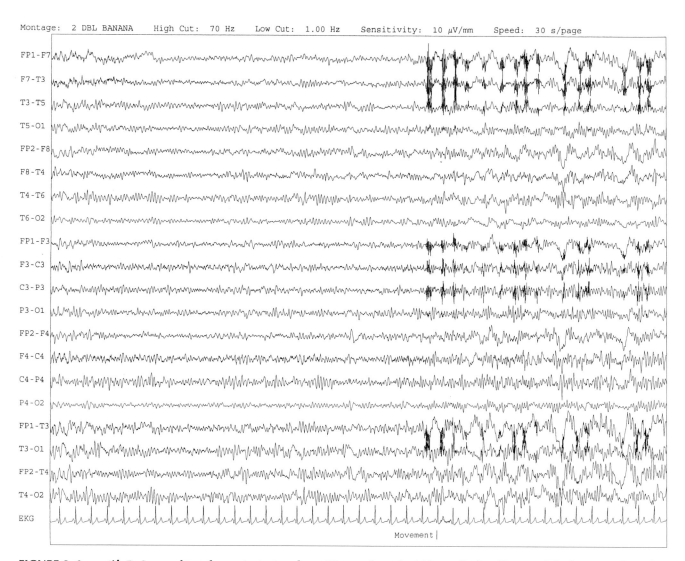

Montage: 2 DBL BANANA   High Cut: 70 Hz   Low Cut: 1.00 Hz   Sensitivity: 10 μV/mm   Speed: 30 s/page

Movement

FIGURE 2–6, cont'd B: *Same subject data as in* **A** *viewed at a 30-second epoch. Additionally, brief bursts of rhythmic muscle artifact are noted on the left side toward the end of the epoch. Mild diffuse slowing of the background rhythm may be missed during conventional polysomnography scoring. The clue is in that the epoch looks like an awake recording without the characteristic alpha rhythm. This necessitates viewing the segment as a 10-second epoch.*

Montage: 4 Ref Cz   High Cut: 70 Hz   Low Cut: 1.00 Hz   Sensitivity: 10 μV/mm   Speed: 10 s/page

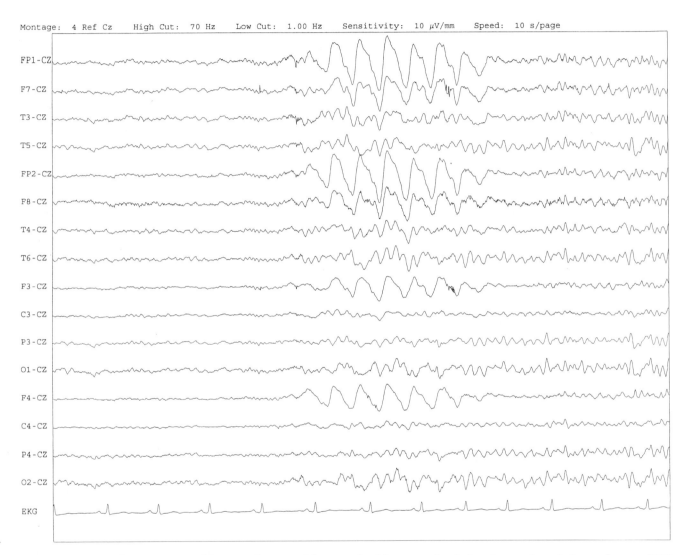

FIGURE 2–6, cont'd C: *A 27-year-old man with a 3-week history of sudden severe headaches diagnosed as pituitary adenoma. EEG shows evidence of a brief burst of frontal intermittent rhythmic delta activity (FIRDA), synchronously recorded over both hemispheres. FIRDA was originally believed to arise from deep midline pathology, which is demonstrated in this case. However, FIRDA is now believed to be anatomically nonlocalizing and indicates diffuse cerebral dysfunction secondary to metabolic or structural involvement.*

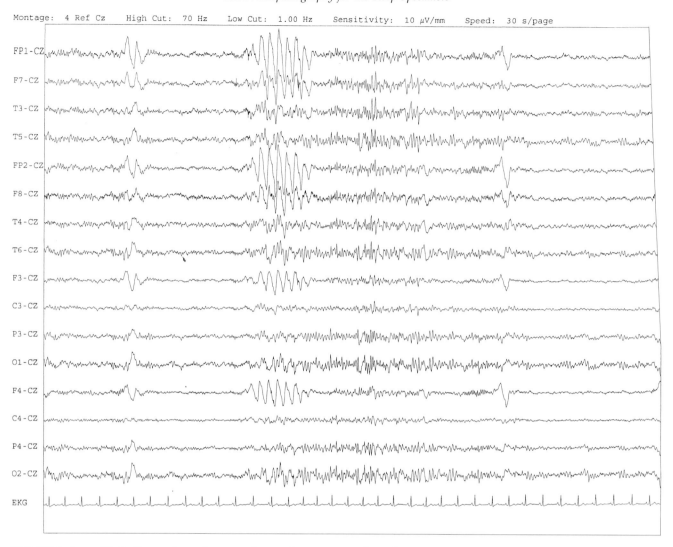

FIGURE 2–6, cont'd D: *Same subject data as in* **C** *viewed at a 30-second epoch.*

is referred to the sleep laboratory with a suspected diagnosis of nocturnal seizure. The history must include ictal, preictal, postictal, and interictal periods, family and drug histories, as well as history of any significant medical or surgical illnesses that might be responsible for triggering the seizures. Physical examination must be conducted to find any evidence of neurological or other medical disorders before PSG recording in the laboratory.

EEG SIGNS OF EPILEPSY

EEG is the single most important diagnostic laboratory test for patients with suspected seizure disorders. Certain characteristic EEG waveforms correlate with a high percentage of patients with clinical seizures and therefore

can be considered of potentially epileptogenic significance. These epileptiform patterns consist of spikes, sharp waves, spike and waves, sharp- and slow-wave complexes, as well as evolving pattern of rhythmic focal activities, particularly in neonatal seizures. Another pattern that correlates highly with complex partial seizure is the temporal intermittent rhythmic delta activity (TIRDA) (Figure 2–7).

Recognition of a spike or a sharp wave depends on the presence of certain characteristics. A spike is defined as a waveform, which suddenly appears out of the background rhythm with a brief duration of 20 to 70 milliseconds showing a field of distribution and is often followed by an after-going slow wave (Figure 2–8A). The characteristic feature of a true epileptiform spike or sharp wave is a biphasic or triphasic appearance with a sharp ascending limb followed by a slow descending limb in contrast to aug-

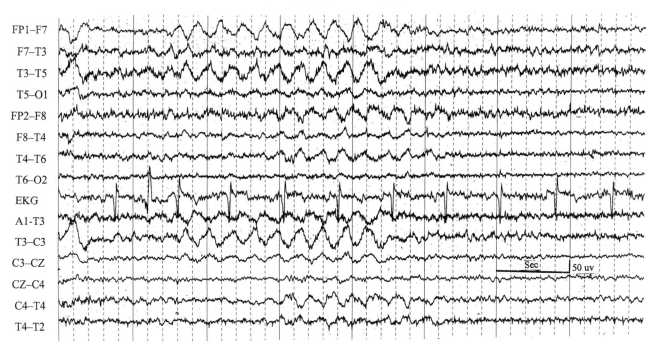

FP1–F7
F7–T3
T3–T5
T5–O1
FP2–F8
F8–T4
T4–T6
T6–O2
EKG
A1–T3
T3–C3
C3–CZ
CZ–C4
C4–T4
T4–T2

Sec   50 uv

FIGURE 2–7. *Left temporal intermittent rhythmic delta activity (TIRDA) during wakefulness in a 30-year-old woman with partial complex seizures.*

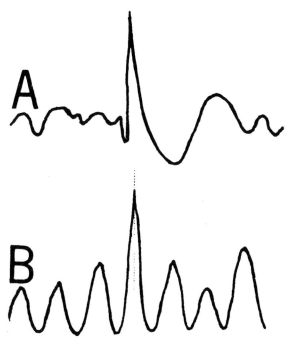

FIGURE 2–8. *Diagram of epileptic spike (A) and an augmented background sharp rhythm (B). (From Ajmone-Marsan C. Encephalographic studies in seizure disorders: Additional considerations. J Clin Neurophysiol 1984;1:143, with permission.)*

mented background rhythm of sharp contour, which is generally monophasic and has uniform ascending and descending limbs (Figure 2–8B). The amplitude of a true epileptiform spike or sharp wave is at least 30 percent higher than the background activity, and often there is a disturbance in the background rhythm in the neighboring region of the spikes or the sharp waves. Generally, the spike or sharp waves are surface negative. A sharp wave fulfills all the criteria described for a spike except that the duration is 70 to 200 milliseconds. Spike and waves, and sharp- and slow-wave complexes may be transient or may repeat for several seconds or longer, and in some patients these repeat in a rhythmic manner such as may

be seen in patients with absence seizure showing 3-hertz spike and wave complexes in the EEG (Figure 2–9).

An EEG showing all the characteristic features of sharp waves or spikes and accompanied by the behavioral correlates simultaneously during the recording in the laboratory makes the diagnosis of epilepsy positive. However, it is rare to observe the occurrence of a clinical seizure during an EEG recording (Figures 2–10 and 2–11). Therefore a definitive statement about the diagnosis of epilepsy in a particular patient cannot be made even in the presence of the characteristic EEG signs of epilepsy. In patients suspected of seizure disorder, it is advantageous to include activation procedures such as sleep, hyperventilation and

Text continued on p. 52

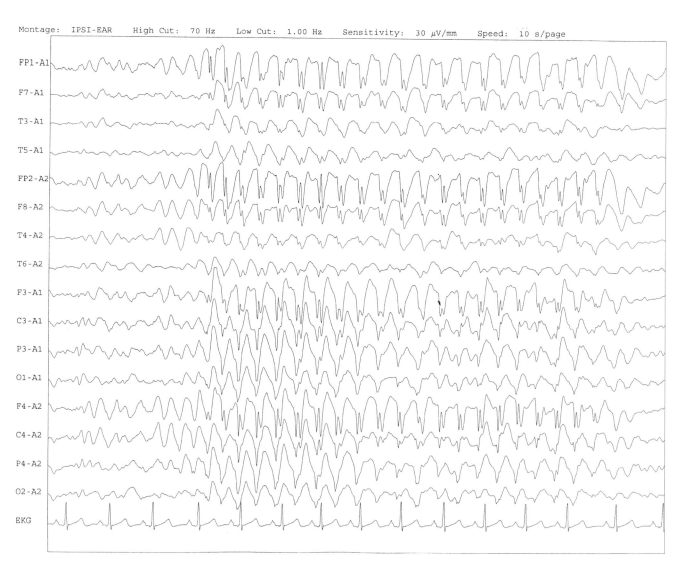

FIGURE 2–9. A: *An 11-year-old girl with history of staring spells, suspected to have petit mal seizures. EEG shows a burst of synchronous, anteriorly dominant spike and wave activity at 3 hertz lasting for approximately 7 seconds.*

Montage: IPSI-EAR   High Cut: 70 Hz   Low Cut: 1.00 Hz   Sensitivity: 30 μV/mm   Speed: 30 s/page

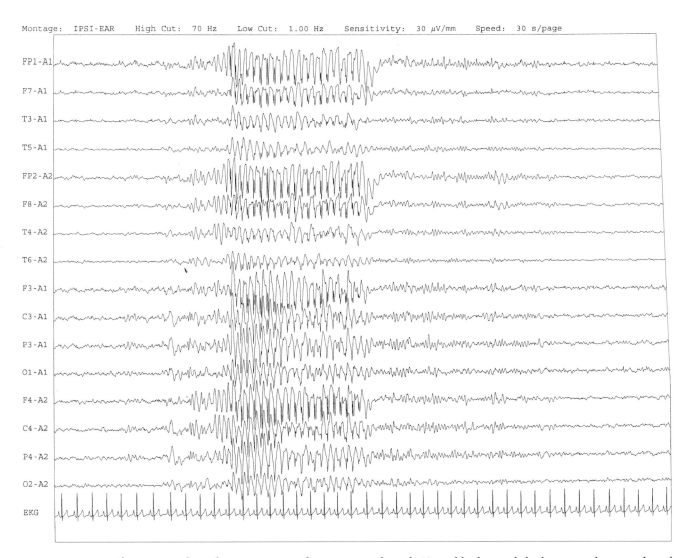

FIGURE 2–9, cont'd B: *Same subject data as in* **A** *viewed at a 30-second epoch. Normal background rhythm is noted to precede and follow the brief burst of spike and wave activity.*

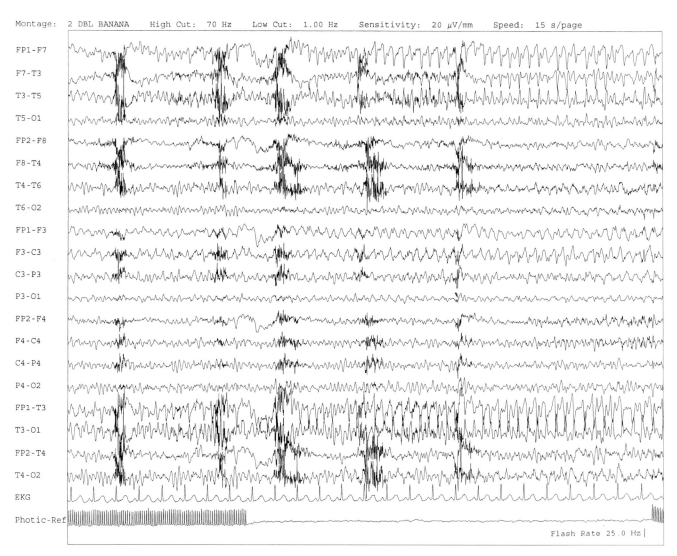

FIGURE 2–10. *A:* A 61-year-old woman with a history of insomnia and one episode of screaming at night. The EEG shows four sequential epochs at 15 seconds per page at sensitivities ranging from 20 microvolts to 50 microvolts per millimeter. The figure shows onset of left temporofrontal rhythmic spike and wave activity during photic stimulation at 17 hertz. The spike and wave activity is incremental in nature with increasing frequency and amplitude noted.

Montage: 2 DBL BANANA   High Cut: 70 Hz   Low Cut: 1.00 Hz   Sensitivity: 30 µV/mm   Speed: 15 s/page

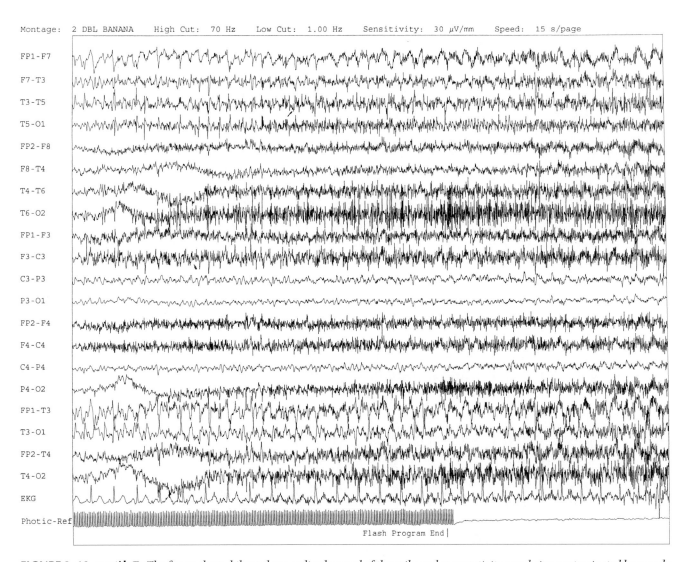

FIGURE 2–10, cont'd B: *The figure shows bilateral generalized spread of the spike and wave activity now being contaminated by muscle activity.*

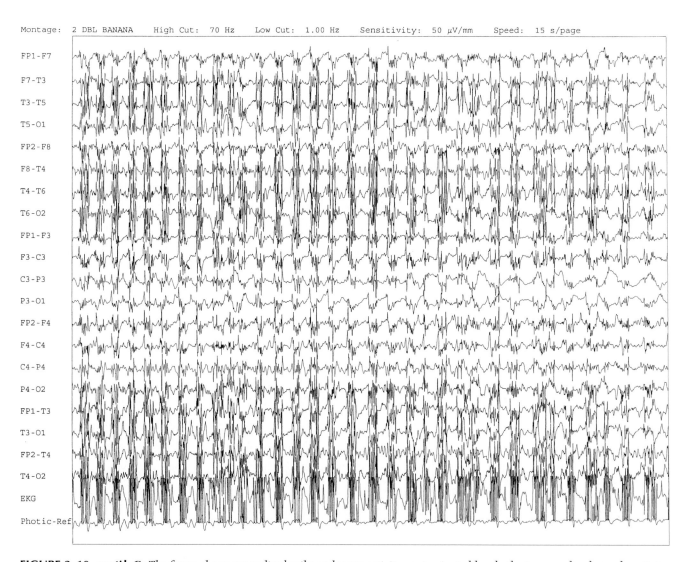

FIGURE 2–10, cont'd C: *The figure shows generalized spike and wave activity contaminated by rhythmic generalized muscle activity.*

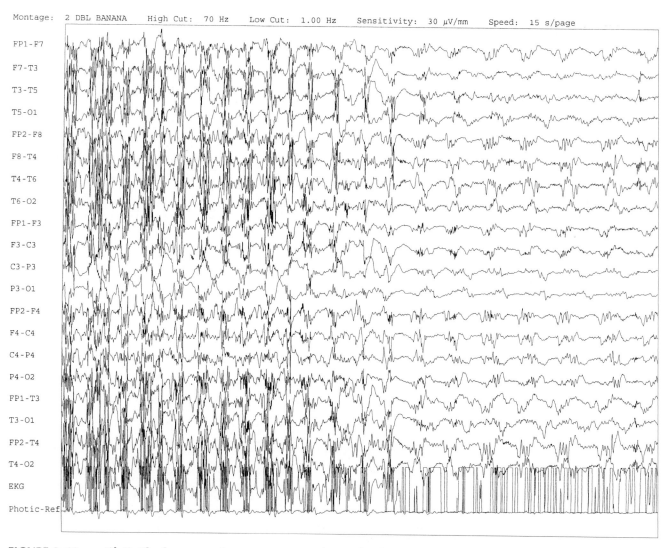

FIGURE 2–10, cont'd D: *The figure now shows continuation of generalized spike and wave activity contaminated by muscle activity followed by postictal EEG depression of the amplitudes and slowing of the background. The EEG development of the ictus was clinically accompanied by a loud scream and sudden turning of the head to the right, followed by shaking of both arms, frothing at the mouth, and fixed and dilated pupils. The entire episode lasted for about 60 seconds. The patient was in a postictal state for approximately 10 minutes.*

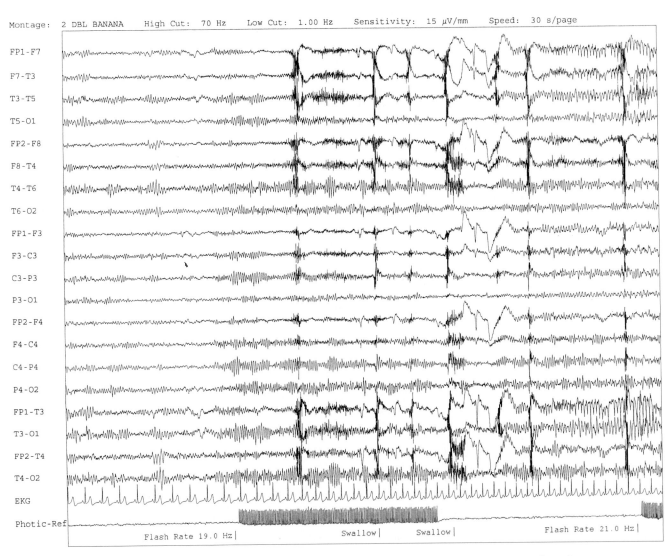

FIGURE 2–11. *The same subject data as in Figure 2–10, A, B, C, D viewed over three consecutive 30-second epochs.*

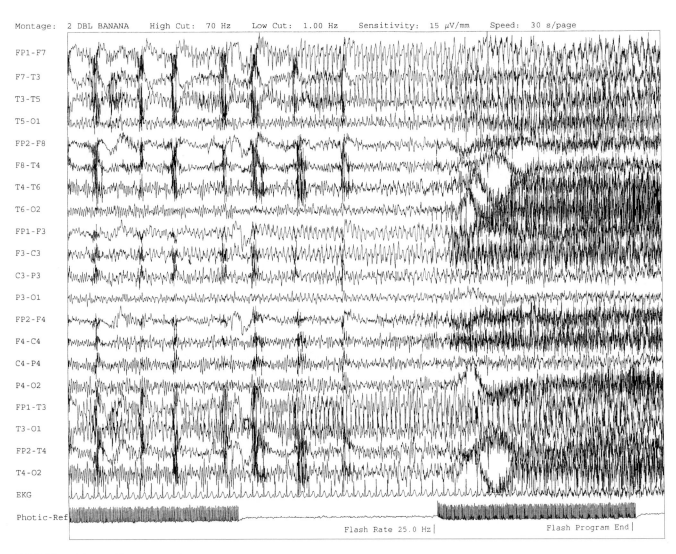

Montage: 2 DBL BANANA   High Cut: 70 Hz   Low Cut: 1.00 Hz   Sensitivity: 15 μV/mm   Speed: 30 s/page

FIGURE 2–11, cont'd.

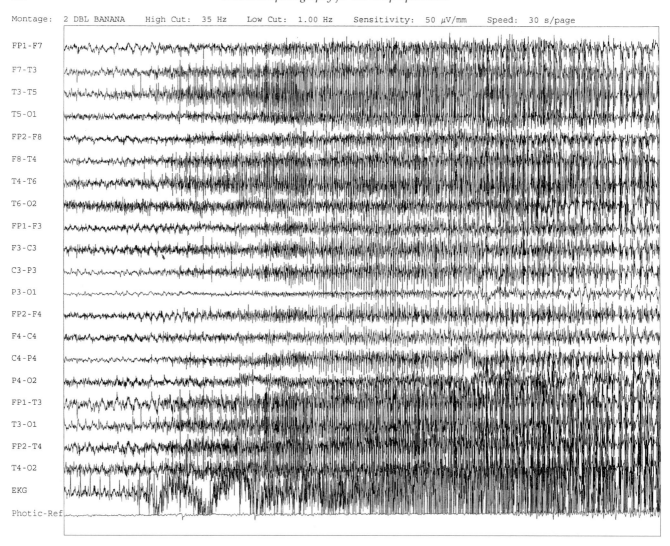

Montage: 2 DBL BANANA   High Cut: 35 Hz   Low Cut: 1.00 Hz   Sensitivity: 50 μV/mm   Speed: 30 s/page

FIGURE 2–11, cont'd.

photic stimulation during routine EEG recording in the daytime in order to bring out the ictal or interictal epileptiform patterns. Special basal temporal electrodes (T1, T2, nasopharyngeal, and sphenoidal electrodes) should be used in addition to the routine electrode placement in patients suspected of partial complex seizure. Furthermore, in such patients, the PSG study must include multiple EEG channels covering the parasagittal and temporal regions bilaterally.

NONEPILEPTIFORM PATTERNS MIMICKING EPILEPTIFORM DISCHARGES

There are several nonepiletpiform EEG patterns which may mimic epileptiform patterns but are not of epileptogenic significance. Such patterns must be identified in order to determine that the patient has true epilepsy. Following are some of the EEG findings that may mimic true epileptiform patterns.

Sharp Artifacts

Sharp artifacts include electrocardiograph artifacts, electrode pops, and muscle artifacts that are easy to identify from the distribution and morphologic appearance. EKG artifacts (Figure 2–12) can be identified by the findings on a one-lead EKG. Electrode pops are limited to one channel (Figure 2–13) and the artifacts are eliminated after the electrode problems are resolved. Muscle artifacts (Figure 2–14) can be reduced by having the patient relaxed.

Text continued on p. 62

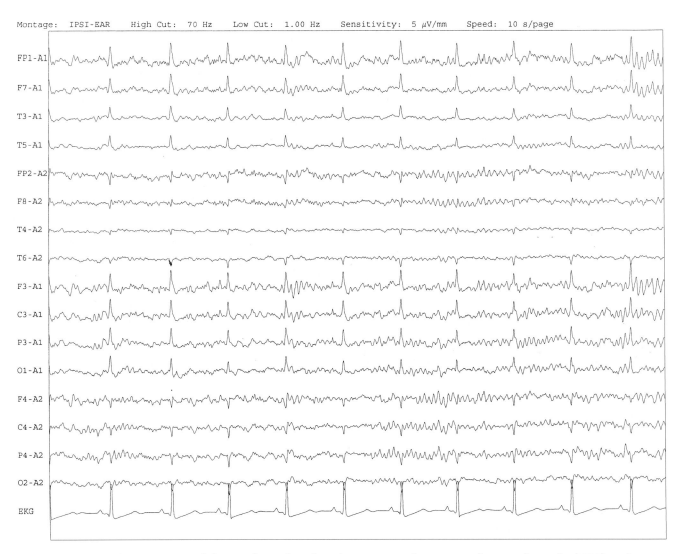

Montage: IPSI-EAR   High Cut: 70 Hz   Low Cut: 1.00 Hz   Sensitivity: 5 μV/mm   Speed: 10 s/page

FIGURE 2–12. A: *This tracing recorded in a referential ipsilateral ear montage demonstrates electrocardiography (EKG) artifact seen diffusely throughout the recording. It is recognized by its morphology, rhythm, and synchrony with simultaneously monitored EKG recording.*

Montage: IPSI-EAR   High Cut: 70 Hz   Low Cut: 1.00 Hz   Sensitivity: 5 µV/mm   Speed: 30 s/page

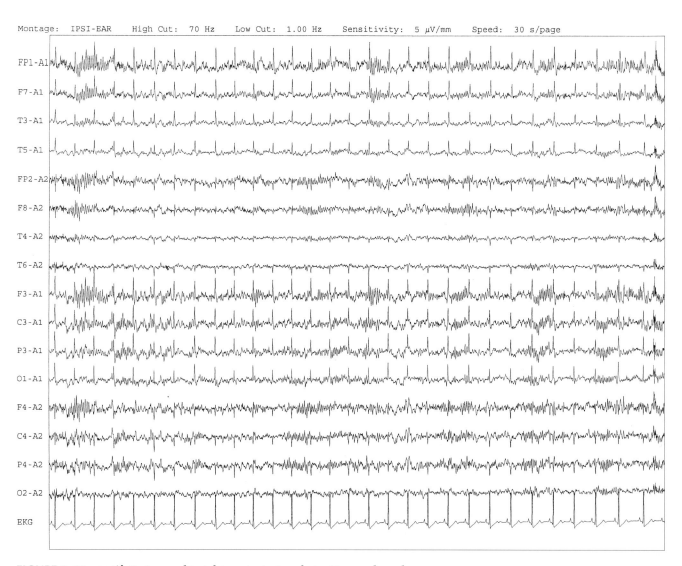

FIGURE 2–12, cont'd B: *Same subject data as in* **A** *viewed at a 30-second epoch.*

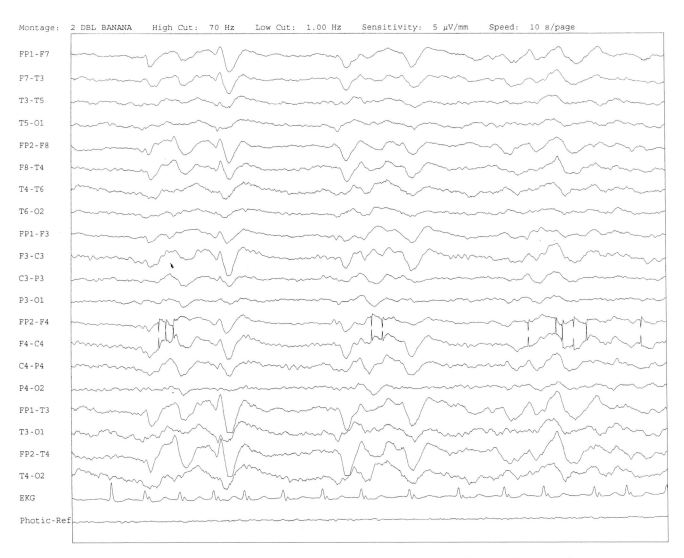

Montage: 2 DBL BANANA   High Cut: 70 Hz   Low Cut: 1.00 Hz   Sensitivity: 5 μV/mm   Speed: 10 s/page

FIGURE 2–13. **A:** *An electrode pop artifact resulting from poor F4 electrode contact, resembling a spike potential.*

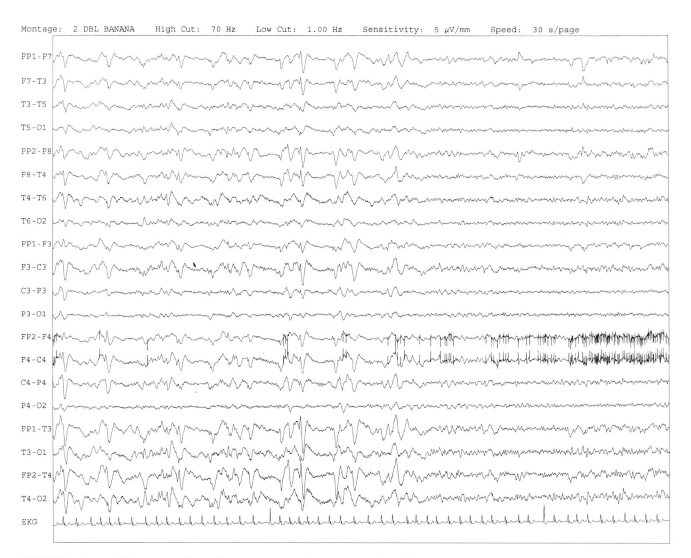

FIGURE 2–13, cont'd B: *Same subject data as in* **A** *viewed at a 30-second epoch.*

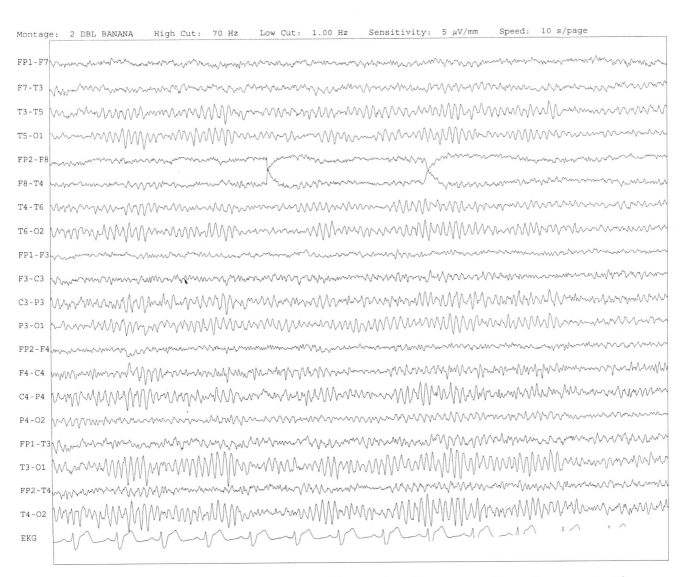

Montage: 2 DBL BANANA   High Cut: 70 Hz   Low Cut: 1.00 Hz   Sensitivity: 5 μV/mm   Speed: 10 s/page

FIGURE 2–13, cont'd C: *An electrode pop artifact at F8 caused by poor electrode contact, resembling a slow-wave potential.*

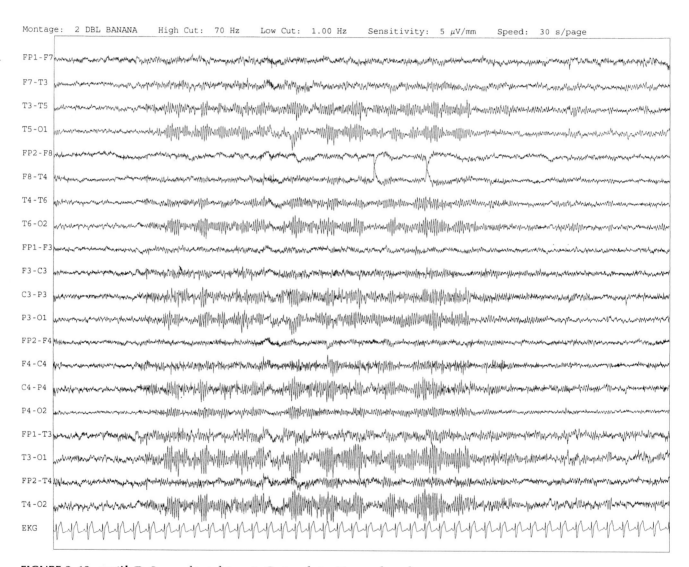

Montage: 2 DBL BANANA   High Cut: 70 Hz   Low Cut: 1.00 Hz   Sensitivity: 5 μV/mm   Speed: 30 s/page

FIGURE 2–13, cont'd D: *Same subject data as in* **C** *viewed at a 30-second epoch.*

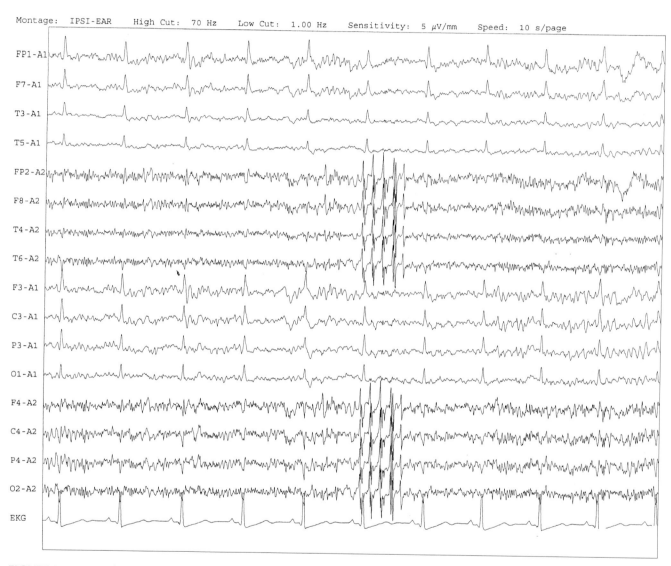

FIGURE 2–13, cont'd E: *An electrode pop artifact, resembling spike activity in all the right-sided electrodes resulting from poor right ear (A2) electrode contact.*

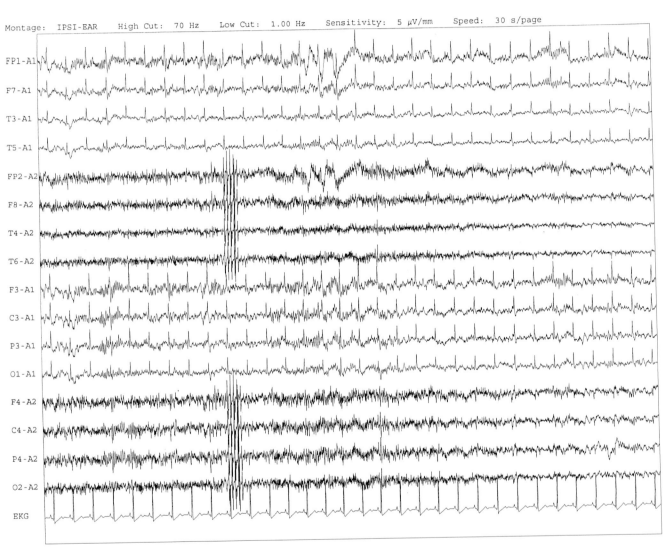

FIGURE 2–13, cont'd *F: Same subject data as in E viewed at a 30-second epoch.*

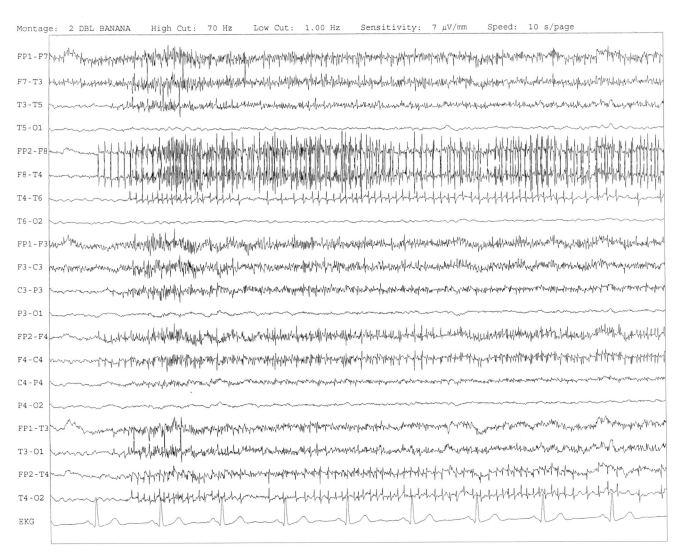

Montage: 2 DBL BANANA   High Cut: 70 Hz   Low Cut: 1.00 Hz   Sensitivity: 7 μV/mm   Speed: 10 s/page

FIGURE 2–14. A: *Muscle artifact resembling very brief spike potentials at varying amplitudes and frequencies diffusely present bilaterally. It is most prominent and of highest amplitude at F8 electrode.*

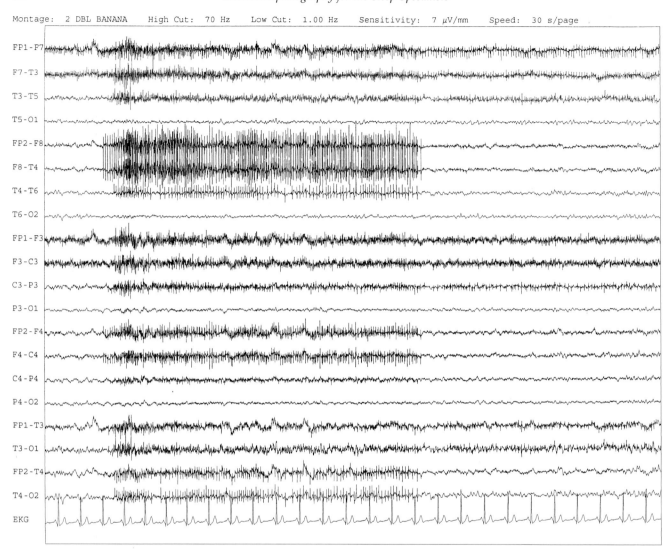

Montage: 2 DBL BANANA   High Cut: 70 Hz   Low Cut: 1.00 Hz   Sensitivity: 7 µV/mm   Speed: 30 s/page

FIGURE 2–14, cont'd   ***B:*** *Same subject data as in* **A** *viewed at a 30-second epoch.*

Sharp Transients Seen during Sleep and Wakefulness

Sharp transients seen during sleep and wakefulness may include positive occipital sharp transients (POSTS) (Figures 2–15 and 2–16), Mu rhythms (Figure 2–17) posterior slow waves of youth (Figure 2–18), vertex sharp waves (Figure 2–19), K-complexes (Figure 2–20), sharp appearing spindles, hypnagogic or hypnopomping hypersynchrony resembling spike-wave complexes (Figure 2–21), benign epileptiform transients of sleep (BETS) (Figure 2–22), photic driving responses that may resemble spikes or sharp waves (Figure 2–23), and augmentation of ongoing background rhythm assuming a sharp or spike-like appearance (see Figure 2–8B). These sharp transients can

be differentiated by paying attention to their distribution and morphology, the background activities, and the state of the patient's alertness. Vertex sharp waves, sharp-appearing K complexes, spindles, POSTs, and hypnagogic hypersynchrony are state dependent and have characteristic distribution. Some are age-dependent such as hypnagogic hypersynchrony and posterior slow wave of youth. Mu rhythms (see Figure 2–17) consist of brief bursts of 7 to 11 hertz over the central regions, which show attenuation on active or passive movements of the limbs or even an intention to move the limbs, usually contralaterally. Similar rhythms located in the temporal regions are called *wicket rhythms* (Fgiure 2–24), and these have no specific significance but may sometimes be mistaken for epileptiform discharges.

Text continued on p. 80

Montage: 2 DBL BANANA   High Cut: 70 Hz   Low Cut: 1.00 Hz   Sensitivity: 3 μV/mm   Speed: 10 s/page

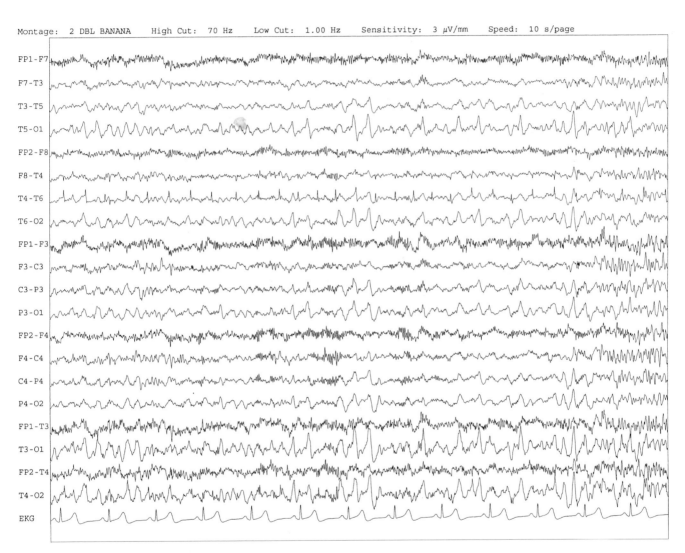

FIGURE 2–15. A: *Positive occipital sharp transients (POSTs) of sleep seen bilaterally in posterior temporal and occipital electrodes in non–rapid eye movement (NREM) sleep. POSTs occur predominantly in stage I and II NREM; they are characterized by monophasic positive polarity in occipital electrodes and may be recorded synchronously or asynchronously.*

Montage: 2 DBL BANANA   High Cut: 70 Hz   Low Cut: 1.00 Hz   Sensitivity: 3 μV/mm   Speed: 30 s/page

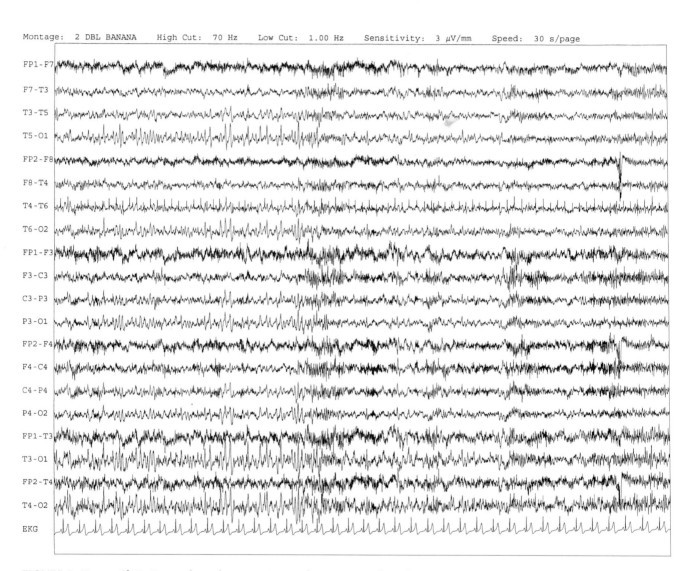

FIGURE 2–15, cont'd B: *Same subject data as in* **A** *viewed at a 30-second epoch.*

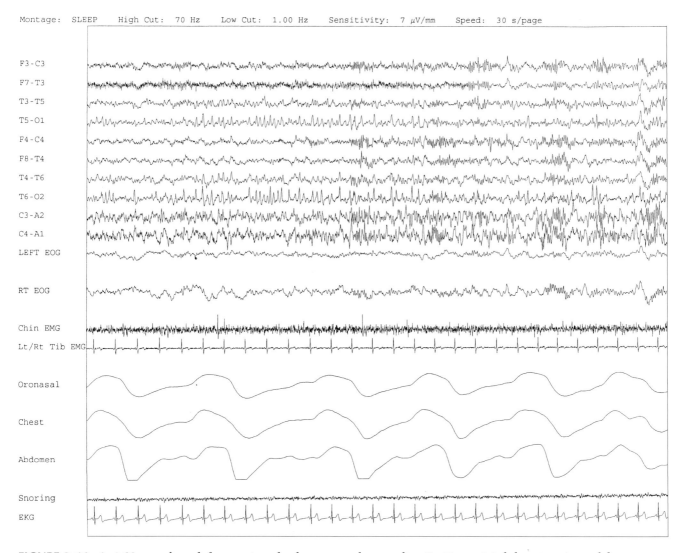

Montage: SLEEP   High Cut: 70 Hz   Low Cut: 1.00 Hz   Sensitivity: 7 μV/mm   Speed: 30 s/page

FIGURE 2–16. **A:** *A 30-second epoch from nocturnal polysomnography recording. Positive occipital sharp transients of sleep are seen bilaterally in posterior temporal and occipital electrodes recorded during stage II non–rapid eye movement sleep.*

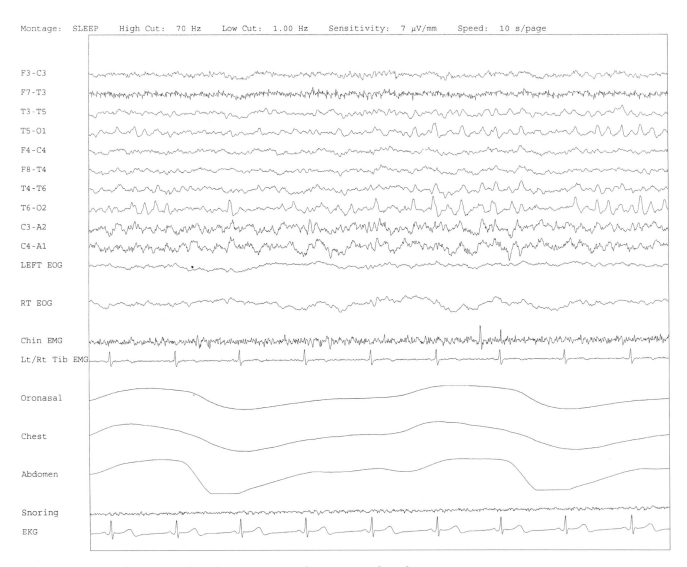

FIGURE 2–16, cont'd *B: Same subject data as in* **A** *viewed at a 10-second epoch.*

Montage: MSLT-NEW   High Cut: 70 Hz   Low Cut: 0.53 Hz   Sensitivity: 5 µV/mm   Speed: 10 s/page

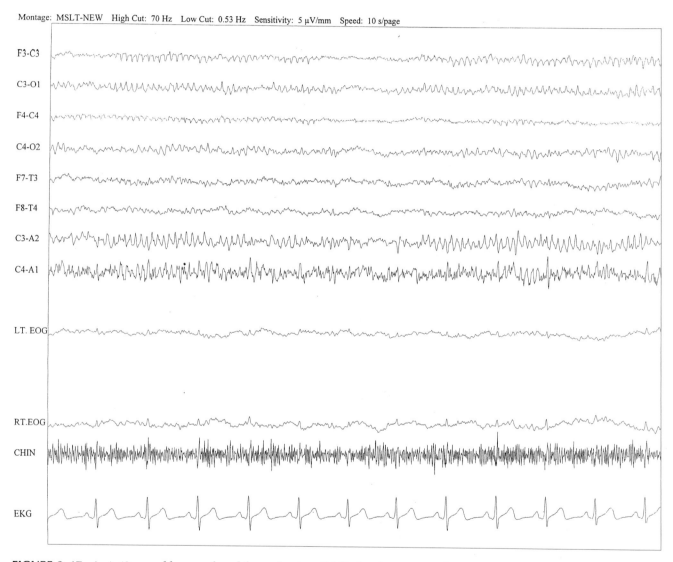

FIGURE 2–17. **A:** *A 40-year-old man referred for evaluation of difficulty sleeping at night, snoring, and excessive daytime sleepiness. The epoch is taken from multiple sleep latency test in stage I non–rapid eye movement sleep. Mu rhythm is seen bilaterally over the central regions (C3-C4 electrodes), but it is better defined on the left than on the right central regions.*

Montage: MSLT-NEW   High Cut: 70 Hz   Low Cut: 0.53 Hz   Sensitivity: 5 μV/mm   Speed: 30 s/page

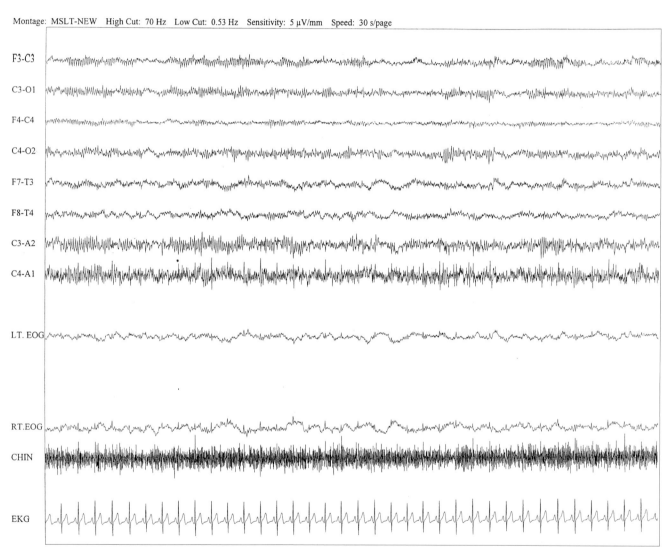

FIGURE 2–17, cont'd B: *Same subject data as in* **A** *viewed at a 30-second epoch.*

Montage: 2 DBL BANANA   High Cut: 70 Hz   Low Cut: 1.00 Hz   Sensitivity: 10 μV/mm   Speed: 10 s/page

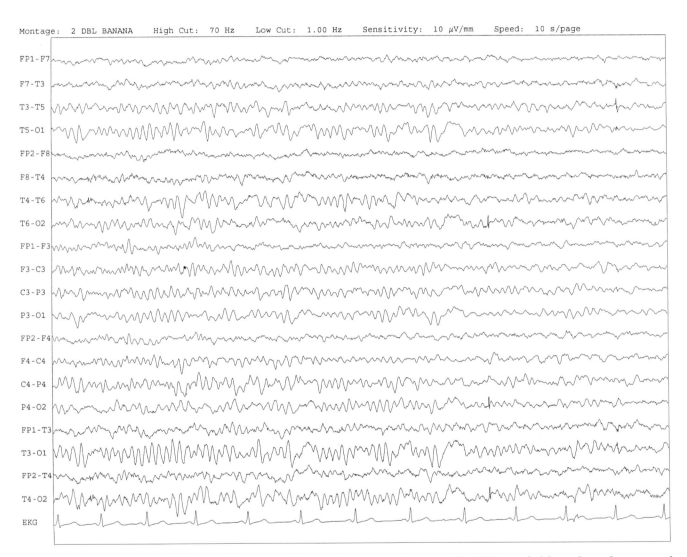

FIGURE 2–18. A: *A 15-year-old female adolescent with history of new onset of seizures. The EEG in wakefulness shows slow waves of youth at 2 to 3 hertz superimposed intermittently on occipital alpha rhythm at 9 to 10 hertz bilaterally. This is a normal finding between ages 2 and 21 years of age, most commonly occurring between 8 and 14 years of age, and attenuates with eye opening.*

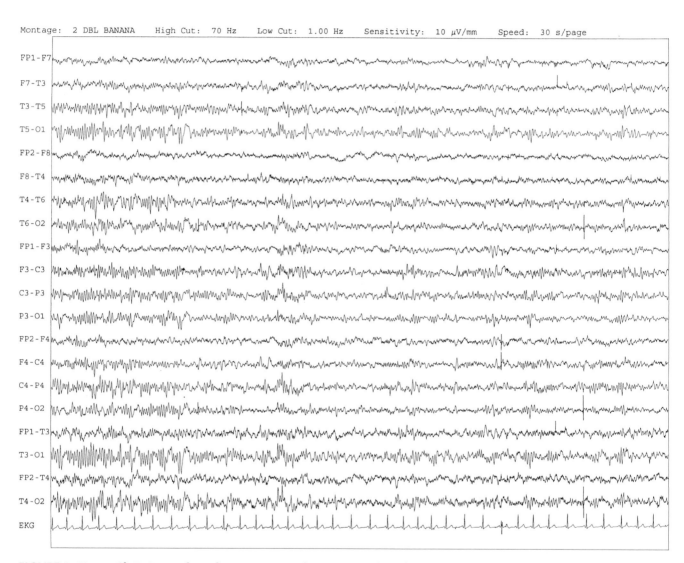

FIGURE 2–18, cont'd B: *Same subject data as in* **A** *viewed at a 30-second epoch.*

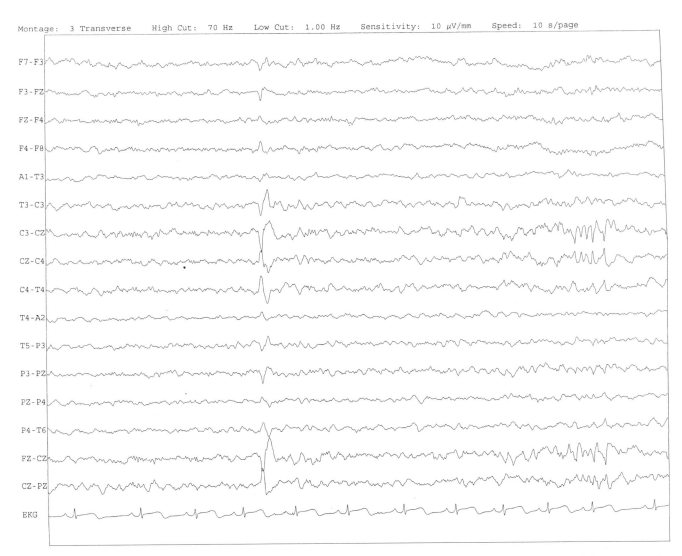

FIGURE 2–19. A: *This tracing shows vertex sharp waves seen as negative potentials with a wide distribution around the vertex. In this segment, V waves are seen at C3, C4, and CZ with spread of activities to F3, F4, P3, P4, PZ and FZ.*

Montage: 3 Transverse   High Cut: 70 Hz   Low Cut: 1.00 Hz   Sensitivity: 10 μV/mm   Speed: 30 s/page

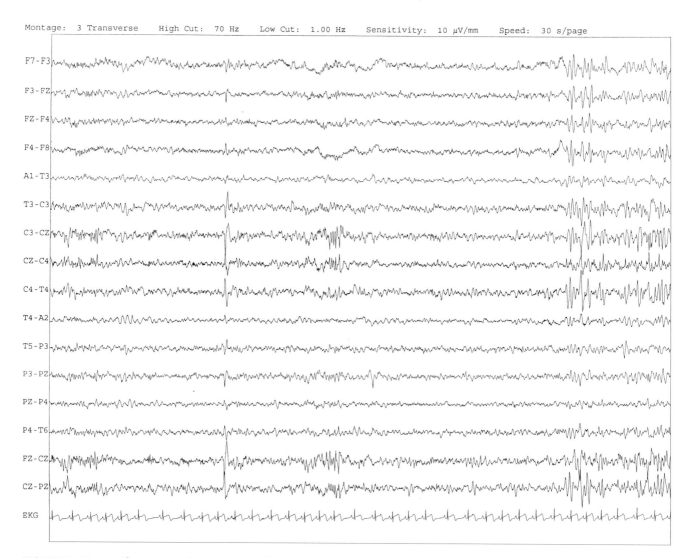

FIGURE 2–19, cont'd B: *Same subject as in* **A** *with data viewed over a 30-second epoch.*

Montage: 4 Ref Cz   High Cut: 70 Hz   Low Cut: 1.00 Hz   Sensitivity: 7 µV/mm   Speed: 10 s/page

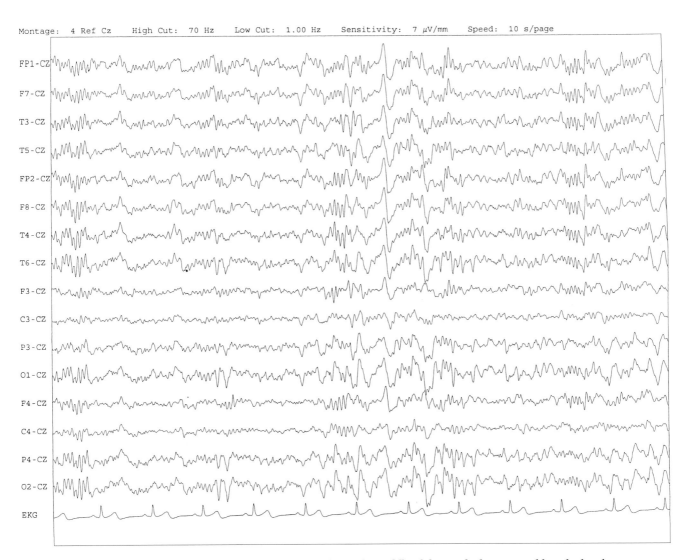

FIGURE 2–20. **A:** *The tracing shows the presence of a K complex in the middle of the epoch characterized by a high-voltage negative-positive potential followed by sleep spindles.*

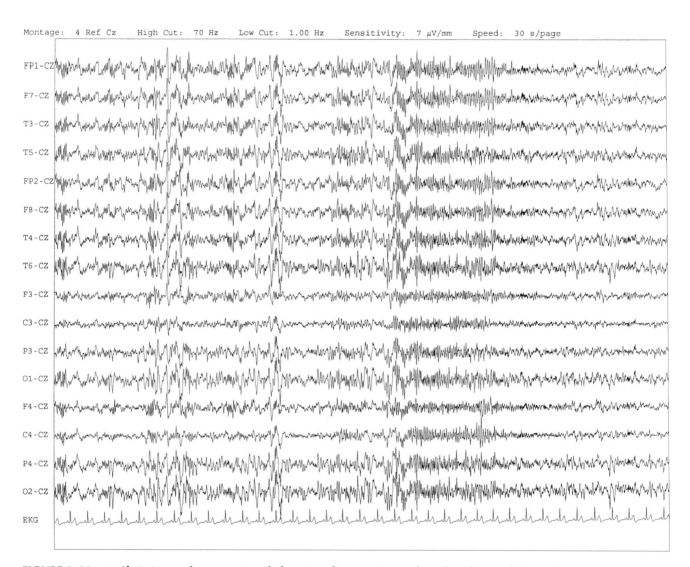

```
Montage:  4 Ref Cz    High Cut:  70 Hz    Low Cut:  1.00 Hz    Sensitivity:  7 µV/mm    Speed:  30 s/page
```

FIGURE 2–20, cont'd B: *Same subject as in* **A** *with data viewed over a 30-second epoch with several K complexes.*

Montage: 4 Ref Cz   High Cut: 70 Hz   Low Cut: 1.00 Hz   Sensitivity: 20 μV/mm   Speed: 10 s/page

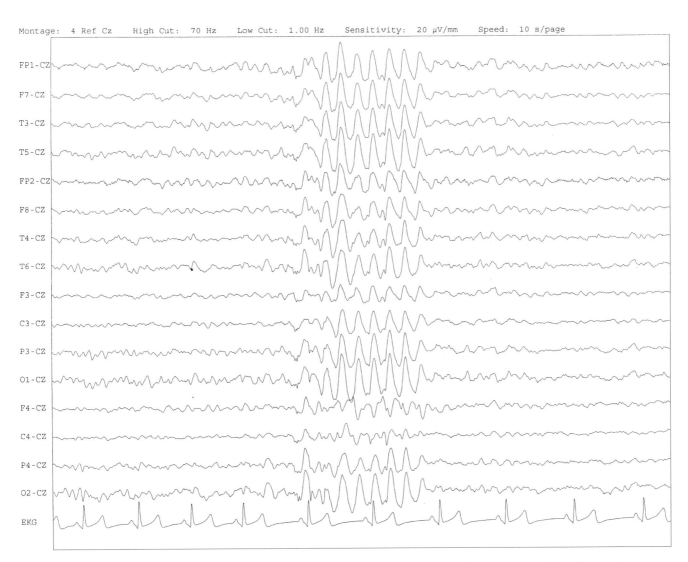

FIGURE 2–21. A: *This epoch was recorded in a 9-year-old girl during stage II non–rapid eye movement sleep showing hypnagogic hypersynchrony characterized by a brief burst of synchronous high-voltage slow activity at 4- to 5-hertz activity.*

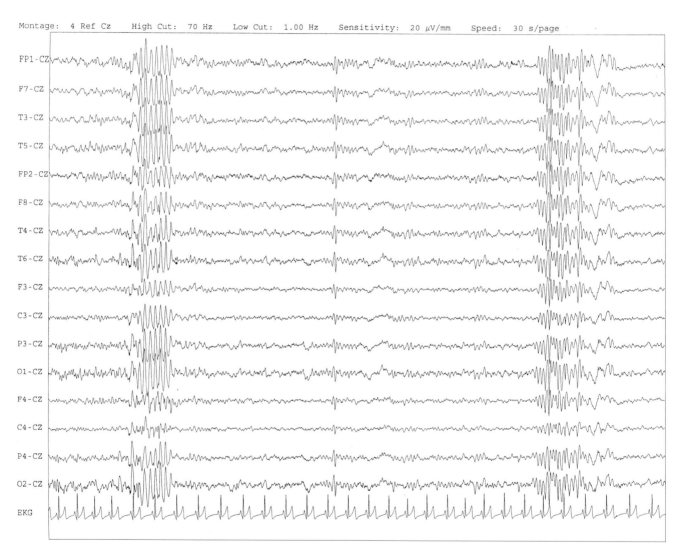

FIGURE 2–21, cont'd B: *Same subject data as in* **A** *viewed over a 30-second epoch. At end of the epoch, a sleep spindle burst is seen in all channels referred to the CZ electrode.*

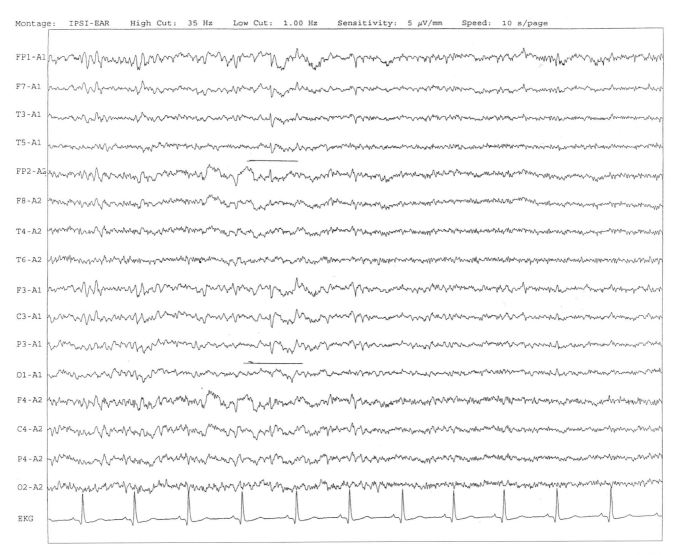

FIGURE 2–22. A: *Benign epileptiform transients of sleep or small sharp spikes (SSS) are seen bilaterally, more prominent on the left side in channels (as underlined) 1 to 5 and 9 to 11 in a 67-year-old man. SSS are best recorded in ipsilateral ear montage during stage I non–rapid eye movement sleep as shown in this epoch. SSS may be seen asynchronously on either side as well.*

Montage: IPSI-EAR   High Cut: 35 Hz   Low Cut: 1.00 Hz   Sensitivity: 5 μV/mm   Speed: 30 s/page

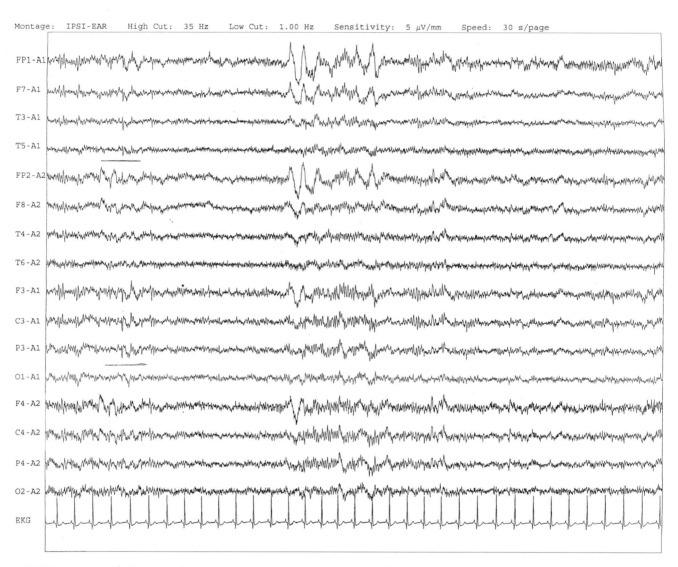

FIGURE 2–22, cont'd B: *Same subject as in* **A** *viewed over a 30-second epoch.*

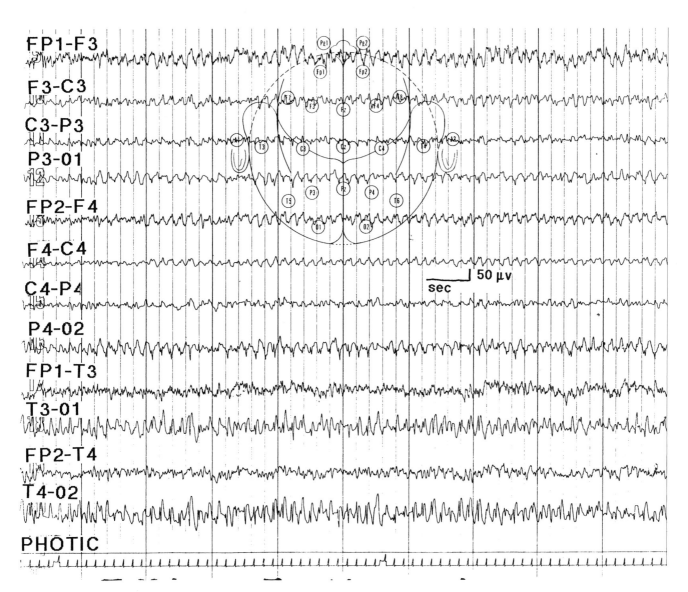

FIGURE 2–23. *Photic driving responses seen diffusely at 7 hertz resembling spike and wave bursts. (From Chokroverty S. Role of electroencephalography in epilepsy. In Management of Epilepsy. Boston: Butterworth-Heinemann, 1996, with permission.)*

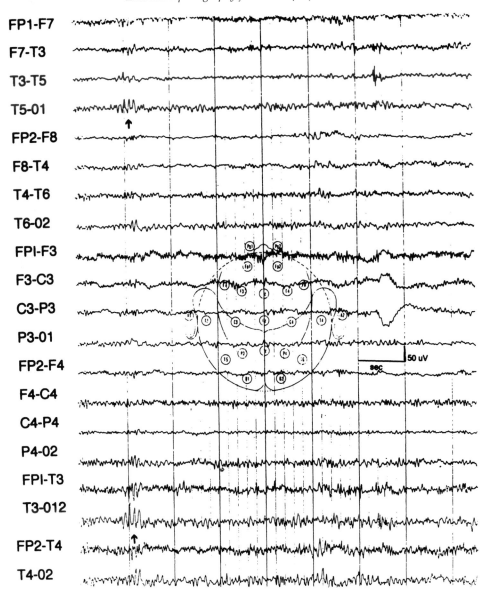

FIGURE 2–24. *Several spike-like waves (wicket spikes) repeating rhythmically at T3-T5 (arrows) as well as in T4 with reduced amplitude in an adult without any history of seizures. (From Chokroverty S. Role of electroencephalography in epilepsy. In Management of Epilepsy. Boston: Butterworth-Heinemann, 1996, with permission.)*

Sharp Transients of Doubtful Significance

These transients include small sharp spikes (2–22) or BETS, 6-hertz spike and waves (Figure 2–25) or phantom spike-waves, and psychomotor variant pattern or rhythmic midtemporal discharges (Figure 2–26). Midtemporal rhythmic discharge of drowsiness has characteristic square-topped appearance and is usually seen during stages I and II of NREM sleep, maximally in the midtemporal region.

Epileptiform-like Patterns without Epileptogenic Significance

These patterns include the following: Triphasic waves (Figure 2–27), periodic or pseudoperiodic lateralized epileptiform discharges (PLEDs) (Figure 2–28), periodic complexes (Figure 2–29), subclinical rhythmic epileptiform discharge of adults, and burst suppression patterns (Figure 2–30).

Text continued on p. 91

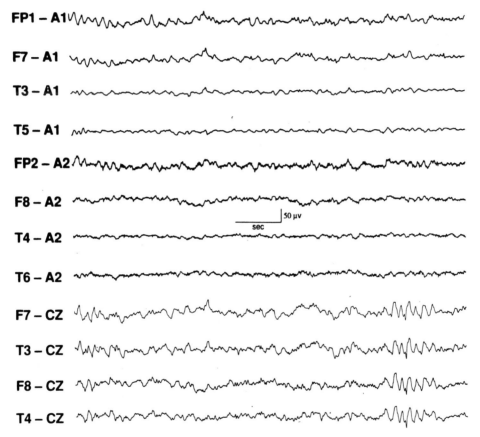

FIGURE 2–25. *Six-hertz spike and wave pattern seen in the last four channels. (From Walczak T, Chokroverty S. Electroencephalography, electromyography and electrooculography: General principles and basic technology. In Chokroverty S, ed. Sleep Disorders Medicine. Boston: Butterworth-Heinemann, 1999:191, with permission.)*

Montage: PSG limbs-PFLOW   High Cut: 70 Hz   Low Cut: 1.00 Hz   Sensitivity: 7 μV/mm   Speed: 10 s/page

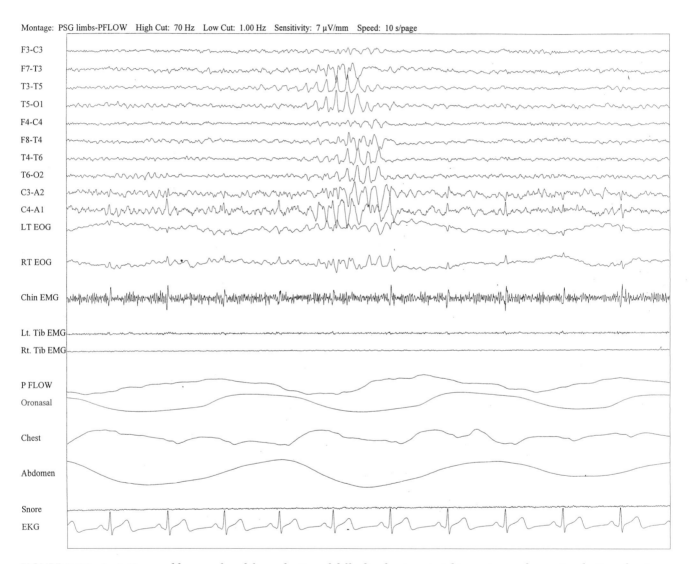

FIGURE 2–26. A: *A 40-year-old man referred for evaluation of difficulty sleeping at night, snoring, and excessive daytime sleepiness. This 10-second epoch is taken from nocturnal polysomnography in stage I non–rapid eye movement sleep. Rhythmic mid-temporal theta of drowsiness (RMTD) is seen as a brief burst of rhythmic theta activity at 6 to 7 hertz recorded asynchronously over left and right temporal electrodes.*

Montage: PSG limbs-PFLOW   High Cut: 70 Hz   Low Cut: 0.53 Hz   Sensitivity: 7 μV/mm   Speed: 30 s/page

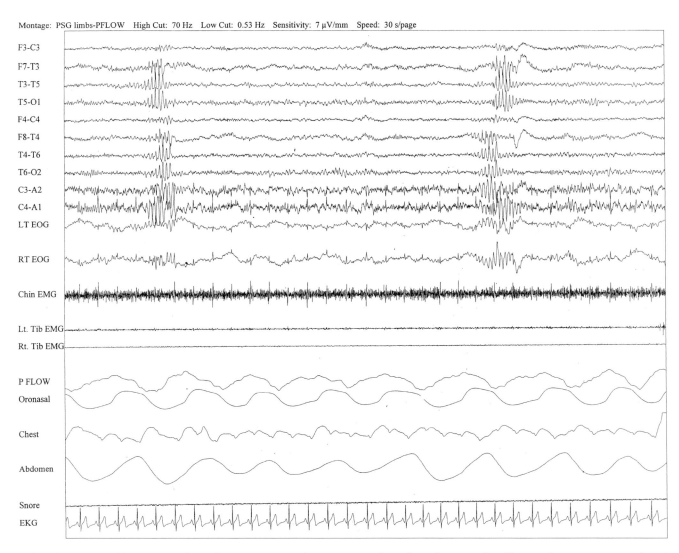

FIGURE 2–26, cont'd B: *Same subject data as in* **A** *viewed over 30-second epoch. It shows two brief bursts of RMTD, one at each end of the epoch.*

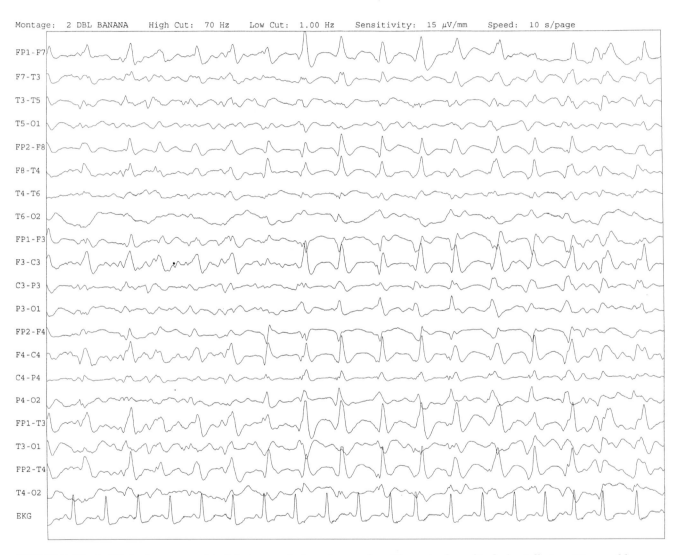

FIGURE 2–27. A: *Triphasic waves at 1 to 2 hertz recorded synchronously, with maximal amplitude frontally in a 67-year-old woman with a history of end-stage renal disease and hepatitis.*

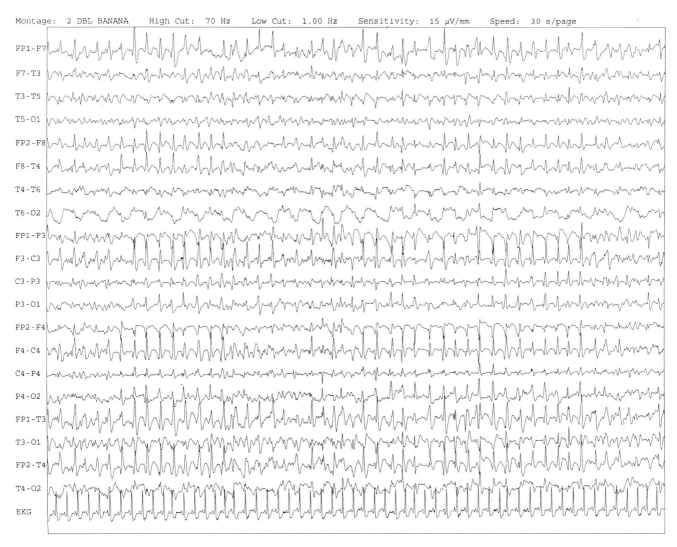

Montage: 2 DBL BANANA   High Cut: 70 Hz   Low Cut: 1.00 Hz   Sensitivity: 15 μV/mm   Speed: 30 s/page

FIGURE 2–27, cont'd B: *Same subject data as in* **A** *viewed over a 30-second epoch.*

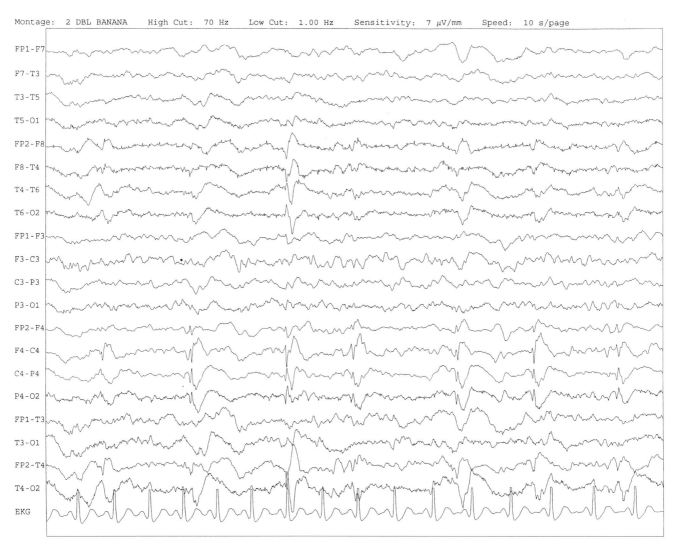

Montage: 2 DBL BANANA   High Cut: 70 Hz   Low Cut: 1.00 Hz   Sensitivity: 7 µV/mm   Speed: 10 s/page

FIGURE 2–28. A: *A 49-year-old woman with a history of right frontal subdural hematoma, ovarian cancer, colon cancer, and seizures. Periodic lateralizing epileptiform discharges are characterized by spike and wave activity recurring at 1.5 to 2 seconds over the right central region and spreading to the right temporal region. The background shows diffuse slowing.*

Montage: 2 DBL BANANA   High Cut: 70 Hz   Low Cut: 1.00 Hz   Sensitivity: 7 μV/mm   Speed: 30 s/page

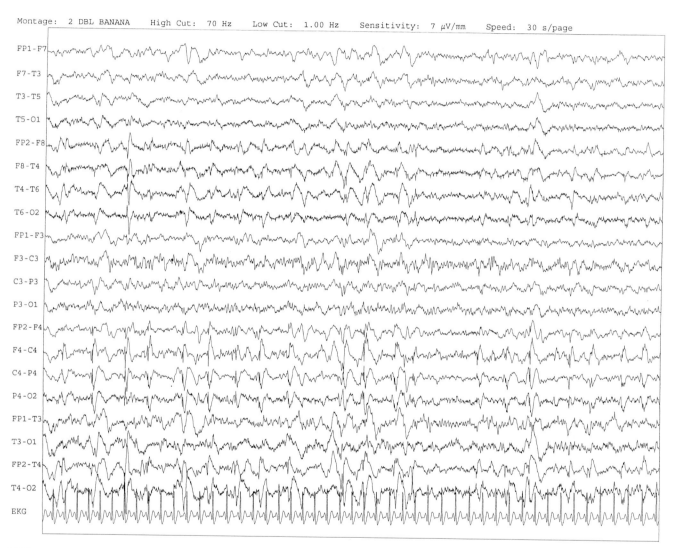

FIGURE 2–28, cont'd B: *Same subject data as in* **A** *viewed over 30-second epochs.*

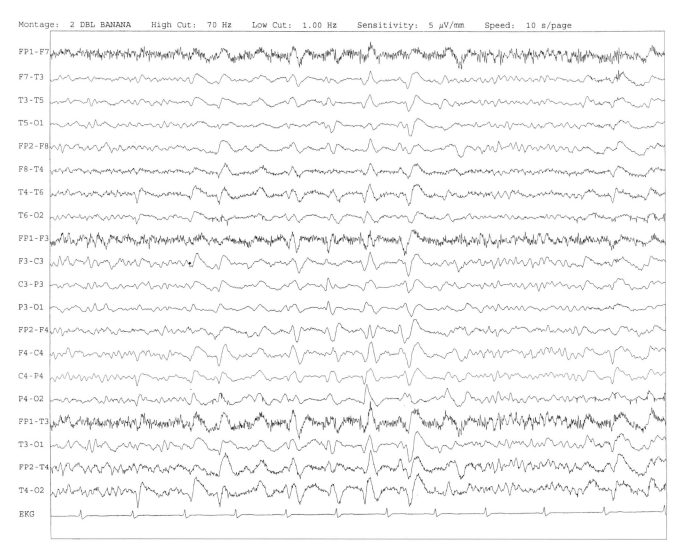

FIGURE 2–29. A: *An 81-year-old man with history of dementia and transient ischemic attacks. EEG shows the presence of generalized, intermittent, periodic or pseudoperiodic sharp- and slow-wave discharges at 1 to 2 hertz.*

Montage: 3 Transverse   High Cut: 70 Hz   Low Cut: 1.00 Hz   Sensitivity: 7 μV/mm   Speed: 30 s/page

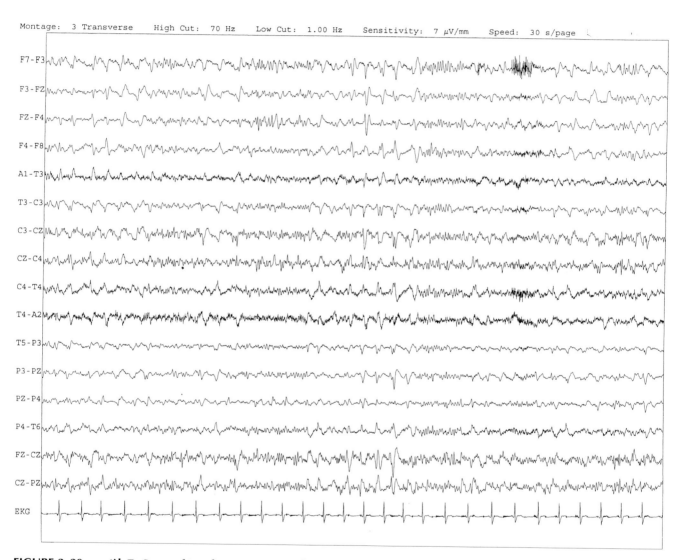

FIGURE 2–29, cont'd B: *Same subject data as in **A** viewed at a 30-second epoch.*

Montage: 2 DBL BANANA   High Cut: 70 Hz   Low Cut: 1.00 Hz   Sensitivity: 20 µV/mm   Speed: 10 s/page

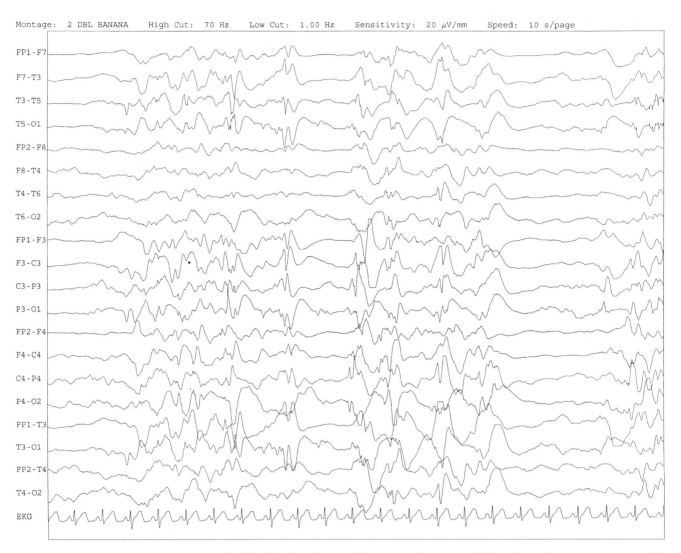

FIGURE 2–30. A: *The patient is a 6-month-old girl with a history of hypoxic ischemic encephalopathy and recurrent seizures. The recording shows a burst suppression pattern characterized by bursts of generalized spike and wave and polyspike and wave discharges lasting 2 to 3 seconds with intervening periods of relative voltage suppression (quiescence).*

Montage: 2 DBL BANANA   High Cut: 70 Hz   Low Cut: 1.00 Hz   Sensitivity: 20 μV/mm   Speed: 30 s/page

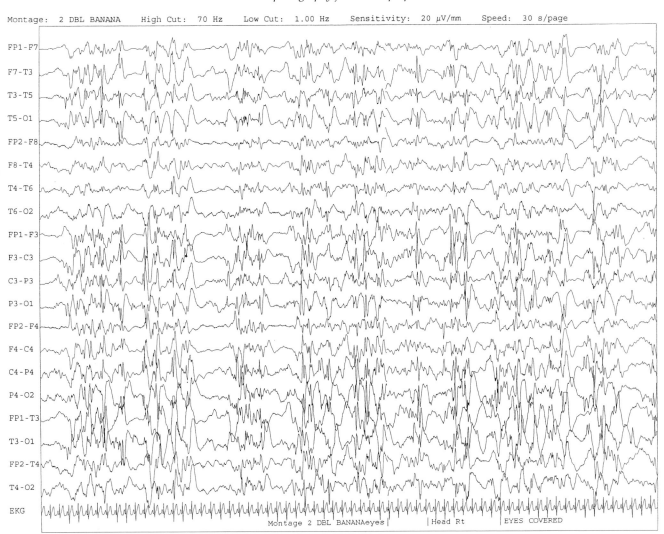

FIGURE 2–30, cont'd **B:** *Same subject data as in* **A** *viewed at a 30-second epoch.*

Triphasic waves have an initial positive configuration and characteristic distribution. These are seen synchronously and symmetrically with frontal dominance of the amplitude with anteroposterior phase shift. Triphasic waves are not of epileptiform significance but may be seen in metabolic or toxic encephalopathies (e.g., hepatic, renal, or respiratory failure). Sometimes these are seen in anoxic encephalopathies also.

Patients with focal or generalized seizures may sometimes present only during night (nocturnal seizures) and may be mistaken for other motor disorders during sleep such as motor parasomnias. Sometimes patients with sleep apnea are mistaken for nocturnal seizures. It is, therefore, important for the sleep specialists to be familiar with the patterns seen in primary generalized seizure (e.g., absence spells or generalized tonic-clonic seizures) and partial

complex seizures of temporal or extratemporal (frontal) origin. Patients with nocturnal frontal lobe epilepsy are often referred to the laboratory for PSG recording (see Chapter 9). The characteristic EEG pattern in the primary generalized epilepsy of the absence type is the presence of symmetrical and synchronous frontally dominant 3-hertz spike and wave discharges (see Figure 2–9) seen either as an ictal or interictal pattern. Patients with tonic-clonic seizure may show a sudden burst of spike and slow waves beginning at a rate of 4 to 6 hertz and then gradually slow down and stop before the postictal period. These discharges are seen in a bilaterally symmetrical and synchronous fashion. Postictal slow waves are followed by gradual recovery to the preictal normal background rhythm after several hours or sometimes after a day or two. Interictal EEG may show generalized synchronous and symmetrical

4- to 6-hertz spike- and slow-wave discharges or multiple spike and waves.

Certain types of seizures are characteristically observed during sleep, including tonic seizures, benign focal epilepsy of childhood with centrotemporal spikes, juvenile myoclonic epilepsy, continuous spike and waves during slow-wave sleep, nocturnal frontal lobe epilepsy, and a subtype of partial complex seizure of temporal lobe origin. Some patients with generalized tonic-clonic and partial complex seizure may also have predominantly nocturnal seizures. It is important to differentiate nocturnal seizures from motor and behavioral parasomnias and other movement disorders persisting during sleep. Tonic seizures are typically activated by sleep, occur frequently during NREM sleep, and are never seen during REM sleep. A typical EEG shows interictal abnormality as slow spike and waves intermixed during sleep with trains of fast spikes. Benign focal epilepsy of childhood with centrotemporal spikes is characterized by the presence of centrotemporal or rolandic spikes or sharp waves (Figure 2–31). Seizures generally stop by the age of 15 to 20 years without any neurologic sequelae. Juvenile myoclonic epilepsy shows typi-

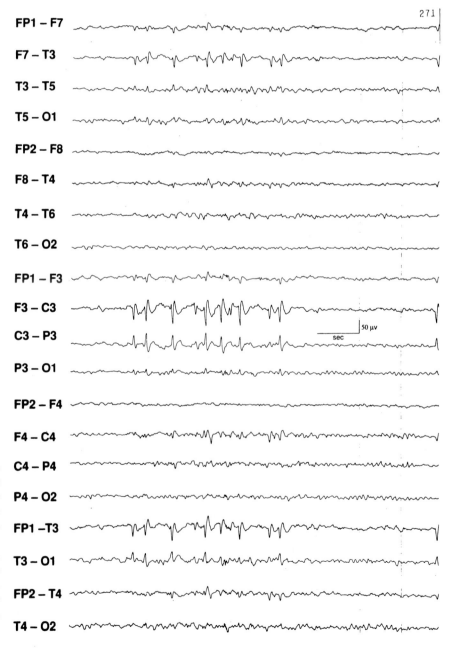

FIGURE 2–31. *EEG showing left centrotemporal spikes and sharp waves in a patient with benign rolandic epilepsy (sylvian seizures). Benign rolandic seizures commonly present in childhood as unilateral tonic or clonic seizures in face or arm, speech arrest, and paresthesias in the mouth or tongue. (From Chokroverty S, Quinto C. Sleep and epilepsy. In Chokroverty S, ed. Sleep Disorders Medicine. Boston: Butterworth-Heinemann, 1999:711, with permission.)*

cally in the EEG synchronous and symmetrical multiple spikes and spike-wave discharges. The EEG in the entity of continuous spike and waves during NREM sleep consists of generalized 2- to 2.5-hertz spike and wave discharges occupying 85 percent of NREM sleep and are suppressed during REM sleep. This entity is generally seen in children. Nocturnal frontal lobe seizures are discussed in Chapter 9.

In a patient suspected of seizure, the patient should have a routine EEG recording with hyperventilation, sleep, and photic stimulation during daytime. If no epileptiform discharge is noted, then the EEG should be repeated after partial or total sleep deprivation. After 3 to 4 negative EEGs in these particular patients suspected of nocturnal seizure, an overnight PSG study, preferably video-PSG, should be obtained for electroclinical correlation. In such patients, appropriately devised seizure montage with full complement of electrodes or special electrode placements (e.g., T1 and T2 electrodes) should be used. If during the recording the technician observes or suspects a seizure, then the recording should be switched during this episode to 10 millimeters per second for better recognition. During the interpretation of PSG study, of course, the montage can be reformatted to study the pattern at 10 millimeters instead of the usual PSG recording speed of 30 millimeters per second because it is easy to recognize the pattern in 10-millimeter-per-second speed.

REFERENCES

1. Walczak T, Chokroverty S. Electroencephalography, electroymyography, and electro-oculography: General principles and basic technology. In: Chokroverty S, ed. *Sleep Disorders Medicine: Basic Science, Technical Considerations, and Clinical Aspects*, 2nd ed. Boston, MA: Butterworth Heinemann; 1999:175–203.
2. Niedermeyer E, Lopes Da Silva, eds. *Electroencephalography: Basic Principles, Clinical Science, and Related Fields*, 4th ed. Philadelphia: Lippincott, Williams and Wilkins, 1999: 858–895.
3. Ebersole J, Pedley T. *Current Practice of Clinical Electroencephalography*, 3rd ed. Philadelphia: Lippincott, Williams and Wilkins, 2003.
4. Fisch BJ. *Fisch and Spehlman's EEG Primer: Basic Principles of Digital and Analog EEG*, 3rd ed. Amsterdam: Elsevier, 1999.
5. Chokroverty S. Role of electroencephalography in epilepsy. In: Chokroverty S, ed. *Management of Epilepsy*. Boston: Butterworth-Heinemann, 1996:67–112.

3

Recognition of Sleep Stages and Adult Scoring Technique

ALON Y. AVIDAN

SLEEP STAGE SCORING

Sleep stage scoring is based on criteria derived from several physiologic signals, usually as outlined by Rechtschaffen and Kales (1968). The Rechtschaffen and Kales (R-K) method divides sleep into five distinct stages: non–rapid eye movement (NREM) I , II, III, and IV and stage rapid eye movement (REM) sleep. Particular signals of interest are generated from the cerebral cortex (electroencephalography [EEG]), eye movements (picked up by the electrooculography [EOG] electrodes), and the muscles of the face (picked up by chin electromyographic [EMG] activity). Sleep stages should not be viewed as distinct entities, but rather as a gradual transition of a waveform. The scoring rules were devised to allow for uniformity between sleep laboratories and conceptual simplicity rather than being a rigid framework. Table 3–1 summarizes sleep stages and lists their characteristics utilizing the R-K criteria.

This chapter will include a discussion of the specific parameters required for staging sleep, and a summary of the various EEG activity needed to score sleep. This discussion will be followed by a discussion of the stages of sleep utilizing specific polysomnographic (PSG) records. Unless otherwise stated, all PSG samples are recorded at a paper speed of 10 millimeters per second, where one page equates to 30 seconds and is defined as one epoch.

The following abbreviations are used in the PSG samples provided in this chapter:
LOC-A2, ROC-A1 = Left and right electrooculogram referred to right and left mastoid leads.
LOC-AVG = Left electrooculogram referred to an average reference electrode.

Chin1-Chin2 = Chin EMG electrode.
EEG Monitoring = The exploring reference electrode (F3, F4, C3, C4, O1, and O2) is chosen on the opposite side of the head from the mastoid electrode (A1, A2) or average (AVG).
LAT1-LAT2, RAT1-RAT2 = Leg (anterior tibialis) EMG electrode (L = Left, R = Right).
ORAL-NASAL = Oral/nasal airflow channel.
THOR1-THOR2 = Thoracic effort channel.
ABD1-ABD2 = Abdominal effort channel.
*Figures are provided with a 1-second ruler.

PARAMETERS FOR STAGING HUMAN SLEEP

Common to all PSG monitoring is the measure of the following three physiologic parameters:

EOG leads: Left eye and right eye.
EEG leads: A minimum of one central EEG lead and one occipital EEG lead.
EMG lead: One submental EMG channel.
Eye movements: EOG activity.

The EOG signals measure changes in the electrical potential of the positive anterior aspect of the eye, the cornea, relative to the negative posterior aspect, the retina. Horizontal axis electrodes are placed near the outer canthi and vertical axis electrodes 1 centimeter below (LOC) and 1 centimeter above (ROC) the eye to measure transient changes in potential during the actual eye movement. During any eye movement, the cornea moves toward one electrode, while the retina moves away. When the eye is

Table 3–1. Summary of Sleep Stages According to Rechtschaffen-Kales Criteria

Properties	Stage Wake (W)	Stage I	Stage II	Stage III & IV Sleep	Stage REM Sleep
EEG	Eyes open: Low voltage, mixed frequency. *Alpha* attenuates. Eyes closed: Low voltage, high frequency. More than 50% *alpha* activity	Low voltage, mixed frequency. *Theta activity*. *Vertex sharp waves*	Low voltage, mixed frequency. At least one *K complex/sleep spindle* Less than 20% high amplitude delta	**Stage III** = 20%–50% high-amplitude delta activity; **Stage IV** = >50% high- amplitude delta activity	Low voltage, mixed frequency. Presence of *sawtooth waves* *Desynchronized EEG* (In all other stages, the EEG is *synchronized*)
EOG	Eye blinks, voluntary control, *SREM* when drowsy	*SREM*	Occasional *SREM*	Mirrors EEG	Phasic REM
EMG	Tonic activity, High EMG activity Under voluntary control	Tonic activity High-medium EMG activity	Tonic activity Low EMG activity	Tonic activity Low EMG activity	*T-REM*: Relatively reduced *P-REM*: Episodic EMG twitching
Duration		10 minutes	20 minutes	30-45 minutes	The first REM period is very short, lasting about 5 minutes, the second is about 10 minutes, and the third is roughly 15 minutes. The final REM period usually lasts for 30 minutes, but sometimes lasts an hour.
Arousal Threshold		Lowest	Lower	Highest	Low
Physiological Changes		Progressive reduction of physiologic activity, heart rate slow down		Progressive reduction of physiologic activity, blood pressure,	*T-REM* = Muscle paralysis, increased cerebral blood flow *P-REM* = Irregular breathing, variable heart rate, REM, phasic muscle twitching
%TST	2–5%	3–8%	44–55%	10–15%	20–25%
Dreaming				Diffuse dreams	Vivid, bizarre and detailed dreams
Parasomnias	Hypnic jerks in transition to stage I	Hypnic jerks	Confusional arousals, Somniliquy	Sleep walking, night terrors	REM sleep behavior disorder, REM nightmares

EEG, Electroencephalography; *EOG,* electrooculography; *MG,* electromyography; *REM,* rapid eye movements; *T-REM,* tonic REM; *P-REM,* phasic REM; *SREM,* slow, rolling eye movements. [For stage MT (movement time), please see text]
Adapted from Rechtschaffen A, Kales A, eds. *A Manual of Standardised Terminology, Techniques and Scoring System for Sleep Stages of Human Subjects.* Los Angeles: Brain Information Service/Brain Research Institute, 1968.

not moving, the change in relative position is zero, and the eye leads do not record a signal.

Slow, rolling eye movements, or SREMs, occur during drowsiness and light sleep, and are recorded as long gentle waves, whereas rapid jerking movements are represented by sharply contoured fast waves. Blinking of the eyes produces rapid vertical movements. During REM sleep, eye movements again become active and jerky. The intensity of the bursts of activity is used to describe the density of REM sleep.

Electrooculogram Recording

EOG voltages are higher than EEG signals. Since the eye is outside of the skull structure, there is no bone to attenuate signal.

The cornea (front) has a positive polarity. The retina (back) has a negative polarity.

EOG placement (LOC and ROC) is on the outer canthus of the eye, offset 1 centimeter below (LOC) and 1 centimeter above (ROC) the horizon.

EOG picks up the inherent voltage of the eye. During eyes-open wakefulness, sharp deflections in the EOG tracing may indicate the presence of eye blinks.

Electroencephalography Recording

Wakefulness and sleep are determined by the characteristic patterns of the scalp EEG signals and are of fundamental importance in interpreting PSG studies. EEG records electrical potentials generated by the cortex but can reflect the influence of deeper brain structures, such as the thalamus. Two centrencephalic and two occipital cortical channels are recorded. Measurement of the EEG signal is possible because of the relative difference in potential between two recording electrodes. A negative discharge, by convention, is represented by an upwardly deflecting wave. The PSG references the left and right centrencephalic electrodes (C3, C4) or the left and right occipital electrodes (O1, O2) to electrodes on the opposite right and left ears (A2, A1). The general rule is to read only from the left cortical channel. However, when the left channel develops artifact or the validity of the signal is suspected, comparison is made with the right cortical channel.

Electroencephalography Recording Criteria

Minimum paper speed of 10 millimeters per second. One page equates to 30 seconds and is defined as one epoch.

Time constant (TC) of 0.3 second or low-frequency filter (LFF) of 0.3 hertz.

Pen deflections of 7.5 to 10 mm for 50 microvolts are recommended.

Electrode impedances should not exceed 10 kilohms.

Electromyographic Recording

The EMG signals are muscle twitch potentials that are used in PSG to distinguish between sleep stages based on the fact that EMG activity diminishes during sleep. Specifically, during REM sleep, muscle activity is minimal. Compounding the problem of interpreting EMG channels is the occasional intrusion of EMG artifact into the record. Some of these intrusions are in the form of yawns, swallows, and teeth grinding (bruxism).

Submental Electromyographic Recording Criteria

Mental, submental, and masseter placements are acceptable.

They are used to detect muscle tone changes for scoring REM versus NREM sleep.

Muscle tone is high during wakefulness and NREM sleep. It is lower in NREM sleep than in wakefulness. It is generally lower in slow-wave sleep than in stage I or II.

Muscle tone is lowest during stage REM.

Submental EMG records muscle tone. This is a mandatory recording parameter for staging sleep.

ELECTROENCEPHALOGRAPHIC ACTIVITY DURING WAKEFULNESS AND SLEEP

Cortical activity can be characterized by their specific frequencies. Frequency is defined as the number of times a repetitive wave recurs in a specific time period (typically 1 second). Frequency is noted as cycles per second (i.e., hertz). EEG activity has been divided into four bands based on the frequency and amplitude of the waveform and are assigned Greek letters (alpha, beta, theta, and delta). The following conventions for EEG frequencies are used: Beta is greater than 13 hertz; alpha is between 8 and 13 hertz; theta is between 4 and less than 8 hertz, and delta is the slowest activity at less than 4 hertz. Another EEG activity is gamma, which ranges from 30–45 Hz.

Beta Activity

Beta EEG is defined as a waveform between 14–30 hertz. But is usually between 18–25 hertz.

Originates in the frontal and central regions; can also occur more diffusely.

Present during wakefulness and drowsiness.

May be more persistent during drowsiness, diminish during deeper sleep, and reemerge during REM sleep.

The amplitude over the two hemispheres should not vary by more than 50 percent.

Enhanced or persistent activity suggests use of sedative-hypnotic medications.

Alpha Activity

Alpha EEG: 8 to 13 hertz.

Originates in the parietooccipital regions bilaterally.

A normal alpha rhythm is synchronous and symmetric over the cerebral hemispheres.

Seen during quiet alertness with eyes closed.

Eye opening causes the alpha waves to "react" or decrease in amplitude.

Has a crescendo-decrescendo appearance.

Decrease in frequency occurs with aging.

Theta Activity

Theta EEG: A frequency of 4 to 8 hertz.

Originates in the central vertex region.

There are no amplitude criteria for theta activity.

It is the most common sleep frequency.

Sleep Spindles

EEG frequency: 12 to 18 hertz, most commonly 14 hertz.

Originates in the central vertex region.

Has a duration criterion of 0.5 to 2 to 3 seconds.

Typically occurs in stage II sleep, but can be seen in other stages.

K Complexes

Are sharp, slow waves, with a biphasic morphology (negative then positive deflection).

Predominantly central-vertex in origin.

Duration must be at least 0.5 seconds.

Does not have an amplitude criterion.

Indicative of stage II sleep.

Delta Activity

Delta activity has a frequency of 0.5 to 2 hertz.

Clinical EEG: frequency of >.5 to <4 hertz.

Seen predominantly in the frontal region.

Delta activity has an amplitude criterion of greater than or equal to 75 microvolts.

There is no duration criterion.

Stage II sleep: Less than 20 percent delta activity is seen.

Stage III sleep: 20 percent to 50 percent delta activity is seen.

Stage IV sleep: More than 50 percent delta activity is seen.

EOG leads will only pick up the EEG activity.

EMG may be slightly lower than that of stage II.

STAGES OF SLEEP

When scoring a record for stage of sleep, the reader should initially scroll through the entire record quickly to evaluate the quality of the recording and the usefulness of specific channels. He or she should observe the specific shape of the features that represent the stages in that particular individual and to gain an overall picture of the cycles for that record. Specifically observe for sleep spindles, K complexes, slow waves, and REM.

Stage Wake (Figures 3–1 through 3–3)

Typically, the first several minutes of the record consists of wake (W) stage. Stage W is recorded when more than 50 percent of the epoch has scorable alpha EEG activity. The EEG shows mixed beta and alpha activities as the eyes open and close, and predominantly alpha activity when the eyes remain closed. Submental EMG is relatively high tone and reflects the high-amplitude muscle contractions and movement artifacts. The EOG channels show eye blinking and rapid movement. The record slows in frequency and amplitude as the subject stops moving and becomes drowsy.

As the patient becomes drowsy, with the eyes closed, the EEG shows predominant alpha activity, while the EMG activity becomes less prominent. The EOG channels may show SREM. If the patient moves in bed or rolls, the record reflects this as a paroxysmal event characterized by high-amplitude activity with sustained increased artifact. The patient may enter stage I of sleep for one or two epochs and then reawaken. Transitions may be difficult to score. From stage W, patients typically proceed to stage I, but infrequently they may enter REM sleep or stage II sleep directly, if the pressure to do so is high (reflecting a state of pathological sleep deprivation).

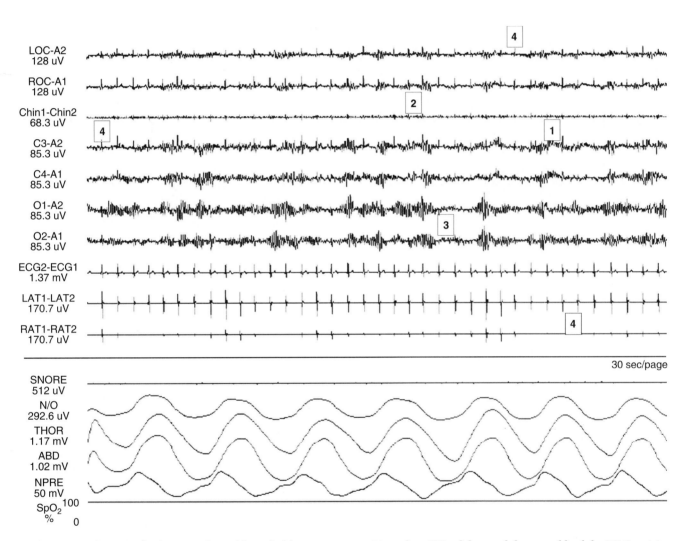

FIGURE 3–1. *Stage Wake* (30-second epoch). *Wakefulness, eyes open. More than 50% of the epoch has scorable alpha EEG activity (1). EMG activity is reduced, consistent with relaxed wakefulness (2). Note the posterior dominant alpha frequency in the O1-A2 and O2-A1 leads (3). An EKG artifact is noted in the EOG, EEG and EMG leads (4). N/O = Nasal/oral airflow, NPRE = Nasal pressure recording effort, SPO₂ = Pulse oxymetry.*

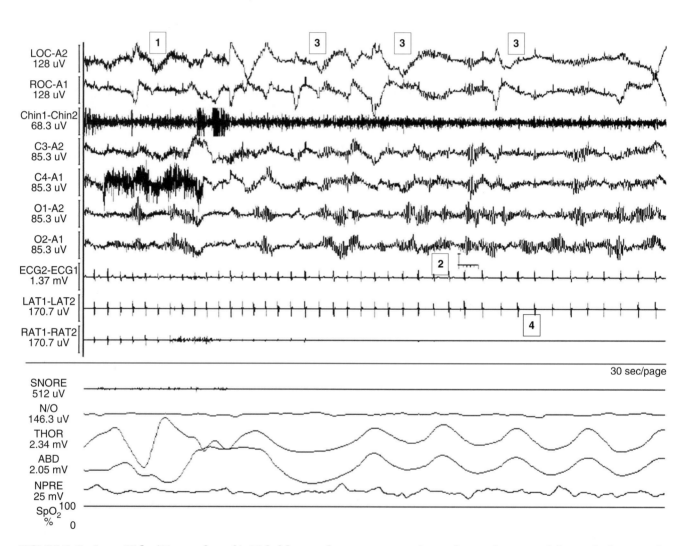

FIGURE 3–2. *Stage Wake* (30-second epoch). *Wakefulness with a movement artifact in the initial portion of the epoch obscuring the recording (1). There is evidence of posterior dominant alpha frequency (>50% of the record) in the O1-A2 and O2-A1 leads (2) next to the 1-second ruler. The EOG leads confirm that the eyes are open and blink (3). An EKG artifact is seen most prominently in the EMG and EOG leads (4).*

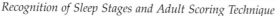

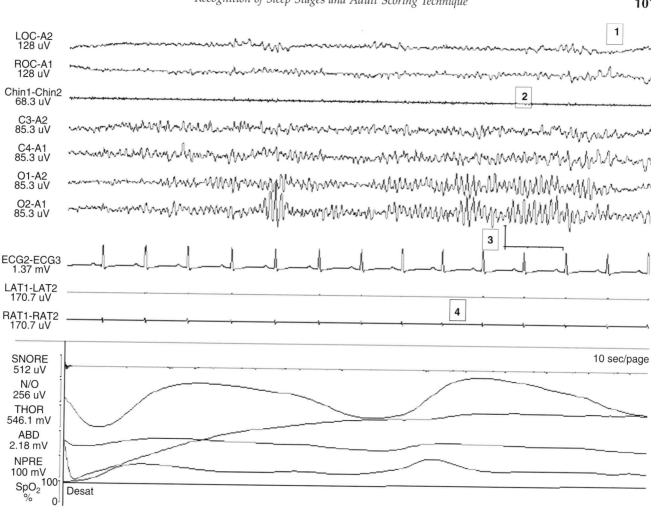

FIGURE 3–3. ***Stage Wake*** *(10-second epoch). Wakefulness with SREM (1). The EMG activity is reduced consistent with relaxed wakefulness (2). There is evidence of posterior dominant alpha frequency (>50% of the record) in the O1-A2 and O2-A1 leads. On this epoch, a 10-second ruler (3) was added to make the reader appreciate the 11 Hz alpha activity visible on the O2-A1 lead (3). An EKG artifact is seen most prominently in the EMG lead (right anterior tibialis surface-4).*

Stage I NREM Sleep (Figures 3–4 through 3–6)

Stage I NREM sleep, may also be termed as *transitional sleep* or *light sleep*. Transition into sleep occurs following stage W sleep. Stage I NREM sleep is transitional state characterized by low-voltage fast EEG activity. The EEG patterns may be quite variable and may shift rapidly, making it sometimes difficult to interpret. Stage I sleep is scored when more than 15 seconds (≥50 percent) of the epoch is made up of theta activity (4 to 7 hertz), sometimes intermixed with low-amplitude delta activity replacing the alpha activity of wakefulness. Amplitudes of EEG activity are less than 50 to 75 microvolts. Paroxysms of 2 to 7 hertz less than 75 microvolts may occur. The alpha activity in the EEG drops to less than 50 percent. Stage I sleep is considered a transitional sleep stage of very short duration, lasting for 1 to 7 minutes.

Vertex sharp waves may occur, but sleep spindles or K complexes are never a part of stage I sleep and neither are REM. Vertex waves are typically present toward the end of stage I sleep. They have a characteristic high-voltage sharp surface-negative followed by a surface-positive component and are maximal over the Cz electrode. The EMG shows less activity than in W stage, but the transition is gradual and of little assistance in scoring. Arousals are paroxysms of activity lasting at least 3 seconds but less than 15 seconds. If an arousal occurs in stage I sleep and if the burst results in alpha activity for greater than 50 percent of the record, then the epoch is scored as stage W.

During drowsiness and stage I sleep, the eyes begin to slowly roll (SREMs). Sometimes, eye movements during drowsiness and stage I NREM sleep may be jerky, irregular, or gently rolling. Theta activity may start to enter into

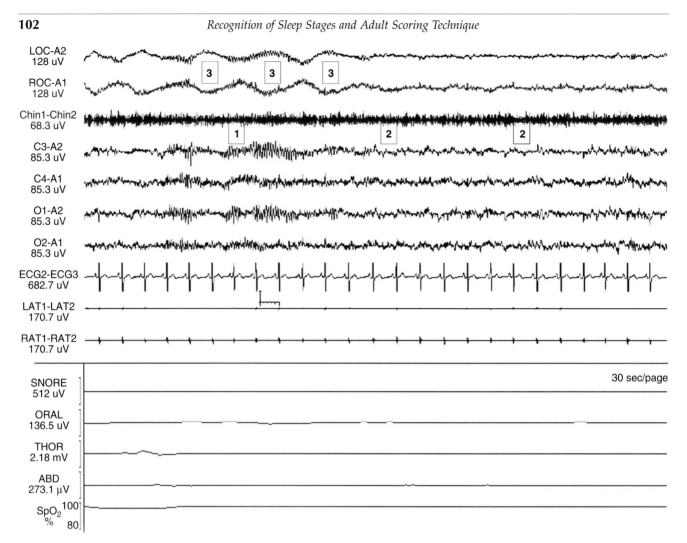

FIGURE 3–4. *Stage I Sleep* (30-second epoch). *The record depicts stage 1 sleep. Alpha activity (1) is present during the initial 10 seconds of the epoch and is gradually replaced by low voltage, mixed frequency theta activity (2). Slow rolling eye movements become more prominent (3).*

the EOG tracing as an artifact. The submental EMG tone is relatively high.

Physiologically, patient's breathing becomes shallow, heart rate becomes regular, blood pressure falls, and the patient exhibits little or no body movement. It lasts for up to ten minutes in most patients. This portion of sleep is distinguished by drifting thoughts and dreams that move from the real to the fantastic, along with a kind of floating feeling. The sleeper is still easily awakened and might even deny having slept.

In general, the time spent in stage I sleep increases with age.

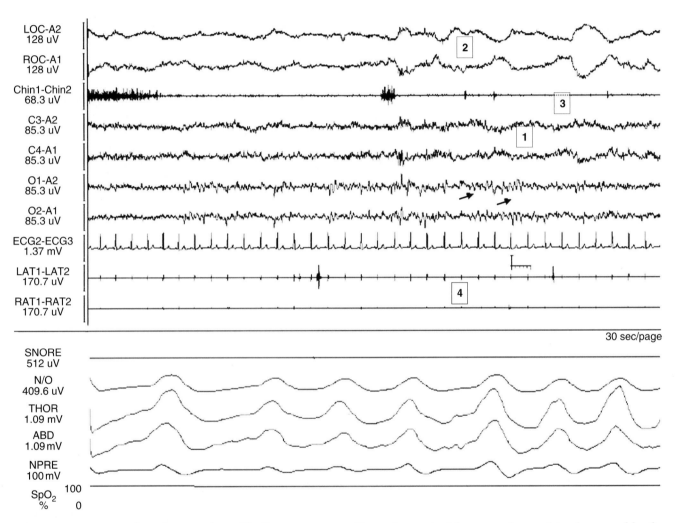

FIGURE 3–5. *Stage I Sleep* (30-second epoch). *There is presence of low-voltage, mixed-frequency theta activity demarcated by the arrows (1). Slow-rolling eye movements are evident (2) and so is a more substantial reduction in chin EMG tone (3), which happens to capture activity from the EKG leads in the form of an EKG artifact (4).*

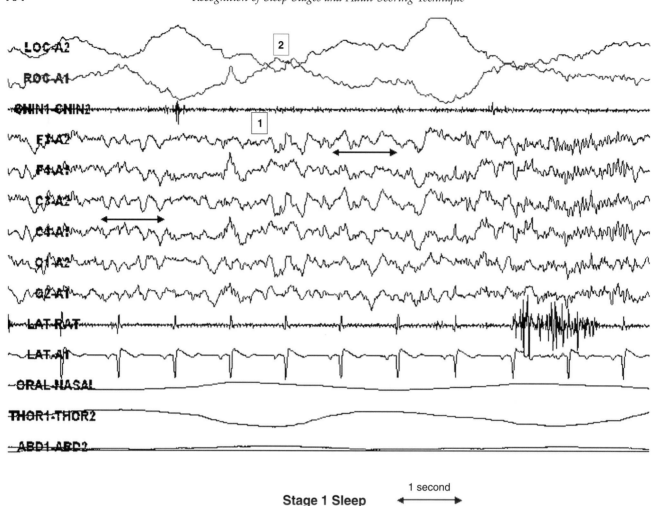

Stage 1 Sleep   ◄─ 1 second ─►

FIGURE 3–6. *Stage I Sleep* (10-second epoch). *This is a 10-second epoch from stage-1 sleep designed to assist the reader in appreciating the low-voltage, mixed-frequency theta activity demarcated by the 1-second arrows (1). Slow-rolling eye movements are noted (2).*

Stage II NREM Sleep
(Figures 3–7 through 3–10)

Stage II NREM sleep may also be termed *spindle*, or *intermediate sleep*. It is an intermediate stage of sleep, but it also accounts for the bulk of a typical PSG recording (up to 50 percent in adult patients). It follows stage I NREM sleep and initially lasts about 20 minutes. It is characterized by predominant theta activity (3- to 7-hertz EEG activity) and occasional quick bursts of fast activity. The EEG shows no alpha activity. Amplitude may increase from that seen in stage I sleep. Delta is only allowed to occur for less than 20 percent of the epoch. The threshold triggering slow-wave sleep scoring is reached if 20 percent of the epoch is comprised of delta activity.

K complexes and sleep spindles occur for the first time and are typically episodic. The EOG leads mirror EEG activity. Submental EMG activity is tonically low. Exces-sive spindle activity may indicate the presence of medications (such as benzodiazepines). K complexes are sharp, monophasic or polyphasic slow waves, with a sharply negative (upward) deflection followed by a slower positive (downward) deflection. They characteristically stand out from the rest of the background. K complexes have a duration criterion and must persist for at least 0.5 second. No minimum amplitude criterion exists for K complexes. K complexes, even without the presence of sleep spindles, are sufficient for scoring stage II sleep. They are predominantly central-vertex in origin.

K complexes may occur with or without stimuli such as a sudden sound and were so named because they were appreciated as following the *k*nocking sound produced by knuckle rapping. In this respect, they may represent a form of cortical evoked potential in a brain still minimally responsive to external stimuli. K complexes may be labeled as *spontaneous* if they arise within the recording for an

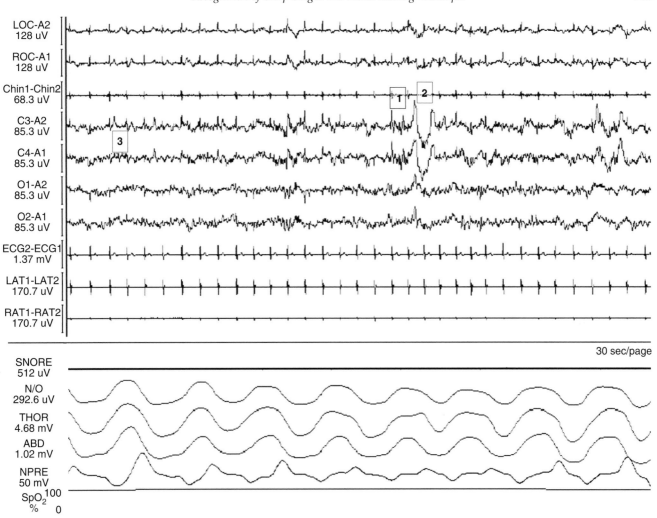

FIGURE 3–7. *Stage-II Sleep* (30-second epoch). *Sleep spindles (1) and K-complexes (2) are the defining characteristics of this sleep stage. No specific criteria exist for EOG and EMG in this stage. There is evidence of theta activity (3).*

unknown reason, indicating that their origin is of an endogenous brain activity. They may be labeled as *evoked* if they are clearly triggered by an external stimulus such as sound or noise. *K-alpha complexes* may be triggered by other entities on the record such as periodic limb movements in sleep (PLMS) or an apneic event. These are typical K complexes and are associated with an arousal (alpha EEG activity) immediately following the complex.

Sleep spindles appear in stage II NREM sleep. They are generated in and controlled by activity within the midline thalamic nuclei and represent an inhibitory activity. Sleep spindles are characterized by 12- to 14-hertz sinusoidal EEG activity in the central vertex region and must persist for at least 0.5 second (i.e., six to seven small waves in 0.5 second), but rarely longer than 1 second. Sleep spindles possess a high degree of synchrony and symmetry between the two hemispheres in patients older than 1 year of age.

Although classically described as spindle shaped, they may be polymorphic and may attach as a tail to a K complex. Normal variant for scoring human sleep is the appearance in stage II sleep of low K-complex quantity and high-amplitude spindle activity. Central nervous system (CNS) depressant drugs (such as benzodiazepines) often increase the frequency of the spindle activity in the record, while advancing age often diminishes their frequency.

No specific criteria exist for EOG and EMG in this stage.

Movement arousal from stage II may default the scoring into stage I or into W stage. If the arousal is 3 seconds or longer and the resulting alpha EEG activity persists for less than 50 percent of the record, than the epoch is scored as stage I sleep. If the alpha persists for greater than 50 percent of the record, the epoch is scored as W stage. If the first half of the following epoch demonstrates stage II

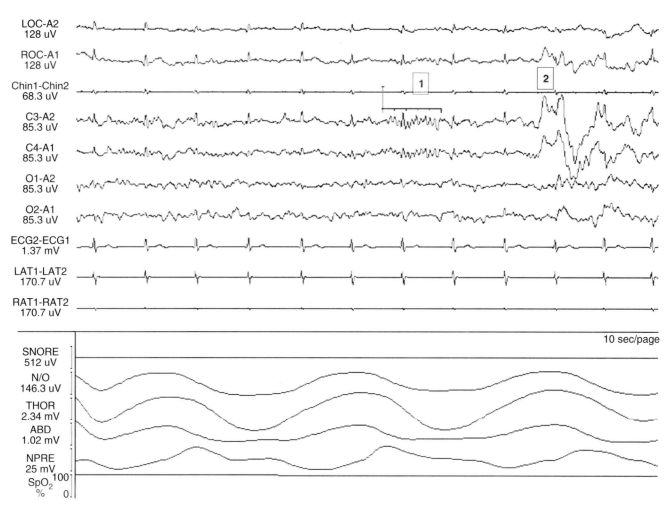

FIGURE 3–8. *Stage-II Sleep* (10-second epoch). *This is a 10-second epoch designed to show the reader the sleep spindles (1) along with K complexes (2). K complexes are sharp, monophasic or polyphasic slow waves, with a sharply negative followed by a slower positive deflection. K complexes have a duration criterion and must persist for at least 0.5 seconds. There is no minimum amplitude criterion for K complexes.*

characteristics (i.e., sleep spindles, K complexes, high-amplitude theta/delta activity), then that epoch is scored as stage II sleep.

Once in stage II, that score is maintained unless a reason to exit presents. One such reason to exit is described as the *Three Minute Rule*. It states that if no specific stage II indicators (such as K complex or sleep spindle) appear, and in the absence of movement arousals and muscle tone changes that would alter the staging, continue to score all epochs as stage II for up to 3 minutes. At 3 minutes, if no specific indicators for stage II have occurred, scroll back 3 minutes and score those epochs as stage I.

Stage II sleep is associated with a relative diminution of physiologic bodily functions. Blood pressure, brain metabolism, gastrointestinal secretions, and cardiac activity decrease. The patient descends deeper into sleep, becoming more and more detached from the outside world and progressively more difficult to arouse.

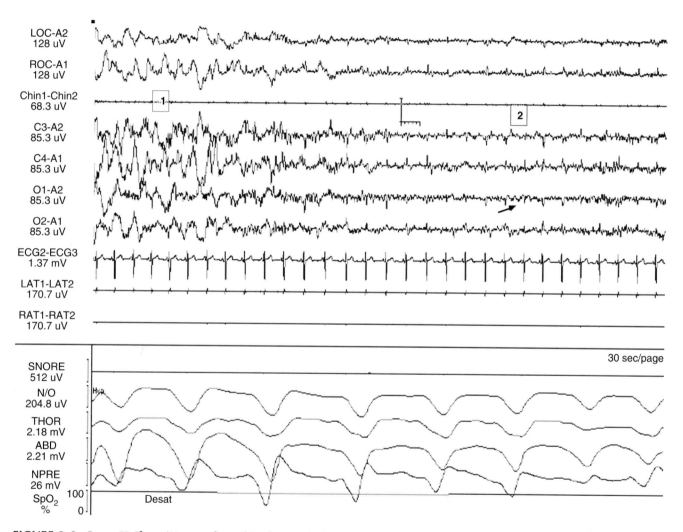

FIGURE 3–9. ***Stage-II Sleep*** (30-second epoch). *This epoch depicts stage II sleep. K-complexes sleep spindles are noted in the early part of the record (1). There is evidence of theta activity (arrow) intermixed with alpha activity (2). According to the* Three Minute Rule, *intervening periods between K complexes and sleep spindles are to be scored as stage II sleep if there are no indications of increased EMG tone, or movement arousals during these intervals. Therefore, this epoch is still scored as stage II sleep.*

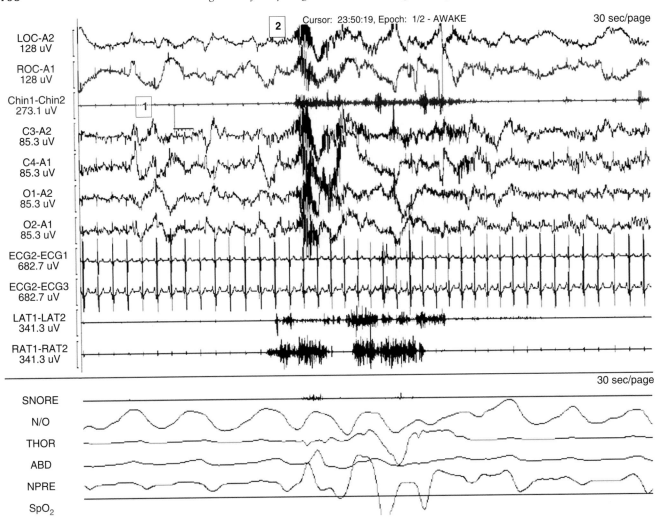

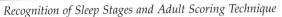

FIGURE 3–10. *Transition of Stage-II Sleep into Wakefulness (30-second epoch). This epoch depicts transition of stage II into stage W. K-complexes sleep spindles are noted in earlier in the record (1). An arousal (2) is 3 seconds or longer in duration, and the resulting alpha EEG activity persists for more than 50% of the record. The epoch is therefore scored as stage W sleep.*

Stages III and IV Non-REM Sleep
(Figures 3–11 through 3–13)

Stage III and IV NREM sleep may also be termed *deep sleep, slow-wave sleep (SWS),* or *delta sleep.* Traditional R-K scoring classifies stage III and IV separately. To distinguish between stage III and IV sleep, one must eliminate frequencies greater than 2 hertz, including K complexes, from consideration. Stage III is scored when 20 percent to 50 percent of the epoch is made of delta activity. Stage IV is scored when greater than 50 percent of the record is comprised of delta activity. However, many clinical sleep laboratories classify stage III and IV together and do not make a distinction between them because this distinction does not serve clear clinical significance. Slow wave sleep is marked by high-amplitude slow waves. No specific criteria for EOG and EMG exist for SWS, but in general,

muscle tone decreases gradually from stage II to stage IV. The transition from stage III to stage IV may be gradual, and stage III may alternate with stage IV. They comprise the deepest, most refreshing and restorative sleep type. They tend to diminish with age.

Physiologically, a patient going through SWS has the highest threshold for arousal. SWS is typically associated with many parasomnias (sleep terrors, sleep walking) that manifest themselves here. Eye movements may cease altogether in this stage of sleep. Physiologically, SWS is often linked with a peak in growth hormone secretion.

Stage III NREM Sleep
(see Figures 3–11 and 3–12)

Stage III NREM sleep is the beginning of slow-wave (deep) sleep, occurring about 30 to 45 minutes after the patient first falls asleep. It is characterized by slow large-

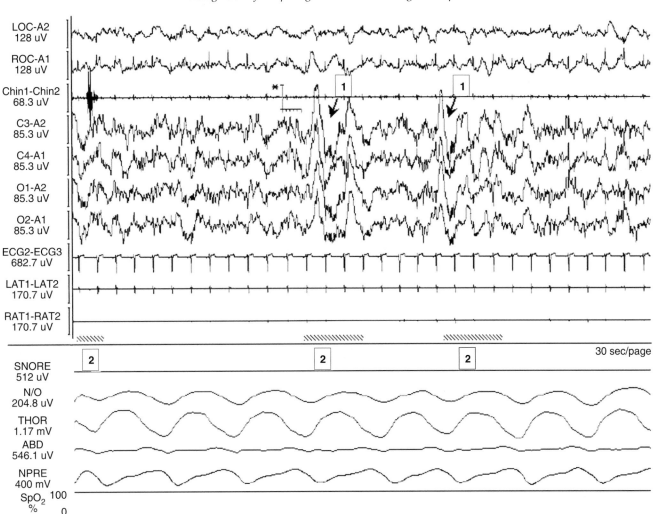

FIGURE 3–11. *Stage-III Sleep* (30-second epoch). *Stage III NREM sleep is characterized by slow large-amplitude delta activity (1) at the rate of 0.5 to 4.0 per second with peak-to-peak amplitudes greater than 75 μV. The ruler provided (°) is at 1-second and 75 uV units. Delta activity should occur for more than 20% but less than 50% of the epoch as demarcated by the patterned lines (2).*

amplitude EEG activity (at the rate of 0.5 to 2 per second; delta wave) with peak-to-peak amplitudes greater than 75 microvolts for between 20 percent and 50 percent of the epoch.

The arousal threshold of this stage of sleep is far greater than for stage I or II sleep. Both K complexes and sleep spindles may be seen in stage III sleep. No specific criteria exist for EOG and EMG. The transition to stage III from stage II may be gradual, and stage III may alternate with stage I.

Stage IV NREM Sleep (see Figure 3–13)

The deepest sleep occurs in stage IV NREM sleep. It is characterized by delta activity of 2 hertz or slower activity,

with peak-to-peak amplitudes greater than 75 microvolts for at least 50 percent of the epoch. Both K complexes and sleep spindles may be seen in stage IV sleep. Stage IV sleep is a stage of deep sleep with a high arousal threshold. During this state, bodily functions continue to decline to the deepest possible state of physical rest. The first period of slow wave sleep is the deepest. If the patient wakes up from slow wave sleep, he or she may appear confused or disoriented. The patient may experience "sleep inertia" or "sleep drunkenness," seeming unable to function normally for several minutes. The duration of sleep inertia depends on prior sleep deprivation and CNS-active medications.

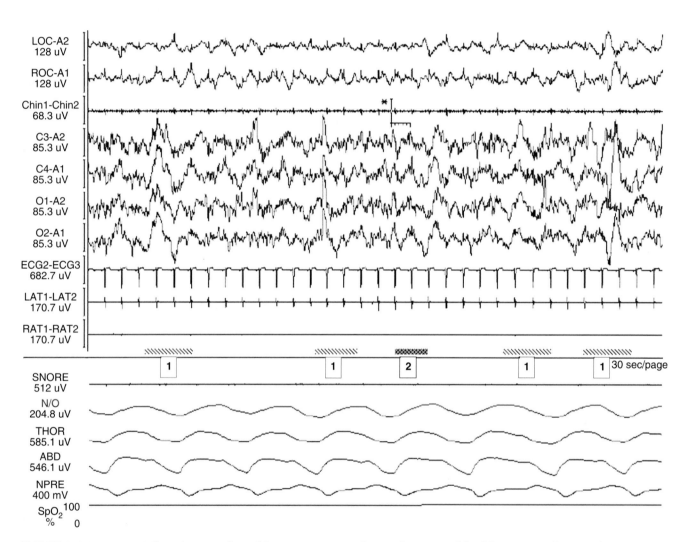

FIGURE 3–12. ***Stage-III Sleep*** *(30-second epoch). Stage III NREM sleep is characterized by delta waves at the rate of 0.5 to 4.0 per second with peak-to-peak amplitudes greater than 75 μV as demarcated by the patterned lines (1). Stage III should consist of delta activity, which occurs for more than 20% but less than 50% of the epoch. Stage IV sleep consists of >50% delta activity in the epoch scored. To further distinguish between stage III and IV sleep, one must eliminate frequencies greater than 2 Hz, including K complexes from consideration (2). The ruler provided (°) is at 1-second and 75 uV units.*

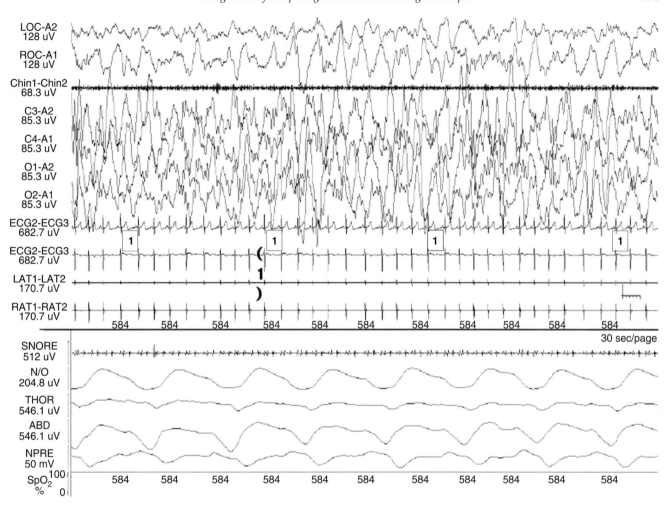

FIGURE 3–13. *Stage-IV Sleep* *(30-second epoch). This epoch is a 30-second epoch depicting stage IV NREM sleep. The predominate feature in this epoch is the that of the high-amplitude delta activity (1).*

Stage REM Sleep (Figures 3–14 through 3–18)

Stage REM sleep may also be termed *paradoxical sleep, D-sleep,* or *dreaming sleep.* REM sleep typically occurs 90 to 120 minutes after sleep onset. It typically occupies 20 percent to 25 percent of the night and is characterized by relatively low-amplitude, mixed frequency EEG theta waves, intermixed with some alpha waves, usually 1 to 2 hertz slower than waking. Brain waves are small and irregular, with big bursts of eye activity (rapid eye movements), which are seen in the EOG leads. During REM sleep, the eyes move rapidly under closed eyelids while dreaming. This produces rapid conjugate eye movements that appear as out-of-phase EOG channel deflections on the PSG. The EOG of REM shows paroxysmal, relatively sharply contoured, high-amplitude activity occurring in all eye leads simultaneously. The EOG activity is not needed to mark the start of an REM period. REM epochs may be recog-

nized by EEG activity before EOG movements start. Small REMs on EOG may serve as a harbinger of REM stage and can indicate the actual onset of REM in another area where interscorer concordance is lower. The first REM period is typically brief with subsequent REM periods becoming progressively more robust.

Stage REM sleep is characterized by a *sawtooth wave* pattern. These are 2- to 6-hertz, sharply contoured triangular EEG patterns that are jagged-like in morphology and evenly formed. They may occur serially for a few seconds and are highest in amplitude over the vertex region (Cz and Fz electrodes). REM sleep may be preceded by a series of sawtooth waves.

REM sleep is sometimes divided into *phasic* (P) and *tonic* (T) components. P-REM sleep is characterized by phasic twitching in the EMG channel occurring concurrently with bursts of REM. This activity has been suggestively correlated with dream content. The phasic EMG

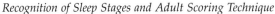

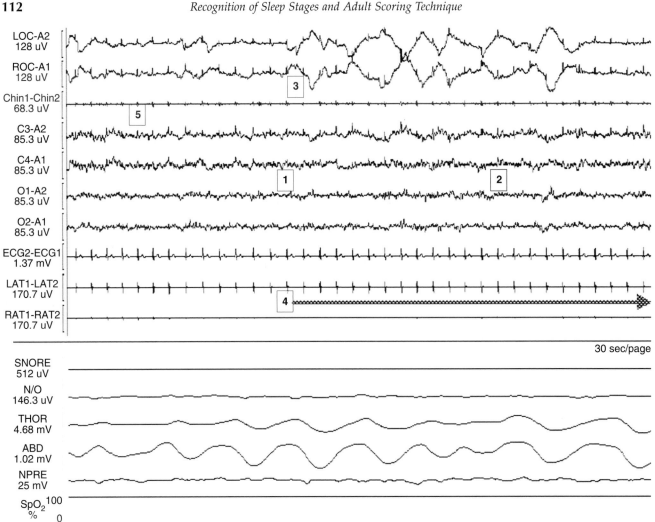

FIGURE 3–14. *Stage-REM Sleep* (30-second epoch). *Stage-REM sleep characterized by relatively low-amplitude, mixed-frequency EEG theta waves (1), intermixed with alpha waves (2). The EOG leads depict Rapid Eye Movements (REM), which are paroxysmal, relatively sharply contoured, high-amplitude activity occurring in all eye leads simultaneously (3) and are demarcated by the arrow (4). EMG tone (5) should show the lowest tone in the record, but no specific amplitude or frequency criteria are in place.*

twitchings in this stage are very short muscle twitches that may occur in the middle ear muscles, genioglossal muscle, facial muscles, and penis (if nocturnal penile tumescence is being monitored). T-REM sleep generally consists of low-voltage activated EEG and is characterized by a marked decrease in skeletal muscle EMG activity, without obvious EOG activity. T-REM appears to be mediated by areas near the locus coeruleus.

The brain wave activity of REM sleep resembles waking state more than it does the sleeping state. The patient's muscles are literally paralyzed and submental EMG should be at its minimum tone. The EMG should show the lowest tone in the record, but no specific amplitude or frequency criteria are in place. Any two of the previous three criteria (mixed frequency EEG, REM, and minimal EMG tone) must be present to score REM sleep.

K complexes and/or spindles may occur while in stage REM. However, to maintain REM sleep, K complexes or spindles must be separated by P-REM. Their presence in this sleep stage is reason to consider moving from stage REM to stage II sleep. While in stage REM, stage II sleep is scored if more than a 3-minute separation period occurs between K complexes or spindles without REM in between. If REM activity occurs on both sides of the K complexes or sleep spindles, then the epoch is scored as REM and the complex is considered to represent a momentary breakthrough into REM rather than a change of stage. No high-amplitude activity may be counted as REM. Bursts of delta activity are also a good reason to reconsider changing sleep stage.

REM can alternate with W stage, stage I, or stage II. Rules to help differentiate intermixing of REM, spindle,

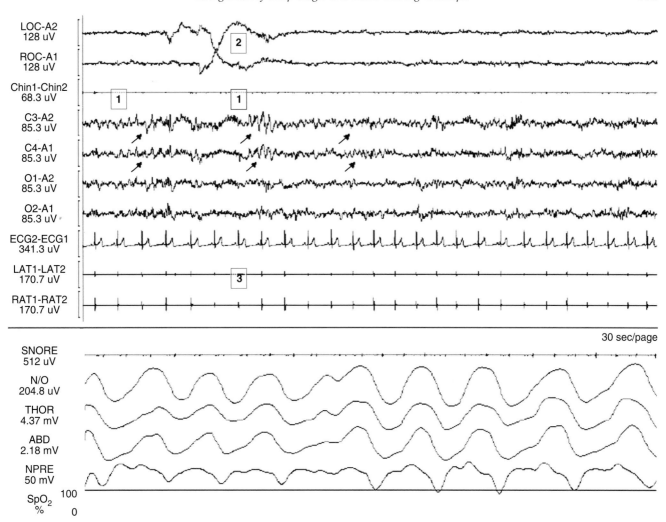

FIGURE 3–15. *Stage-REM Sleep* (30-second epoch). *Stage-REM sleep is also characterized by the unique* <u>sawtooth wave</u> *pattern (1, arrowheads). These are 2–6 Hz, sharply contoured triangular, jagged-like in morphology and evenly formed EEG pattern. They may occur serially for a few seconds and are best visualized, due to its highest amplitude, over the vertex region (Cz and Fz electrodes). REM sleep may be preceded by a series of* sawtooth waves. *Other features of REM sleep shown in this epoch are the rapid eye movements (2) and the muscle atonia reflected in the EMG leads (3).*

and K complex include the following: If a single sleep spindle or K complex occurs during an REM period (REM on both sides of the complex) and the EMG remains unchanged (low amplitude), then the reader should continue to score the epoch as REM. If the EMG amplitude increases with the spindle or K complex and REM is not clearly apparent following the complex, then stage II is scored from that point forward. If two sleep spindles or K complexes occur in the absence of EMG changes (i.e., low amplitude continues), then that epoch and the intervening period should be scored as stage II sleep.

Beginning Scoring REM Sleep

REM periods may begin before the characteristic EOG movements. Occasionally, low-voltage, mixed-activity EEG, sometimes with sawtooth waves and low-amplitude EMG, may begin several epochs before the onset of the characteristic EOG movements. When the EOG movements are recognized clearly as REMs, scroll back to the point where the record became REM-like on both EEG and EMG and score those epochs as REM. REM may begin after a brief arousal.

Ending Scoring REM

REM sleep may end with a brief arousal, after which the EEG looks qualitatively different, with higher amplitude and slower frequency activity. In the absence of arousal, the transition may be subtle.

Because the EEGs of REM, stage I, and stage W can be similar, several criteria are available to help differentiate the stages.

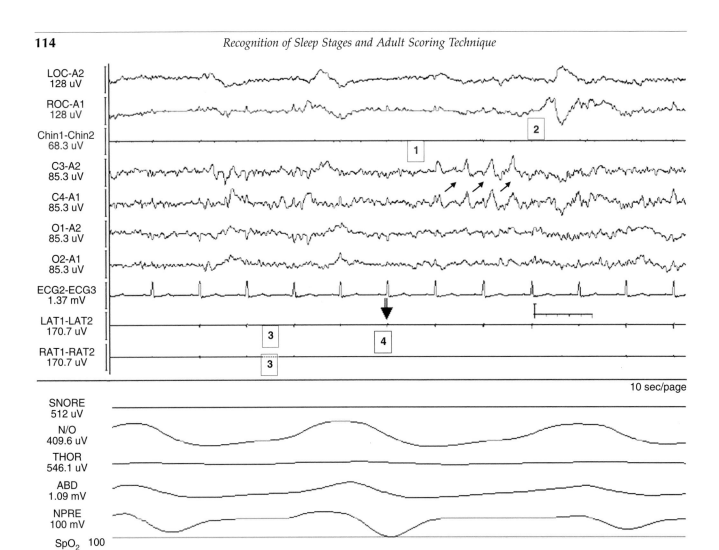

FIGURE 3–16. *Stage-REM Sleep* (10-second epoch). *This 10-second epoch is provided for exemplifying the sharply contoured triangular, jagged-like in morphology of the* <u>sawtooth wave</u> *pattern (1, arrowheads). Also noted are the rapid eye movements (2) and the muscle atonia reflected in the EMG leads (3). The EKG artifact is noted in the EMG lead (4) and originates from the QRS complex from the EKG above (see double arrow showing this relationship).*

First, one must look for development of bursts of higher amplitude and slower frequency EEG activity, which may be associated with EOG eye movements similar in morphology to those of REM. Score the epoch according to the applicable stage criteria from the onset of the EEG bursts of slow activity. Remember that REM does not have high-amplitude, slow EEG activity and that eye movements may occur in all stages. For example, if paroxysms of K complexes begin, then score the stage as II.

Second, refer to the EMG and EOG as adjuncts to help confirm staging. For example, if the EMG increases in amplitude briefly and without warning, the period may be stage I sleep. If higher amplitude EMG discharges persist and are accompanied by increased alpha activity (for more than 50 percent of the record), then the epoch may be scored as stage W.

Other rules to consider include the presence of arousals. One simple rule to follow is that once in a stage, remain in that stage until given an unambiguous reason to change. Arousal of greater than 3 seconds occurring in the first half of the epoch (from stages II, III, IV, or REM) is reason enough to consider changing the stage. Arousals may be observed only on EEG, characterized by the development of theta or alpha activity. Arousals may have EEG activity with EMG activity increases, or they may have EEG, EMG, and EOG activity. For example, if an arousal occurs during stage II sleep, score the epoch as stage II sleep if the arousal is less than half the record, score the epoch as stage I sleep if the arousal is greater than half the record, and score the epoch as stage W if the arousal is greater than half the record and associated with sustained alpha activity. In a given epoch, if a movement occurs from stage

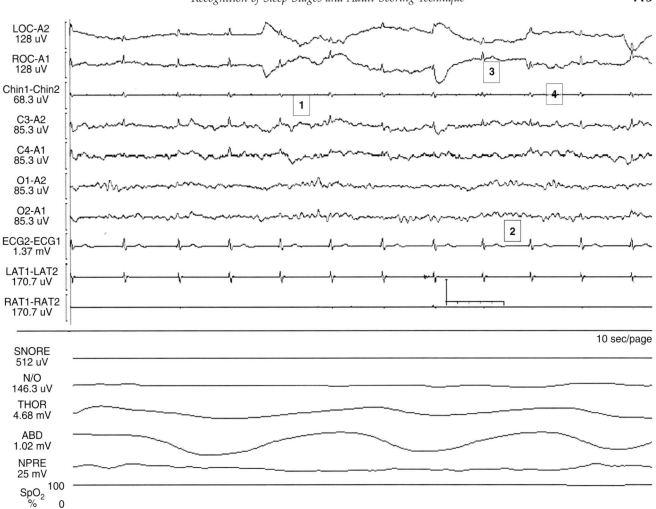

FIGURE 3–17. **Stage-REM Sleep** (10-second epoch). *Stage-REM sleep characterized by relatively low-amplitude, mixed frequency EEG theta waves (1). Intermixed with the theta activity are alpha waves (2) best visualized in the occipital configuration. The epoch shows bursts of REM (3) and absence of muscle activity as reflected in the EMG leads (4).*

II sleep, normally the remaining epoch would be scored as stage I sleep or stage W depending upon the characteristics of the arousal. An exception to this might be if a K complex or a sleep spindle occurs within 15 seconds of the end of the arousal, in which case the epoch is scored as stage II.

Unlike the progressive relaxation noted during the four NREM phases, physiological activity during REM phase is significantly higher. Blood pressure and pulse rate may increase drastically or may show intermittent fluctuations. Breathing becomes irregular and brain oxygen consumption increases. Male patients exhibit penile erections, while women experience clitoral engorgement. The body seems to have abandoned its effort to regulate its temperature

during the REM phase and resembles a state of poikilothermy, drifting gradually toward the temperature of the environment. If patients are awakened from this stage of sleep, they may often recall dreaming. The duration of REM sleep and its latency tend to decrease with advancing age. Pathologically short REM sleep latency may point to a state of acute or cumulative sleep deprivation, may be caused by recent discontinuation of REM sleep–suppressing agents, and may also suggest a major affective disorder. There are a variety of sleep disorders associated with REM sleep including a variety of parasomnias (REM sleep behavior disorder [RBD], REM nightmares) and obstructive sleep apnea, which may be more pronounced in this sleep period.

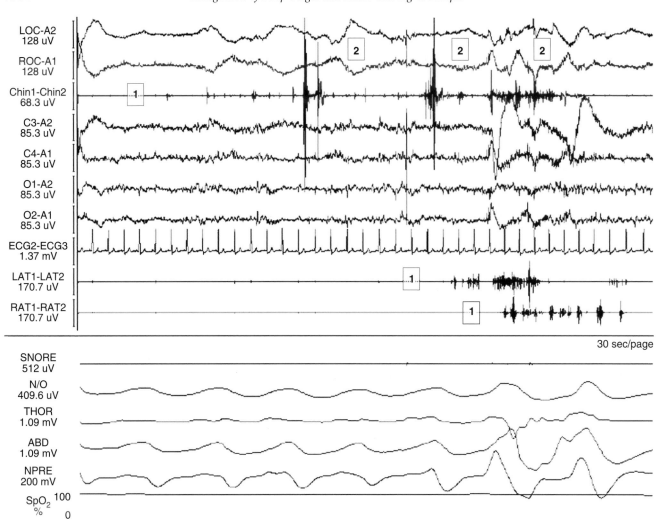

FIGURE 3–18. *Stage-REM Sleep (30-second epoch). Phasic REM sleep: P-REM sleep is characterized by phasic twitching in the chin and limb EMG channels (1) occurring concurrently with bursts of rapid eye movements (2). This activity has been suggestively correlated with dream content. The phasic EMG twitching in this stage are very short muscle twitches that may occur in muscles of the middle ear, tongue, and the face.*

Stage Movement Time (Figure 3–19)

Movement time (MT) is a scorable sleep stage identified by amplifier blocking or excessive EMG activity that obscures the EEG and EOG tracing in more than 50 percent of the epoch. Scorable stage of sleep must occur before and after stage MT. The duration of MT is generally greater than 15 seconds but less than 1 minute. When the MT is immediately preceded and followed by stage W, the epoch is scored as stage W rather than stage MT.

EEG Arousals, Random Body Movements, or Movement Arousal (Figures 3–20 through 3–22)

This is not used as an epoch score as MT, but is intended as an aid in the scoring of sleep stages. Its duration of activity is very short (<15 seconds) with no EEG obscuring. Arousals are paroxysms of activity lasting 3 seconds or longer, but less than 15 seconds of the record. At least 10 seconds of sleep must be maintained before and after the arousal. If an arousal obscuring the record occurs for more than 15 seconds, then the epoch is scored as MT. The minimum arousal is simply a paroxysmal burst in the EEG channel, usually to alpha or theta activity. The arousal itself could result from an isolated muscle contraction, vigorous blink, or a facial grimace. Arousal from stage I is common and usually is represented by a burst of activity on the EEG, EOG, and EMG. If the burst results in alpha activity for greater than 50 percent of the record, then the epoch is scored as W.

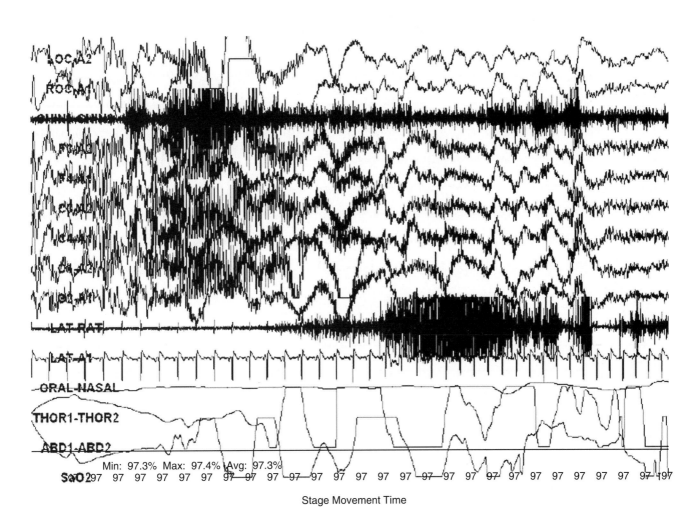

Stage Movement Time

FIGURE 3–19. ***Stage-Movement Time*** (30-second epoch). *Stage Movement time (MT) is characterized by amplifier blocking or excessive EMG activity, which obscures the EEG and EOG tracing in more than 50% of the epoch. Scorable stage of sleep must occur before and after stage MT. The duration of MT is generally greater than 15 seconds but less than 1 minute.*

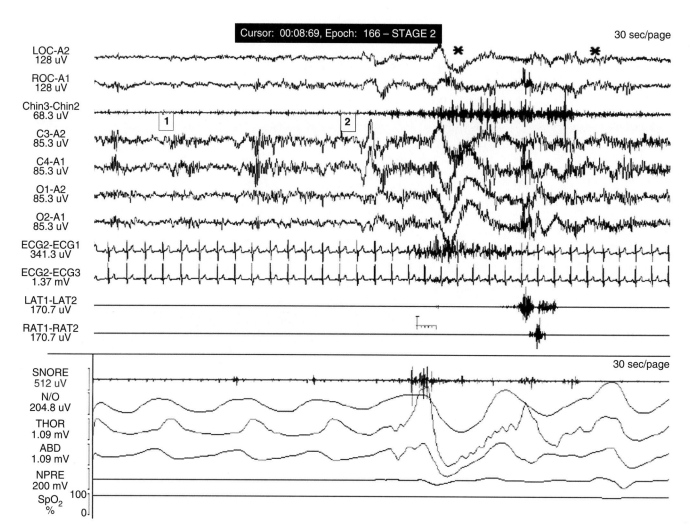

FIGURE 3–20. *EEG Arousal* (30-second epoch). *An EEG arousal is not a scorable epoch of sleep but is intended as an aid in the scoring of sleep stages. Its duration activity is short, and it must take place for longer than 3 seconds but less than 15 seconds. There should be no EEG obscuring. Sleep must be maintained before and after the arousal. In this 30-second epoch, the patient was in stage II sleep just prior to the arousal (°) as noted by the sleep spindles (1) and K complex (2). The EEG leads show a shift to a higher frequency. If an arousal, obscuring the record occurs for longer 15 seconds, then the epoch is scored as MT (Movement Time).*

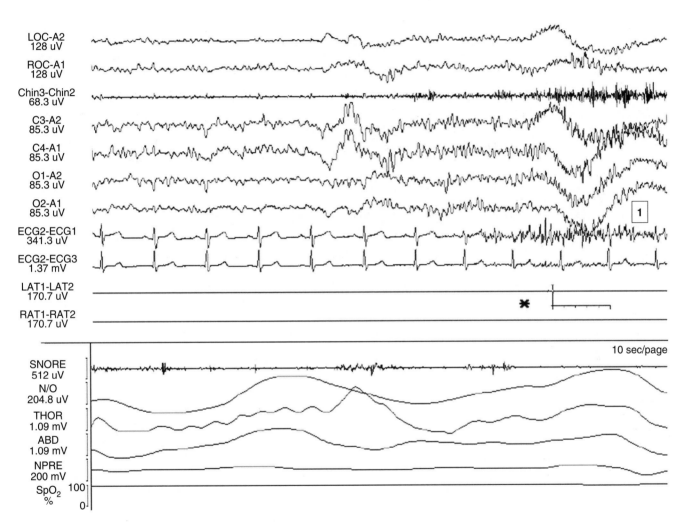

FIGURE 3–21. **EEG Arousal** (10-second epoch). *Arousals are paroxysms of activity lasting 3 seconds or longer, but less than 15 seconds of the record. Sleep (stage-1 here) must be maintained before and after the arousal. The minimum arousal is simply a paroxysmal burst in the EEG channel, usually to alpha activity as in this epoch or theta activity.*

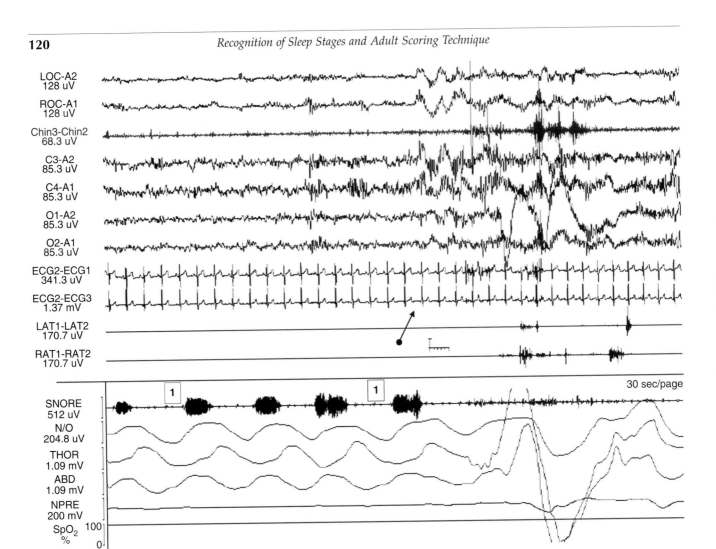

FIGURE 3–22. EEG Arousal *(30-second epoch). Arousals may have obvious causes such as is seen in this epoch of stage I sleep, which illustrates crescendo snoring (1) culminating in an arousal as seen by the arrow.*

BIBLIOGRAPHY

1. Aldrich MS. *Sleep Medicine*, vol 53. New York: Oxford University Press, 1999.
2. Berry RB. *Sleep Medicine Pearls*. Philadelphia: Hanley & Belfus, 1999.
3. Brown CC. A proposed standard nomenclature for psychophysiologic measures. *Psychophysiology* 1967;4:260–264.
4. Butkov N. *Atlas of Clinical Polysomnography*, volume II. Ashland, OR: Synapse Media, 1996:330–362.
5. Geyer JD, Payne TA, Carney PR, Aldrich MS. *Atlas of Digital Polysomnography*. Philadelphia: Lippincott Williams & Wilkins, 2000.
6. Jacobson A, Kales A, Lehmann D, Hoedemaker FS. Muscle tonus in human subjects during sleep and dreaming. *Exp Neurol* 1964;10:418–424.
7. Jasper HH (Committee Chairman). The ten twenty electrode system of the International Federation. *Electroenceph Clin Neurophysiol* 1958;10:371–375.
8. Johnson LC, Nute C, Austin MT, Lubin A. Spectral analysis of the EEG during waking and sleeping. *Electroenceph Clin Neurophysiol* 1967;23:80.
9. McCarley RW. Sleep neurophysiology of basic mechanisms underlying control of wakefulness and sleep. In Chokroverty S, ed. *Sleep Disorders Medicine*, 2nd ed. Boston: Butterworth-Heinemann, 1999.
10. Monroe LJ. Inter-rater reliability of scoring EEG sleep records. Paper read at the Association for Psychophysiological Study of Sleep Meeting, Santa Monica, CA, April 1967. Abstract in *Psychophysiology* 1968;4:370–371.
11. Pampiglione G, Remond A, Storm van Leeuwen W, Walter WG. Preliminary proposal for an EEG terminology by the Terminology Committee of the International Federation for Electroencephalography and Clinical Neurophysiology. *Electroenceph Clin Neurophysiol* 1961;1;3:646–650.
12. Pressman MR. *Primer of Polysomnogram Interpretation*. Boston: Butterworth & Heineman, 2002.
13. Rechtschaffen A, Kales A, eds. *A Manual of Standardised Terminology, Techniques and Scoring System for Sleep*

Stages of Human Subjects. Los Angeles: Brain Information Service/Brain Research Institute, 1968.

14. Roth B. The clinical and theoretical importance of EEG rhythms corresponding to states of lowered vigilance. *Electroenceph Clin Neurophysiol* 1961;13:395–399.

15. Siegel JM. Brainstem mechanisms generating REM sleep. In Kryger MH, Roth T, Dement WC, eds. *Principles and Practice of Sleep Medicine.* Philadelphia: WB Saunders, 2000:112–133.

16. Shepard JW. *Atlas of Sleep Medicine.* Armonk, NY: Futura Publishing, 1991.

17. Walczak T, Chokroverty S. Electroencephalography, electromyography and electrooculography: General principles and basic technology. In Chokroverty S, ed. *Sleep Disorders Medicine*, 2nd ed. Boston: Butterworth-Heinemann, 1999.

4

Sleep-Disordered Breathing and Scoring

Robert J. Thomas, Sudhansu Chokroverty, Meeta Bhatt, and Tammy Goldhammer

Diagnosis and treatment of sleep-disordered breathing is the driving force behind clinical sleep medicine. As understanding and measurement techniques have evolved, so have respiratory event scoring criteria and principles of positive airway pressure titration. A polysomnogram (PSG) is a treasure trove of physiologic data. The electroencephalographic (EEG), respiratory, electrooculographic (EOG), and electromyographic (EMG) patterns are complex, varying, dynamic, and interact in infinite ways, forming complex but recognizable patterns in health and disease. Accurate scoring of sleep studies is central to sleep medicine and research, and will evolve continuously for the decades ahead. Accurate scoring of abnormal respiration is the most critical component of scoring sleep studies in clinical practice. It is also the component that is most controversial. This section of the atlas provides a number of snapshots (Figures 4–1 through 4–36) to illustrate various patterns.

In the 1970s to early 1980s, only apneas were scored. Later, varying percent reductions in signal were included in scoring. The fundamental problem with this is the use of a nonquantitative signal (thermistor) that does not correlate with true flow.

American Academy of Sleep Medicine (AASM) research criteria (Chicago criteria) (1999) include any clear reduction in flow or effort signal associated with an oxygen desaturation or an arousal. The current guidelines are an extension of this statement, incorporating refinements to arousal scoring, pattern recognition, recognizing the importance of sleep stability using cyclic alternating pattern (CAP), and proposing guidelines for difficult situations.

American Academy of Sleep Medicine clinical criteria (2001) include a 30% reduction in airflow or thoracoab-dominal movement associated with a 4 percent oxygen desaturation.

This atlas is not the forum to decide the merits or otherwise of specific scoring criteria, but the pictures speak many thousand words. The reader should simply appreciate the richness of physiologic and pathologic human variability, and incorporate the best evidence into clinical practice. Automated computer-based methods will provide complementary, perhaps non-epoch–based, methods of quantifying disease.

GENERAL CONSIDERATIONS IN SCORING RESPIRATORY EVENTS

- Criteria to score hypopneas that use specific percent reductions in thermistor signals should not be considered valid, as there is a poor correlation between these signals and flow as measured by pneumotachograph. Scoring criteria based on the thermistor alone can seriously underestimate the severity of sleep-disordered breathing.
- Excessive daytime sleepiness may be induced by repetitive arousals and sleep fragmentation.
- Although it has been difficult to establish a clear correlation between indices of poor sleep (desaturation index, arousal index, apnea-hypopnea index) and daytime cognitive abnormalities and mean sleep latencies, these indices remain the basis of quantifying severity of sleep-disordered breathing.
- There is accumulating evidence that sleep-disordered breathing that is characterized by nocturnal desaturations increases the long-term risk of adverse cardiovascular outcomes, but there is no evidence (not studied

Text continued on p. 148

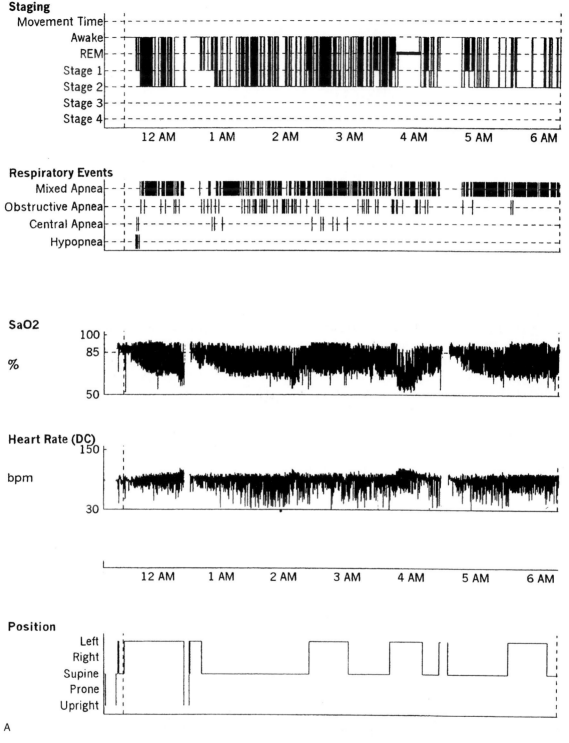

FIGURE 4–1. **A:** *Classic hypoxic sleep-disordered breathing. This is from a 64-year-old man with a history of loud snoring and excessive daytime sleepiness for several years, nocturnal choking, and witnessed apneas. The physical examination is notable for pitting pedal edema, a short neck with a low hairline, weight of 267 pounds, height of 5 feet 11 inches, and blood pressure of 160/98 mm Hg. Oropharyngeal crowding with a large tongue and low hanging uvula are noted. The hypnogram shown in this figure shows severe disorganization of sleep architecture, with frequent sleep stage transitions, absence of stages III and IV NREM sleep, paucity of REM sleep, and a severe reduction in sleep efficiency to 68 percent. The respiratory abnormality is quite extreme, with a dominance of mixed apneas (apnea-hypopnea index of 76) and severe oxygen desaturations. Heart rate variability with tachycardia-bradycardia sequences are also prominent.*

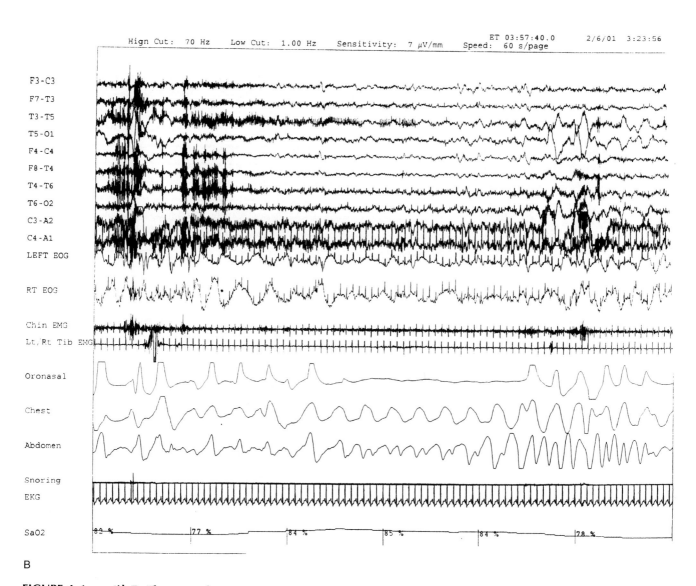

B

FIGURE 4–1, cont'd B: *The same subject as in* **A**. *A 60-second PSG snapshot. An electroencephalographic arousal is noted following the obstructive respiratory event and is associated with oxygen desaturations to the high 70s.*

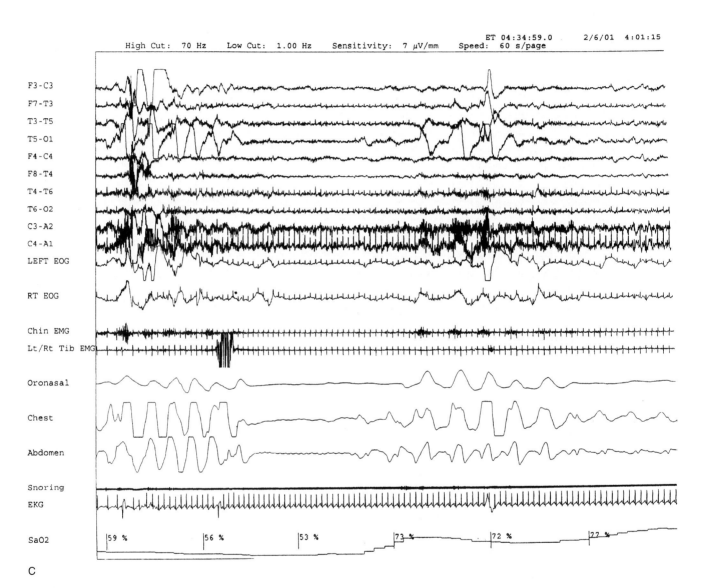

C

FIGURE 4–1, cont'd C: *The same subject as in* **A**. *A 60-second PSG snapshot of a mixed respiratory event associated with ongoing desaturations, which are now in the 50s. The dropout of EMG tone may suggest mixed REM physiology and thus some additional hypoventilation.*

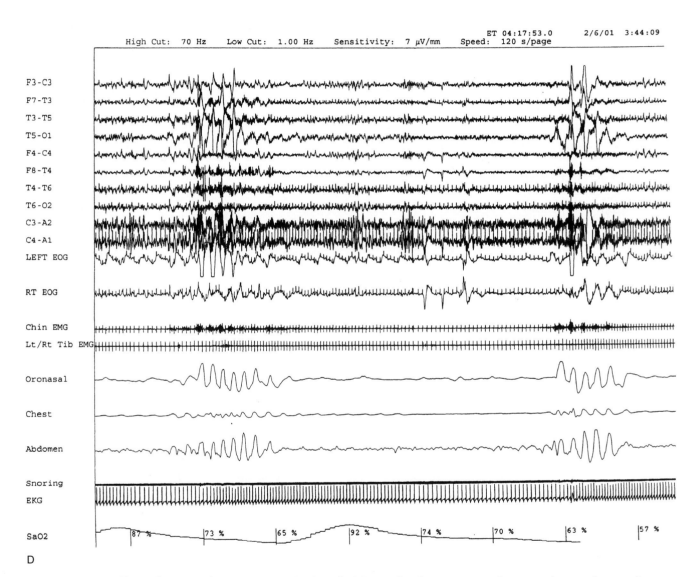

D

FIGURE 4–1, cont'd D: *The same subject as in* **A***. A 120-second PSG snapshot demonstrating a long central apnea during a fragment of REM sleep.*

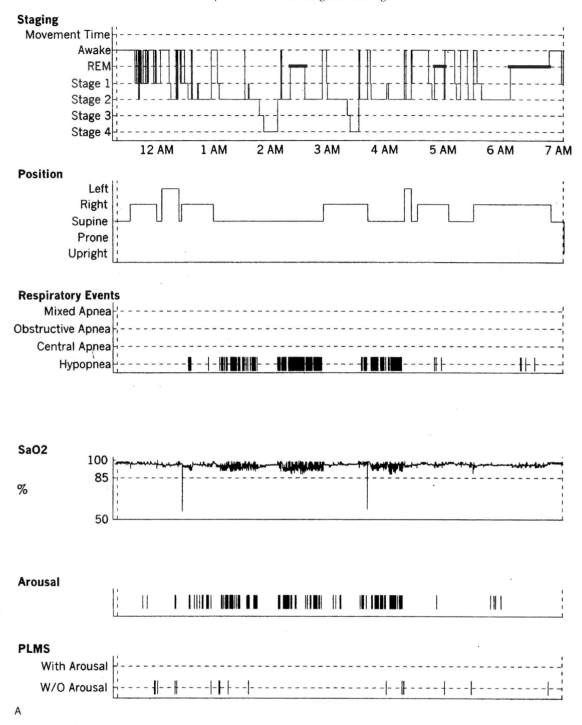

FIGURE 4–2. A: *This hypnogram is from a 5-foot, 7-inch 40-year-old man who weighs 177 pounds. He reports snoring and excessive daytime sleepiness. Physical examination shows a large tongue and low-hanging soft palate. There is supine-dominant disease with relatively mild oxygen desaturations.*

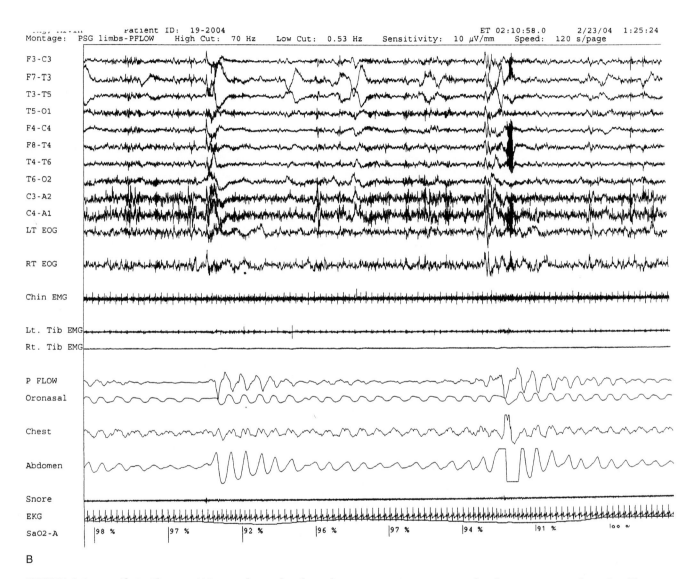

FIGURE 4–2, cont'd B: *This is a 120-second snapshot from the patient in A. Hypopneas, flow limitation, arousals, and mild oxygen desaturation are all seen. The difference in severity at all levels (respiration, sleep architecture, oxygenation) from the patient in A is striking, although the degree of subjective sleepiness may well be similar.*

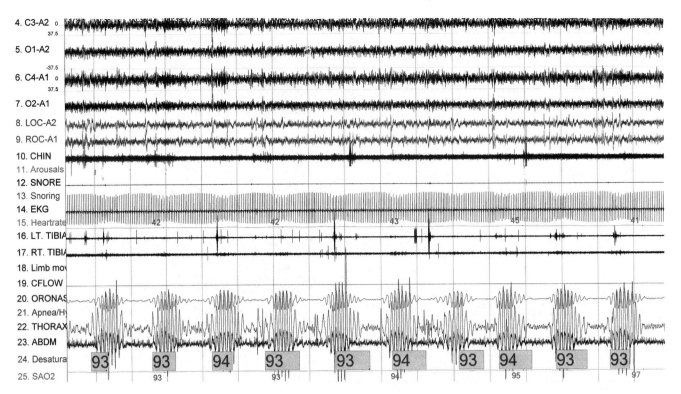

FIGURE 4–3. *This is a 500-second excerpt showing the classic Cheyne-Stokes Breathing (CSB) of crescendo-decrescendo pattern (periodic breathing) from an overnight PSG of a 75-year-old man. The patient has a history of hypertension, excessive daytime sleepiness, and snoring. The presence of CSB throughout most of the NREM sleep (with marked decrement or absence during REM sleep) could suggest incipient left ventricular failure.*

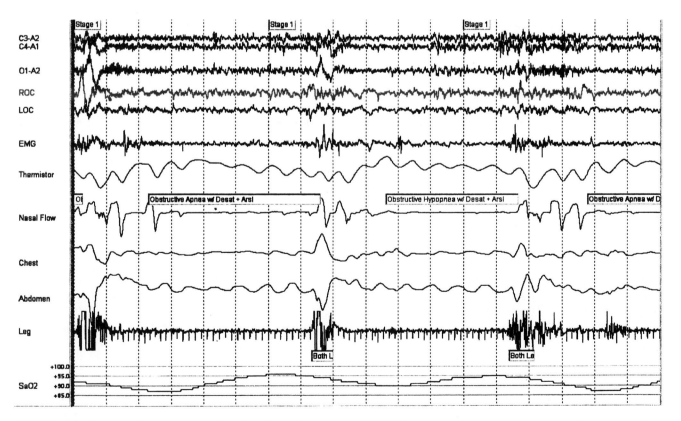

FIGURE 4–4. *Hypoxic obstructive sleep-disordered breathing in stage II NREM sleep, cyclic alternating pattern. Thermistors show recognizable abnormality. The nasal pressure trace amplifies both the abnormality and recovery. Thus, a "flat line" on the trace may not imply a true apnea, if this differentiation is necessary. Periodic limb movement in sleep (PLMS) accompanies each respiratory arousal, and without accurate respiratory monitoring a diagnosis of PLM disorder may result. Arousals show variable durations of alpha/beta intrusion. 90-second epoch.*

131

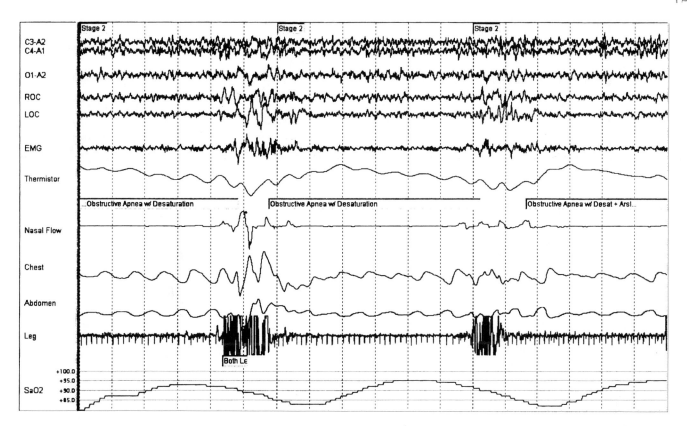

FIGURE 4–5. *Hypoxic obstructive sleep-disordered breathing in stage II NREM sleep, cyclic alternating pattern. Although respiratory events are definitive, the EEG patterns that are associated with event termination and recovery of obstructed breathing demonstrate a paucity of alpha/beta rhythms. Use of medications that enhance slow-wave activities may reduce the number of arousals that have a typical alpha/beta intrusion pattern. 90-second epoch.*

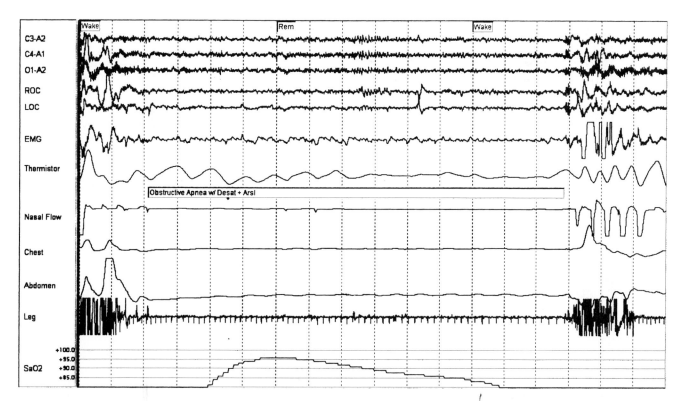

FIGURE 4–6. *Severe hypoxia accompanies this respiratory event during REM sleep. It is probably obstructive, with possibly a component of hypoventilation. Forced oscillation or an intercostal EMG demonstrating diaphragmatic activity could differentiate an obstructive from a central event in this instance. PLMS are unusual in REM sleep, but can accompany repetitive obstructive events. 90-second epoch.*

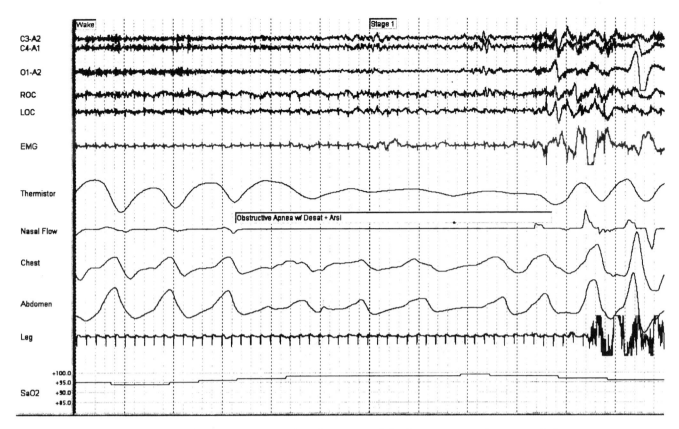

FIGURE 4–7. *Severe obstructive event at sleep onset, evident the moment alpha dropout occurs. Patients with this repetitive pattern at sleep onset may present with a primary insomnia complaint. 60-second epoch.*

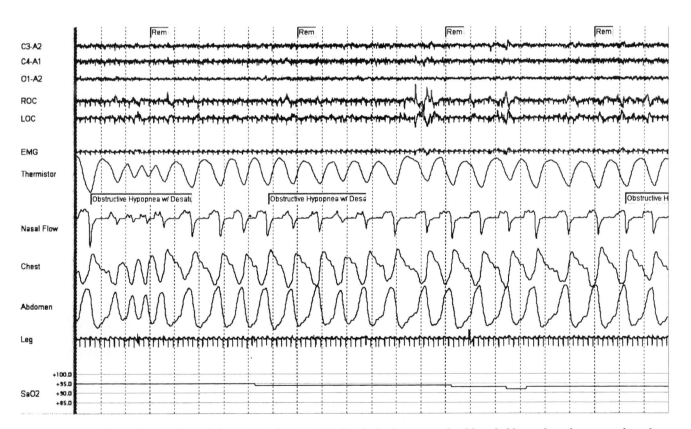

FIGURE 4–8. *What is the boundary of abnormality during REM sleep? The first event should probably not have been scored, as there was no obvious consequence. The second event had a discernible mild desaturation, but even that may be challenged. Intermittent non-progressive flow limitation and hypopneas are normal in REM sleep and should generally not be scored unless there are arousals or desaturations. Electrocardiographic artifact on the EMG interferes with the identification of subtle tone changes. 120-second epoch.*

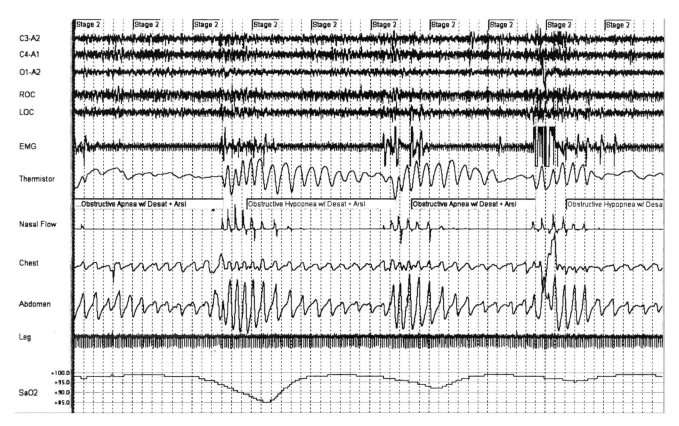

FIGURE 4–9. *Complex respiratory abnormality. The flow channels show clear evidence of reduced flow with persistent effort, making these obstructive events. However, the effort channels have a distinctive periodic pattern. The oxymetry trace shows dips of varying severity and duration. This is more typical of an obstructive disorder. 5-minute epoch.*

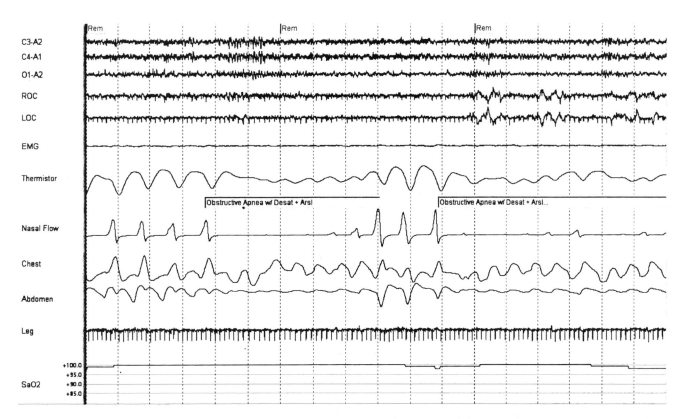

FIGURE 4–10. *Obstructed respiratory event in REM sleep that shows a clear event-recovery correlated alpha/beta intrusion with no increase in EMG tone. It seems clinically logical that such events disrupt sleep. However, most such events in REM sleep do have some increase in EMG tone. 90-second epoch.*

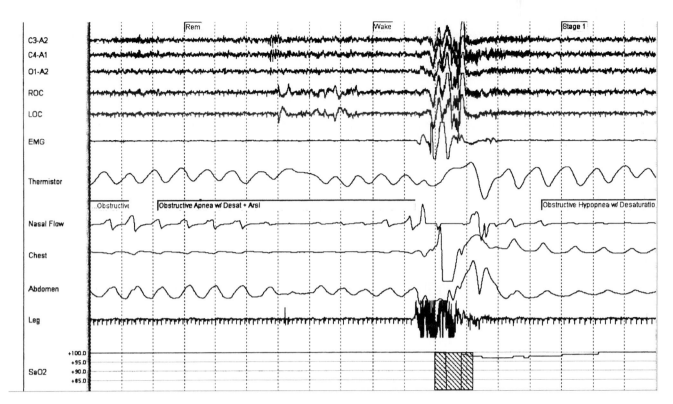

FIGURE 4–11. *Classic obstructive respiratory abnormality in REM sleep. Arousal is accompanied by EMG tone elevation. Hypoxia does not accompany this particular event. 90-second epoch.*

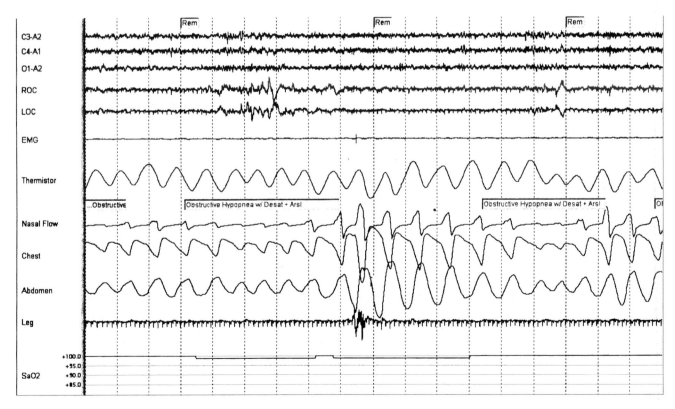

FIGURE 4–12. *Hypopneas in REM sleep with accompanying intermittent alpha/beta intrusions. Flow-limitation suggest that these are obstructive. A leg movement is the major accompanying EMG signature in this case, though the chin EMG possibly shows a single motor unit potential. 90-second epoch.*

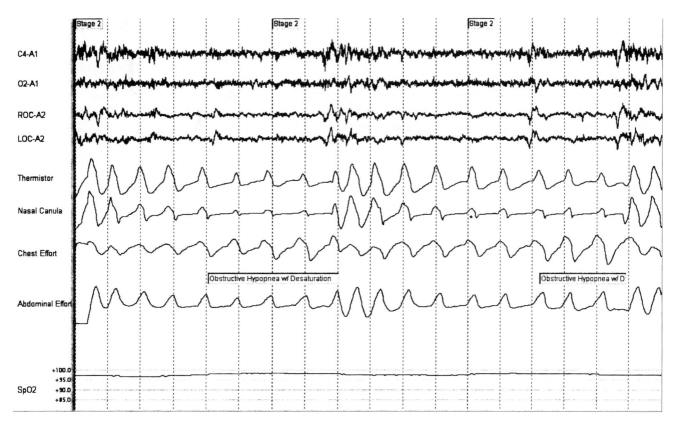

FIGURE 4–13. *Hypopneas in NREM sleep, with minimal saturation alterations. There is a suggestion of periodicity, with the symmetrical "mirror imaging" of respiratory events. 90-second epoch.*

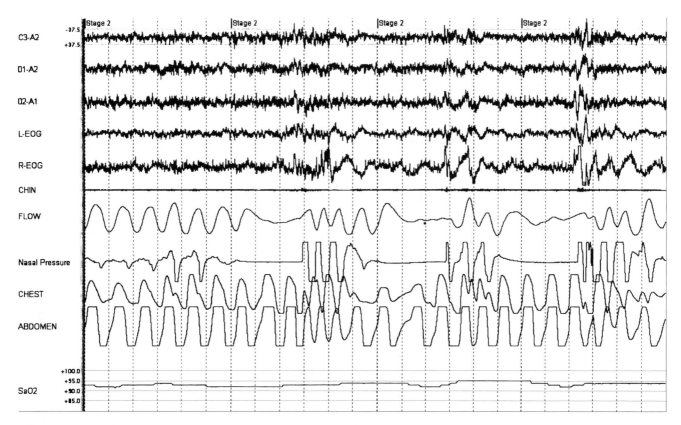

FIGURE 4–14. *Apneas in NREM sleep. The events are associated with mild desaturations, and demonstrate clear arousals and respiratory recovery. 120-second epoch.*

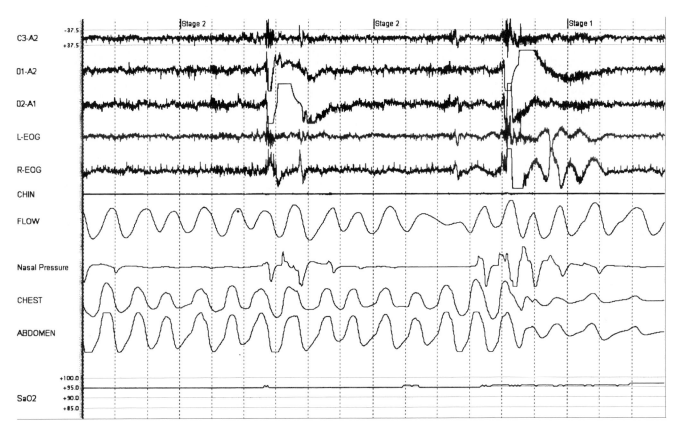

FIGURE 4–15. *Severe non-hypoxic obstructive sleep-disordered breathing. Thermistors do not readily pick up the events in this instance, which cause overt arousals. 90-second epoch.*

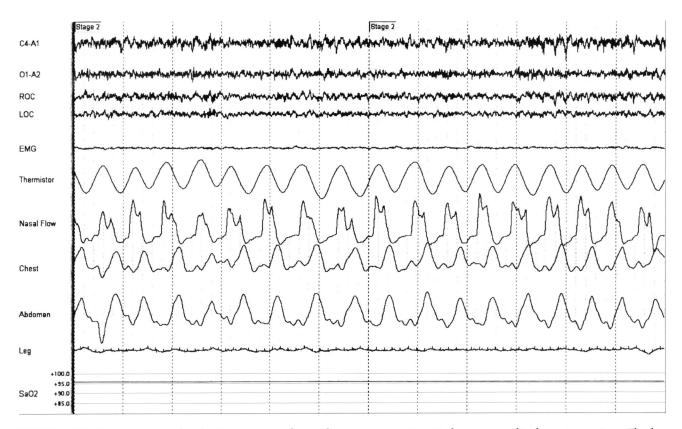

FIGURE 4–16. *Non-progressive flow-limitation seen on the nasal pressure trace. Stage II sleep, non–cyclic alternating pattern. This has also been variously termed* stable *(versus* unstable*), long (versus* short*) flow limitation, and as segments with continuous increases in inspiratory effort. It is not known if such patterns are associated with disrupted sleep. Obstructive hypoventilation may be seen when flow is partially obstructed. 60-second epoch.*

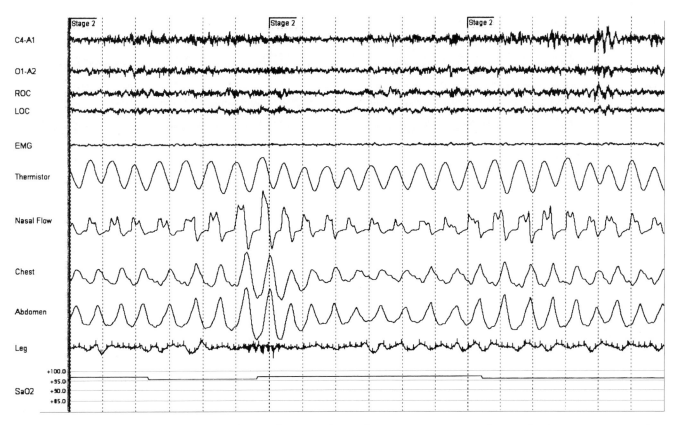

FIGURE 4–17. *Progressive flow-limitation and arousals seen on the nasal pressure trace. Stage II sleep, cyclic alternating pattern. Thermistors cannot provide this information. The effort channels show reductions, but if a 50 percent criterion is used, events will not be scored. 90-second epoch.*

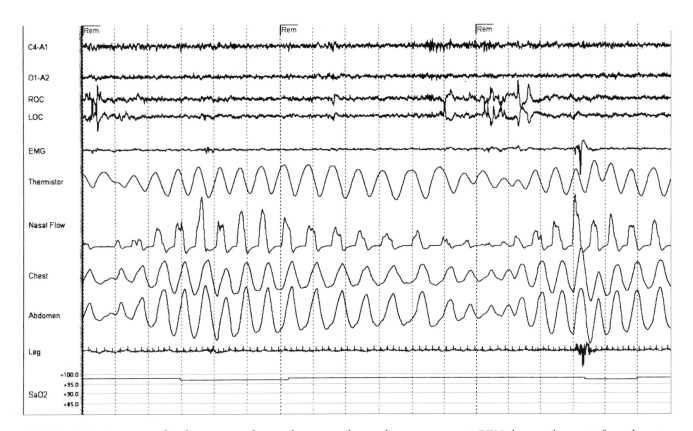

FIGURE 4–18. *Progressive flow-limitation and arousals seen on the nasal pressure trace in REM sleep, without significant hypoxia. EMG elevations are brief (less than 3 seconds). The effort channels also show major reductions. 90-second epoch.*

138

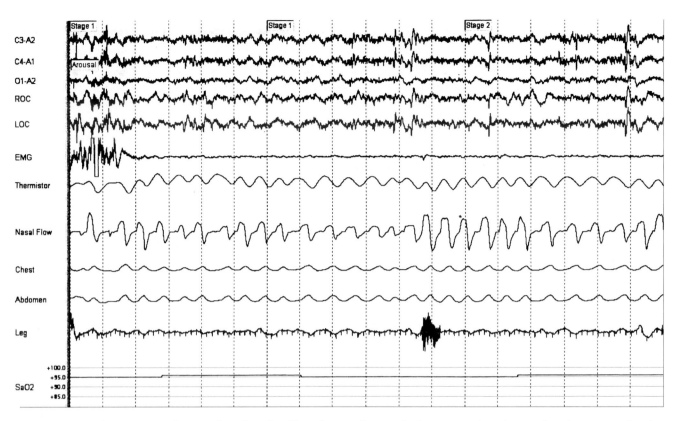

FIGURE 4–19. *Obstructive non-hypoxic sleep-disordered breathing with arousal. The recovery breaths are often the PSG marker that brings our attention to focus on the event. 90-second epoch.*

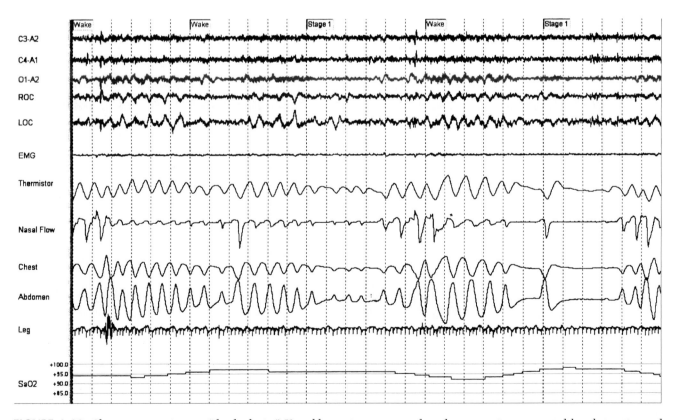

FIGURE 4–20. *Sleep-onset respiratory "dysrhythmia." Unstable respiratory control at sleep onset is exaggerated by obstructive and non-obstructive sleep-disordered breathing. Central apneas, periodic breathing, flow-limitation and desaturations are seen in varying combinations. Standard scoring may have these epochs as "wake." 150-second epoch.*

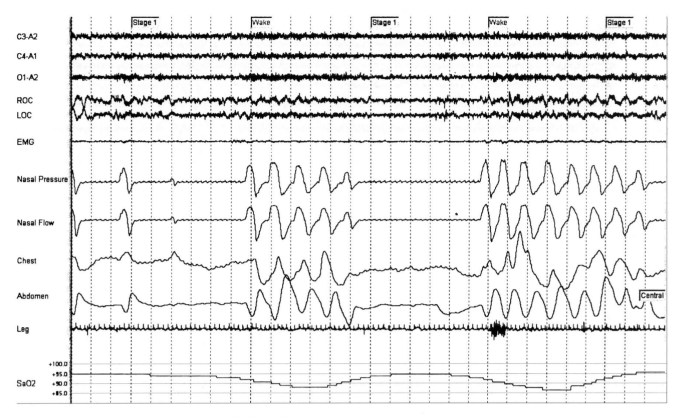

FIGURE 4–21. *Sleep-onset respiratory dysrhythmia during the onset of continuous positive airway pressure (CPAP) titration. Severe respiratory abnormality (central apneas with desaturations) at sleep onset. Cardiogenic oscillations are seen both on the flow and effort signals. 150-second epoch.*

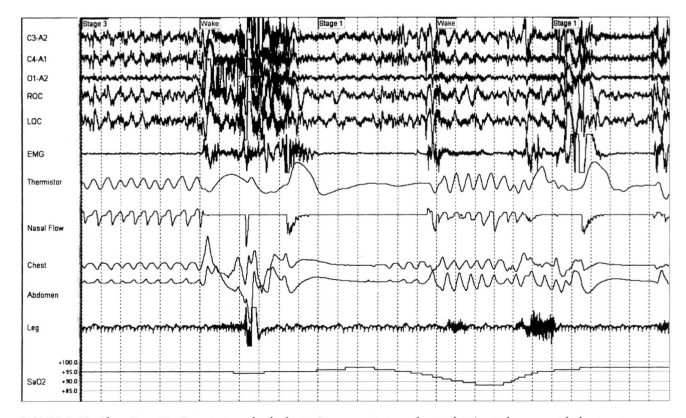

FIGURE 4–22. *Sleep "transition" respiratory dysrhythmia. Severe respiratory abnormality (central apneas with desaturations, some flow-limitation) after an awakening from stable, non-obstructed stage III NREM sleep. This pattern may be a transient or evolve into disordered breathing in lighter NREM sleep. 150-second epoch.*

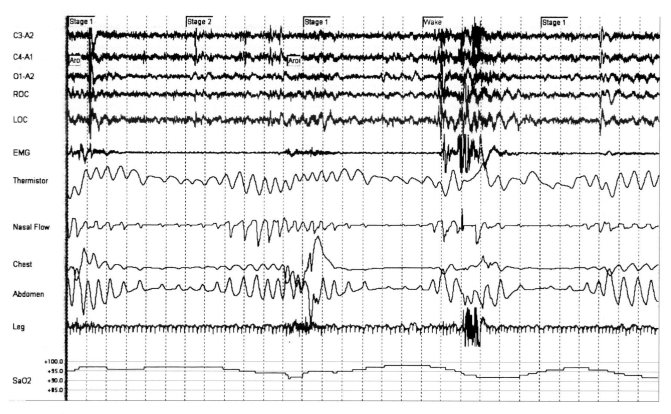

FIGURE 4–23. *Patient X: snapshot-1. Periodic breathing, desaturations, variable flow-limitation and arousals in a patient with severe mixed sleep-disordered breathing. NREM sleep is stage II, cyclic alternating pattern. 150-second epoch.*

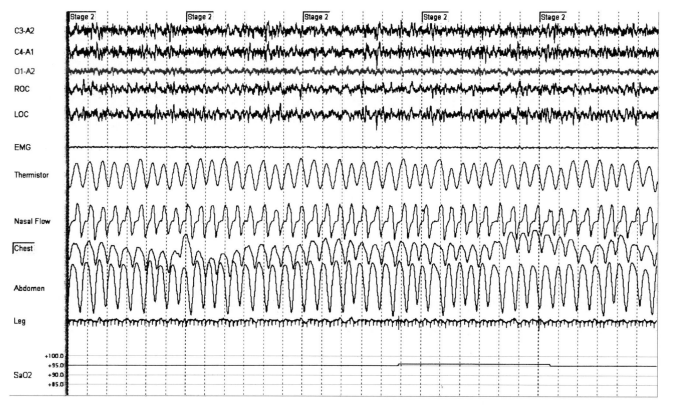

FIGURE 4–24. *Patient X: snapshot-2. Absence of periodic breathing, desaturations, arousals, or flow-limitation in NREM sleep stage II, non–cyclic alternating pattern. This pattern of NREM sleep is associated with sleep and breathing stability, regardless of conventional stages, even in those with significant disease. 150-second epoch.*

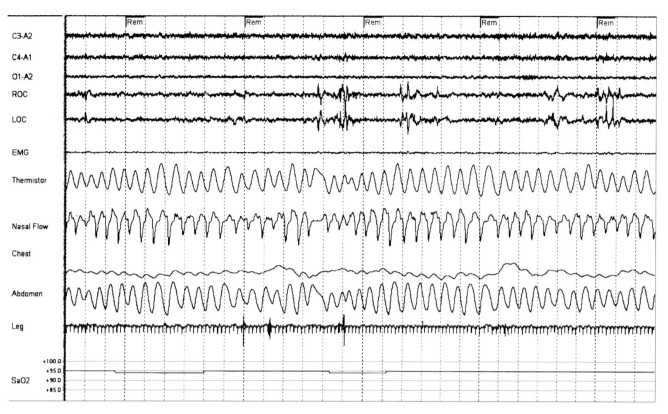

FIGURE 4–25. *Patient X: snapshot-3. Absence of periodic breathing, arousals, or severe desaturations in REM sleep. Intermittent flow-limitation is seen. REM sleep can abolish non-obstructive components of a mixed disorder. The residual obstruction seems to be of minimal consequence in this sample. 150-second epoch.*

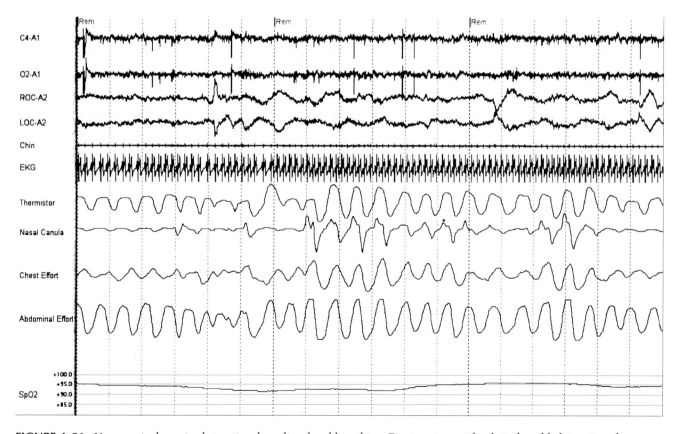

FIGURE 4–26. *Non-apneic, hypoxic obstructive sleep-disordered breathing. Desaturations with relatively mild obstructive phenomena may reflect a baseline reserve abnormality (e.g., chronic obstructive lung disease) or REM hypoventilation. 90-second epoch.*

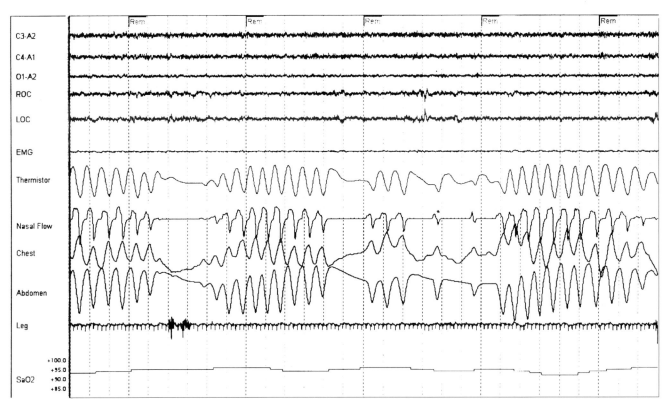

FIGURE 4–27. *Central apneas during REM sleep (especially during phasic REM sleep) are common. If accompanied by arousals or desaturations (as in this case), they should be scored. 150-second epoch.*

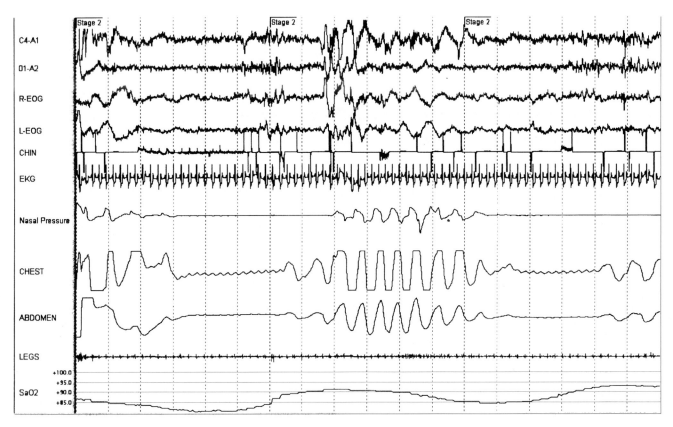

FIGURE 4–28. *Severe "central" sleep-disordered breathing with hypoxia. Cardiogenic oscillations on the effort channels are a useful marker, when present, of the central nature of the event. "Central" is a PSG appearance only, as some of these patients may respond to CPAP and the airway may be demonstrated to be collapsed during this type of event. 90-second epoch.*

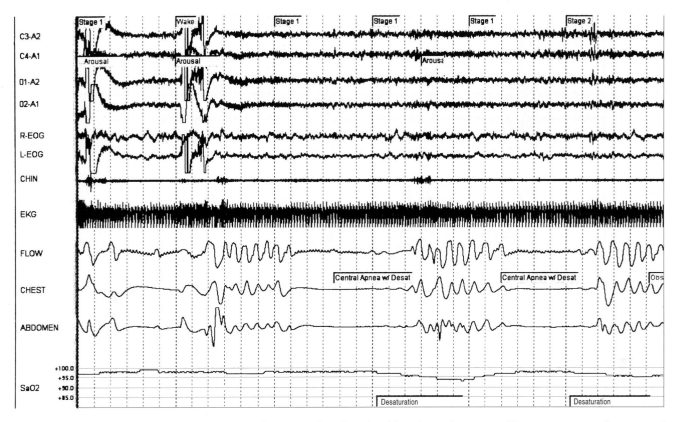

FIGURE 4–29. *Patient Y: snapshot-1. Severe non-obstructive sleep-disordered breathing, characterized by repetitive central apneas and the typically mild desaturations. Cardiogenic oscillation on the flow trace imply an open upper airway. 180-second epoch.*

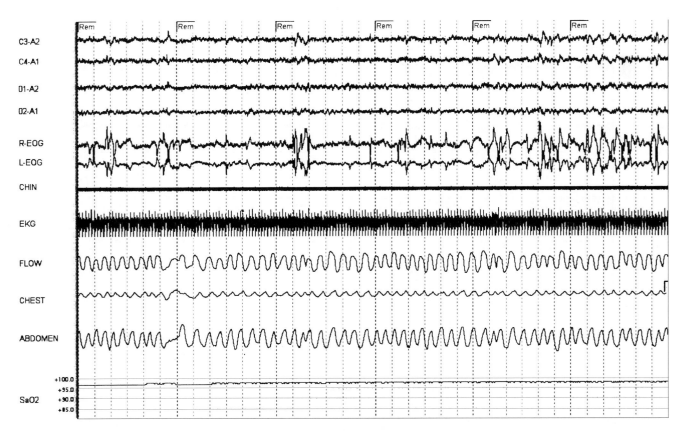

FIGURE 4–30. *Patient Y: snapshot-2. Stable respiration in REM sleep in the same patient. Chin EMG is artifactual. Patients with a dominance of non-obstructive sleep-disordered breathing are often stable during REM sleep. 180-second epoch.*

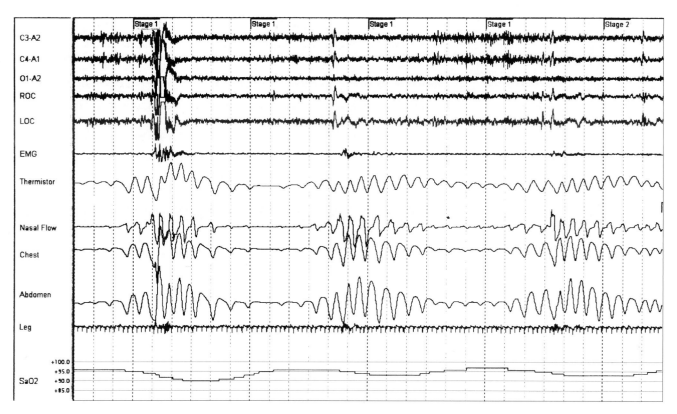

FIGURE 4–31. *Periodic breathing in stage II sleep NREM sleep, cyclic alternating pattern. Flow-limitation (on the nasal flow trace) is most evident during the hyperpnea phase, suggesting some airway collapse at the height of the respiratory drive. This could be secondary to subtle differences in drive or timing between the upper airway and diaphragm. 150-second epoch.*

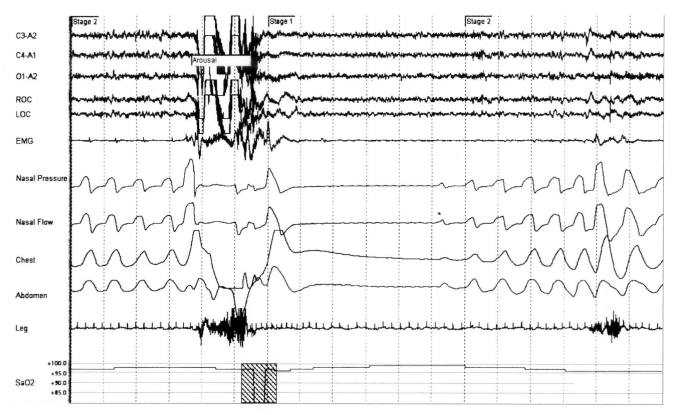

FIGURE 4–32. *Post-arousal central apnea during CPAP titration. Repeated events of this pattern were induced by pressures 1 to 2 centimeters above optimal, and did not occur following an appropriate reduction. Nasal pressure = mask pressure. 90-second epoch.*

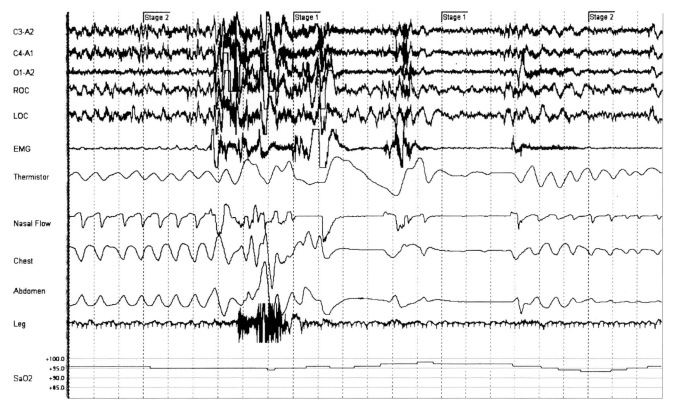

FIGURE 4–33. *Post-arousal central apneas. Respiratory control instability during this transition resulted in two central events before stabilization. The second event probably should be scored. 120-second epoch.*

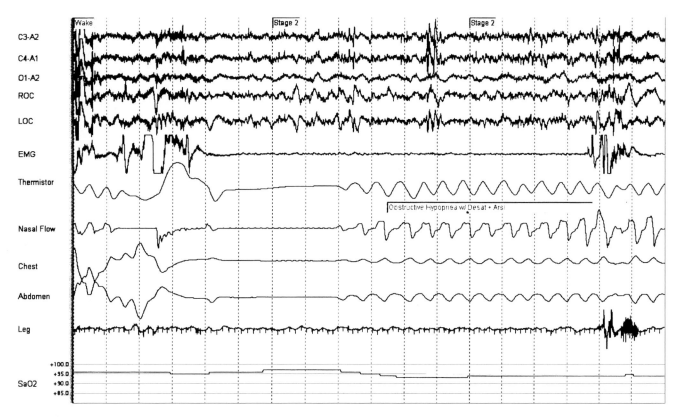

FIGURE 4–34. *Post-arousal central apnea. Flow-limitation on the nasal pressure trace is evident by the first few breaths that follow. The central event is associated with a desaturation and could reasonably be scored. 90-second epoch.*

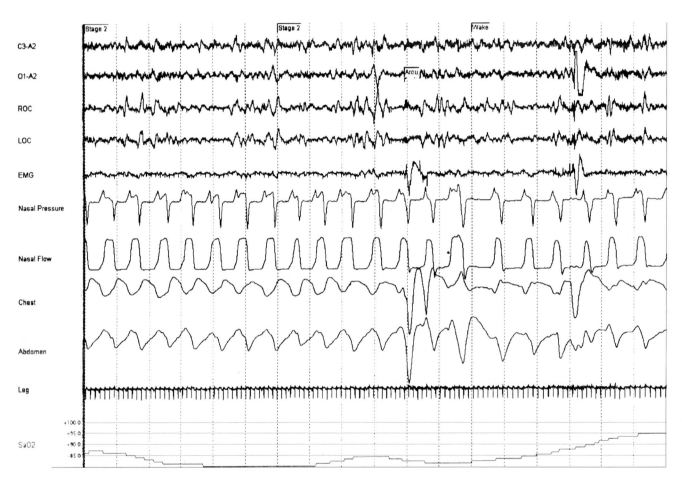

FIGURE 4–35. *Pre-REM-sleep hypoventilation. Flow is only mildly abnormal, while desaturations are severe. Stage II NREM sleep. REM sleep occurred within 2 minutes, where severe hypoventilation was noted, demonstrating that EEG stage shifts are not absolute on-off phenomena. Presumably REM ventilatory physiology was present even before the surface PSG characteristics of REM sleep were visible. 90-second epoch.*

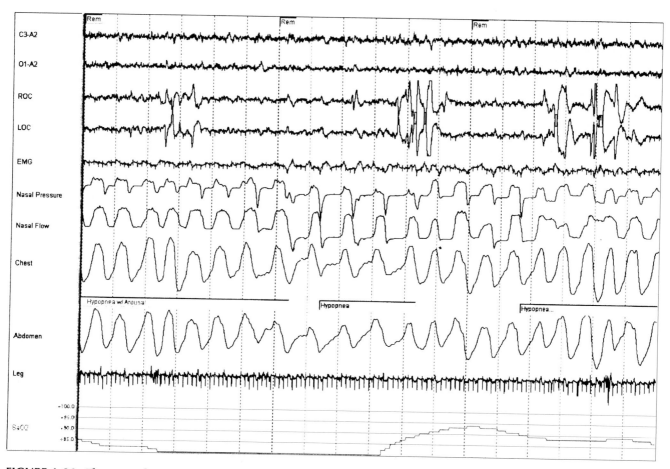

FIGURE 4–36. *The same subject as in Figure 4–35. REM-sleep hypoventilation. Flow is only mildly abnormal, while desaturations are severe. Strictly speaking, a measure of CO_2 is required to establish hypoventilation. In clinical sleep laboratory practice usually dealing with relatively healthy individuals, disproportionate (to obstructions) desaturations are considered an acceptable surrogate marker of hypoventilation. In populations with abnormal cardiopulmonary physiology resulting in ventilation-perfusion mismatch or shunting, this simple assumption will not hold. 90-second epoch.*

yet) that those without desaturations but with severely abnormal breathing and sleep fragmentation are free of risk.

- The requirement for desaturation to score a hypopnea will likely not reflect the full burden of abnormal sleep in every patient with sleep-disordered breathing. The smallest saturation change that can be visually detected is 2 percent to 3 percent. There is no scientific rationale yet proven to prefer any specific degree of reduction (e.g., 3 percent, 4 percent, or 5 percent) in saturation to quantify respiratory events, and requiring a change in saturation (of any degree) will underscore events (worse with higher cutoffs).

- The nasal pressure signal (nasal cannula–pressure transducer system, NC-PT signal) has emerged as a practical and usually tolerable measure that closely correlates with flow as measured by the pneumotachograph. Subtle events that are virtually impossible to clearly define on the thermistor are often clearly seen on the nasal pressure trace. Flow limitation due to increased upper airway resistance is the basic abnormality and is associated with increased respiratory effort ("discomfort") that results in an arousal once the threshold is exceeded for the individual. Nasal pressure flow abnormalities correlate adequately with respiratory effort–related events as noted on esophageal pressure traces. Besides changes evoked by specific neurologic and cardiopulmonary diseases, airflow patterns and arousal thresholds are modulated by sleep macrostructure (rapid eye movement [REM], non-REM sleep, stages of non-REM sleep), sleep microstructure (CAP and non-CAP), sleep deprivation, medication, and age.

- The snapshots in this section (see Figures 4–1 through 4–36) provide several examples, demonstrating some of the spectrum of respiratory events and the superior sensitivity of nasal pressure recordings in the diagnosis of sleep-disordered breathing. Changes in the signal amplitude, an abrupt change in the profile of the inspiratory part of the curve from flat to rounded, a large "recovery" breath, or area under the inspiratory part of the nasal pressure trace may singly or in combination be useful visual guides to determining individual events. Elimination of flow limitation is an important goal of nasal positive pressure therapies.

- *Associated cues.* The recovery breath or breath sequence (more than one large breath) draws attention to a possible event termination. To increase confidence that this event or sequence reflects a transient perturbation of sleep state, associated cues are useful. Other than the arousal, desaturation, and autonomic associations (described later), the following may also be useful: limb movement, brief bursts of slow or rapid eye movements, reversal of paradox on effort channels, and burst of bruxism activity.

- *EEG arousals.* Application of the AASM 3-second arousal rule applies constraints that are not based in biology. In the specific context of respiratory event termination, shorter degrees of alpha/beta intrusion (less than 3 seconds) or K complex and delta bursts may be considered arousal equivalents. However, current AASM guidelines require 3-second arousals for scoring and tabulating arousals. Thus *arousal scoring* implies classic AASM arousals, while *arousal detection* (this is just a suggestion but has not been tested and accepted as valid criteria) implies using a broader spectrum of EEG transients to bias differentiation of significant versus non-significant respiratory events.

SCORING CONCEPTS

- **Apnea.** *Obstructive* apneas should always be scored. *Non-obstructive* apneas (especially during REM sleep and not leading to an arousal or associated with oxygen desaturation), postarousal apneas, and apneas during sleep-wake transition periods should generally not be scored. Prolonged sleep-wake transition respiratory events should be scored if it appears that sleep onset is being interfered with.

- **Obstructive hypopnea.** There is no universally accepted definition for the *minimal clinically significant respiratory event.* It is proposed that identification of an obstructive respiratory event require that two standards be met: One, there must be evidence of upper airway obstruction derived from the flow signal; two, there must be evidence of a physiological consequence of the obstruction, for example, arousal, oxygen desaturation, or autonomic activation. To avoid confusion and impracticality of the clinical usefulness of multiple and possibly overlapping event categories, it is convenient to tabulate events characterized primarily by flow limitation under the general term of *hypopnea.* There is no fundamental pathophysiological difference between an apnea and hypopnea, as obstructed breathing events manifest a continuum of severity. When using the NC-PT signal, obstructed breathing may be seen to evolve for periods much longer or shorter than 10 seconds. What starts as a hypopnea may evolve into apnea level reductions in flow just prior to respiratory event termination. However, arousals terminating an overt apneic event may be more disruptive to sleep than those terminating subtle flow limitation. Continued differentiation of these events will likely remain a useful indicator of severity and be used for comparative purposes. *Central hypopneas* are difficult to score at the current time and may be best avoided. *Central apneas* can have an obstructive pathogenesis. Careful analysis of the nasal pressure inspiratory flow profile (looking for evidence of even subtle degrees of flattening that could suggest flow limitation) should be done and may be useful. Use of techniques that reflect airway impedance such as forced oscillation, if readily adaptable to the diagnostic mode outside the research setting, may also help provide this (obstructive versus non-obstructive) differentiation.

- Measures of autonomic activation could be useful additions to the PSG to help with the identification of the significance of subtle events. These include pulse transit time, peripheral arterial tonometry, heart rate acceleration-deceleration sequences (visible to the human eye or in real-time on several current digital systems), skin blood flow, and skin sympathetic responses, and they may be useful to monitor "autonomic arousals." None of these are yet used in routine clinical practice, and it is not clear that with the use of the NC-PT it will have a significant impact outside research protocols.

SCORING RULES FOR RESPIRATORY EVENTS

1. **Apneas.** These are scored without regard to oxygen saturation changes or EEG evidence of arousal (see exceptions noted above).

   Obstructive/mixed apnea is scored when there is an absence (reduction to less than 10 percent to 15 percent of the baseline) of airflow with continued respiratory effort, lasting 10 seconds or more, derived from the nasal pressure and the thermistor signal. If the nasal pressure signal is flat, an apnea will be scored only if the thermistor signal is also less than 10 percent of its baseline. This is to make allowance for predominantly mouth breathers and the fact that the untransformed NC-PT signal exaggerates the abnormality. The practical utility of differentiating mixed from obstructive apneas is not clear.

   Central apnea is scored as an absence (reduction to less than 10 percent to 15 percent of baseline) of airflow without continued respiratory effort, lasting 10 seconds or more, derived from the nasal pressure and the thermistor signal. If the nasal pressure signal is flat, an apnea will be scored only if the thermistor signal is also less than 10 percent of its baseline. "Central" refers to the PSG pattern, as noted; upper airway obstruction may also cause this pattern.

2. **Hypopneas.** These are scored only when there are arousals or desaturations associated with the event. The standards of autonomic activation are not defined adequately to use them other than to bias scoring an event

when the arousal or desaturation is not definitive. For example, use of benzodiazepines may not allow a clear identification of overt EEG transients, but identification of cyclic variations in heart rate may allow detection of subtle EEG changes.

The primary scoring channel is the NC-PT signal. An event is scored if there is any clear reduction (usually 15 percent to 20 percent) in signal amplitude or progressive flow limitation that is abruptly terminated by a return to a sinusoidal pattern of flow or large recovery breath. If this signal is poor or not available, any clear reduction in the thermistor signal or thoracoabdominal effort that is terminated by an arousal or associated with oxygen desaturation is acceptable. For scoring hypopneas, the signal reduction need only be present in the nasal pressure channel. Thermistor signals provide a useful indicator of mouth breathing, which may occur in 10 percent of individuals during sleep. Reliance on the nasal pressure alone may overscore apneas in these individuals.

The only evidence of upper airways obstruction may be brief (even 2–3 breaths) intermittent flattening or flow limitation of the nasal pressure flow profile. Normal individuals may have intermittent mild flattening up to 10 percent to 15 percent of breaths during sleep, and these flattening contour events should not be scored (as hypopneas) if not associated with desaturations or a pattern of progressive-flow limitation leading to an arousal. No attempt is made to differentiate obstructive from central hypopneas in routine clinical practice. The nasal pressure often records subtle respiratory "events" in slow-wave sleep or REM sleep. These should not be scored unless associated with arousals, desaturation, or a major reduction in signal with an abrupt recovery (approximately 50 percent or more). Utilization of sleep microstructure based on CAP could improve scoring. Respiration is often remarkably stable in non-CAP regardless of severity of the abnormality in CAP, and mild fluctuations in signal should not be scored. A 4% desaturation index is a reasonable estimate of the hypoxic burden, but should be calculated independent of the respiratory disturbance index (RDI).

3. **Cheyne-Stokes breathing (CSB) event.** A CSB event is a breathing pattern characterized by a cyclical fluctuation in ventilation with periods of central apnea or hypopnea alternating with periods of hyperpnea in a gradual crescendo and decrescendo fashion. A CSB event is defined as one cycle of crescendo breathing (hyperpnea) followed by decrescendo breathing, terminating in an apnea or hypopnea. A minimum of three consecutive events is required to identify the characteristic regular periodicity of this breathing pattern. CSB is maximal in CAP and minimal in non-CAP and

Table 4–1. Difficult Clinical Situations and Suggested Mechanisms and Solutions

Problem	Mechanism	Suggestion for resolution
Medication effects or baseline EEG abnormalities make it hard to see discrete EEG transients	Drugs that increase slow-wave activity may increase the slow-wave (delta, K complex) component of arousals. Benzodiazepines may increase beta activity enough to obscure alpha intrusions. Alpha-delta sleep can make it almost impossible to apply standard rules.	Score events based on abrupt reversals of periods of abnormal flow, and use the desaturation criteria as usual. It is usually possible to appreciate a pattern of EEG transients that accompany these events, for the given patients, and this may be helpful. Autonomic activation markers may help.
Obviously abnormal breathing, but sleep scoring is "wake."	Severely abnormal breathing can disrupt sleep so badly that it is completely below the resolution (30-second epochs) of the standard scoring.	Score events, which will not be subtle. Desaturation links are valid, and often arousals are seen, e.g., repetitive K-alpha bursts separated by scored "wake."
Sleep-onset or sleep-wake transition events continue for several (more than 1–2) minutes.	Sleep-onset respiratory "instability" in normal individual consists of brief period of central apnea, flow limitation, and periodic breathing, but this stabilizes quickly. Sleep-disordered breathing may prolong this unstable phase and may significantly prevent entry into continuous sleep.	Score events using usual criteria if this phase is more than 1–2 minutes.
Apply the 4% AASM rule.	The saturation may drop progressively (e.g., 92-90-88-85-83-80) or into a medically significant range (e.g., from 85% to 82%), but each individual event is associated with less than a 4% change. This suggests clinically important sleep hypoventilation.	Score events that have less than 4% desaturation change but the baseline oxygen saturation between events do not return to $\geq 90\%$.

AASM, American Academy of Sleep Medicine.

REM sleep. Separate scoring of CSB events is not generally done outside the research setting.

4. **Sleep (often REM) hypoventilation.** This is a state characterized by a sustained reduction in alveolar ventilation and hypoxemia not associated with phasic breathing events such as apneas and hypopneas. If measured, there is an increase in $PaCO_2$ during sleep greater than or equal to 10 torr from the awake supine value.

DIFFICULT SITUATIONS

There are inevitably situations when the rules do not apply easily. Examples and suggestions for resolution are provided in Table 4–1.

BIBLIOGRAPHY

1. Ayappa I, Norman RG, Krieger AC, Rosen A, O'Malley RL, Rapoport DM. Non-invasive detection of respiratory effort-related arousals (RERA's) by a nasal cannula/pressure transducer system. *Sleep* 2000;23:763–771.

2. Condos R, Norman RG, Krishnasamy I, Peduzzi N, Goldring RM, Rapoport DM. Flow limitation as a noninvasive assessment of residual upper-airway resistance during continuous positive airway pressure therapy of obstructive sleep apnea. *Am J Respir Crit Care Med* 1994;150:475–480.

3. Tkacova R, Niroumand M, Lorenzi-Filho G, Bradley TD. Overnight shift from obstructive to central apneas in patients with heart failure: role of PCO2 and circulatory delay. *Circulation* 2001;103:238–243.

4. Hall MJ, Xie A, Rutherford R, Ando S, Floras JS, Bradley TD. Cycle length of periodic breathing in patients with and without heart failure. *Am J Respir Crit Care Med* 1996;154:376–381.

5. Thomas RJ. Arousals in sleep-disordered breathing: patterns and implications. *Sleep* 2003;26:1042–1047.

6. Bao G, Guilleminault C. Upper airway resistance syndrome—one decade later. *Curr Opin Pulm Med* 2004;10:461–467.

7. Thomas RJ, Terzano MG, Parrino L, Weiss JW. Obstructive sleep-disordered breathing with a dominant cyclic alternating pattern—a recognizable polysomnographic variant with practical clinical implications. *Sleep* 2004;27:229–234.

8. Collop NA. Scoring variability between polysomnography technologists in different sleep laboratories. *Sleep Med* 2002;3:43–47.

9. Whitney CW, Gottlieb DJ, Redline S, Norman RG, Dodge RR, Shahar E, Surovec S, Nieto FJ. Reliability of scoring res-

piratory disturbance indices and sleep staging. *Sleep* 1998;21:749–757.

10. Sanders MH, Givelber R. Sleep disordered breathing may not be an independent risk factor for diabetes, but diabetes may contribute to the occurrence of periodic breathing in sleep. *Sleep Med* 2003;4:349–350.

11. Younes M. Role of arousals in the pathogenesis of obstructive sleep apnea. *Am J Respir Crit Care Med* 2004;169:623–633.

12. Younes M. Contributions of upper airway mechanics and control mechanisms to severity of obstructive apnea. *Am J Respir Crit Care Med* 2003;168:645–658.

13. Johnson PL, Edwards N, Burgess KR, Sullivan CE. Detection of Increased Upper Airway Resistence During Overnight Polysomnography. *Sleep* 2005;28:85–90.

5

*Hypnogram Analysis**

Robert J. Thomas and Sudhansu Chokroverty

The hypnogram is traditionally the compressed graphic summary of sleep stages for the sleep period. In the context of clinical polysomnography (PSG), sleep stages are only one of the many physiological parameters recorded, providing an "extended hypnogram." This allows on a single page a representation of variables including sleep stages, respiration, positive airway pressure if used, motor movements, oxymetry, end-tidal or transcutaneous CO_2, heart rate variability measures, electroencephalographic (EEG) power spectrum, and body position.

Information in a hypnogram has two dimensions—horizontal and vertical. Examples of the horizontal dimension are the flow of sleep stages across the night, the oxymetry profile, and the occurrence of respiratory events.

Examples of the vertical dimension are the effect of body position and sleep stage on respiration and oxygenation. Some patterns are characteristic, such as a sleep-onset rapid eye movement (REM) period, REM-dominant hypoxic sleep-disordered breathing, and central sleep apnea (associated with minimal disease in REM sleep and smooth-symmetrical moderate oxygen desaturations in non-REM [NREM] sleep). Fragmentation of the sleep cycle can be secondary to a severe first night effect or poor sleep hygiene. A prolonged sleep onset latency followed by consolidated sleep suggests delayed circadian phase. The possible combinations of pathophysiology are many, and the following snapshots show some of the patterns that are commonly seen (Figures 5–1 through 5–17).

---

*Also see Chapter 10.

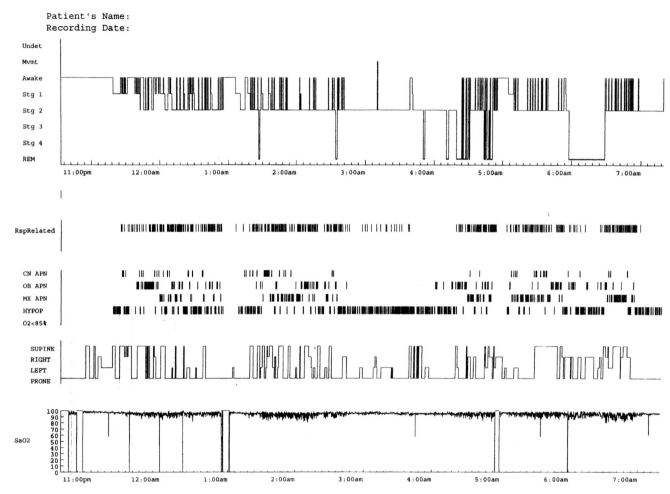

FIGURE 5–1. *Mixed sleep-disordered breathing. A 56-year-old man with hypertension, snoring, daytime fatigue, and nocturnal awakenings. Severe sleep fragmentation manifests as remarkably frequent body position changes and transitions between sleep and wake. REM cycling and distribution is surprisingly well maintained. Obstructive, central, and mixed events occur throughout the night except during a period of relative quiet in the middle of the sleep period (3 AM to 4 AM), when sleep was in non–cyclic alternating pattern (non-CAP). Note that the oxymetry trace dips show some symmetry, typical of those who have underlying periodic breathing. The patient is clearly not worse in REM sleep, which is also a marker of a non-obstructive component in the disorder. Leg movements are periodic, but linked to respiratory events. During titration, BiPAP (bilevel positive airway pressure) was superior to CPAP (continuous positive airway pressure) in stabilizing breathing and sleep.*

Patient's Name:
Recording Date:

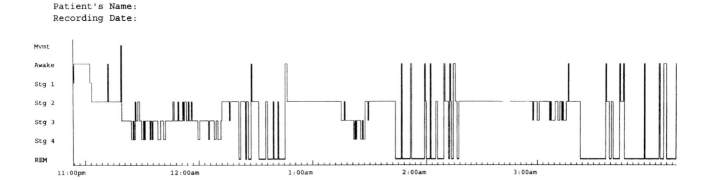

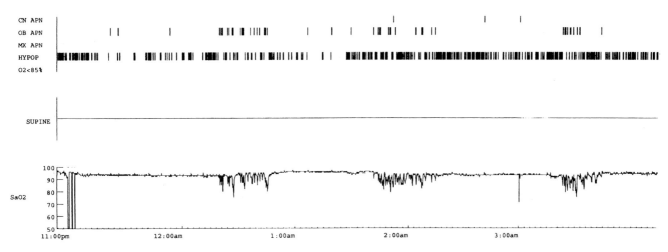

FIGURE 5–2. *REM-dominant obstructive sleep-disordered breathing. A 48-year-old mildly overweight (body mass index [BMI]: 27) man with refractory bipolar disorder, who denies daytime sleepiness, but expresses severe fatigue that peaks in the mid-afternoon. Medications are gabapentin, lithium, fluoxetine, and clonazepam. Sleep architecture is notable for some excess and redistribution of delta sleep into the latter half of the study, unusual when a benzodiazepine is used. Changes in delta sleep may reflect medication effects (lithium + gabapentin) or chronic sleep fragmentation. REM sleep is also increased, in spite of the use of fluoxetine. This may be secondary to increased REM sleep drive from chronic REM sleep fragmentation. Sleep-disordered breathing is maximal during REM sleep. BiPAP better controlled desaturation during REM sleep, when the patient was treated.*

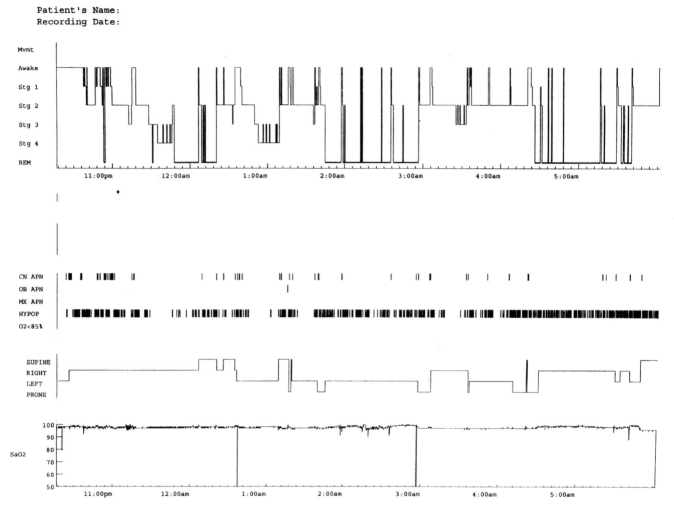

FIGURE 5–3. *Sleep-onset REM sleep (SOREM). A 56-year-old woman with lifelong severe (ESS: 20/24) excessive daytime sleepiness but no cataplexy. There is no snoring; nocturnal sleep is assessed as being chronically unrefreshing. Sleep-disordered breathing was quite overt, being best visualized on the nasal cannula–pressure transducer (NC-PT) trace. Complete resolution of all symptoms are noted on CPAP. Note lack of significant oxygenation abnormality. Markedly increased REM sleep, perhaps from chronic sleep fragmentation. SOREM is an abnormal but diagnostically non-specific PSG finding. Causes include narcolepsy, sleep fragmentation, depression (uncommon), sleep deprivation, circadian rhythm disorders, and abrupt withdrawal of REM-suppressing medications. If airflow was not monitored by NC-PT or if event-linked oxygen desaturation was a requirement for scoring, the diagnosis in this case would have been missed. ESS: Epworth Sleepiness Scale.*

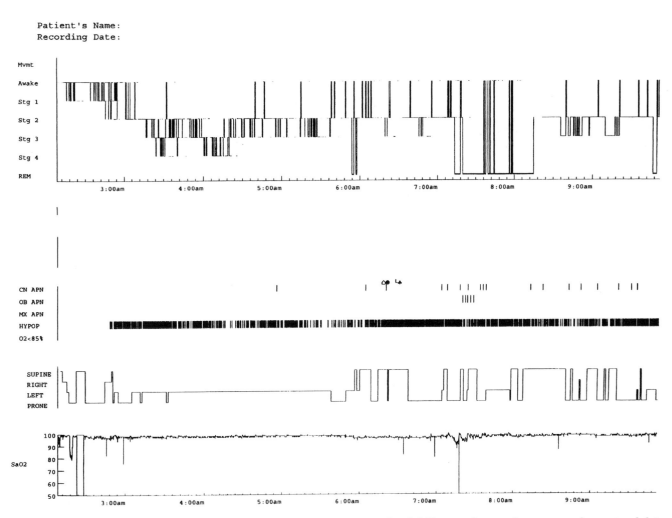

FIGURE 5–4. *Delayed sleep phase syndrome. A 32-year-old woman presented with lifelong "refractory depression and attention deficit disorder." Spontaneous sleep onset was usually between 2 AM and 3 AM, and offset between noon and 2 PM. Severe non-hypoxic sleep-disordered breathing was noted. Treatment with CPAP and morning bright light resulted in treatment responsiveness of depression and resolution of "ADHD" symptoms. Compliance with light treatment has been poor on follow-up.*

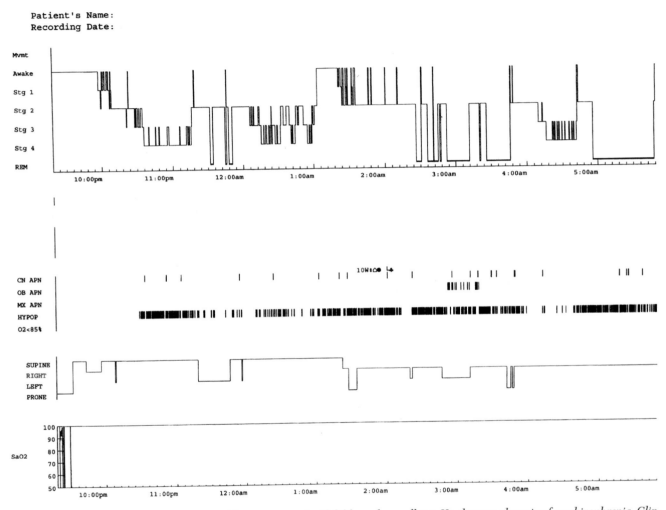

FIGURE 5–5. *Delta sleep excess. A 32-year-old man presented with lifelong sleepwalking. He also uses clozapine for schizophrenia. Clinically significant sleep-disordered breathing was noted (note dysfunctional oxymetry on this study), and CPAP resulted in improved subjective sleep quality and reduced daytime fatigue previously attributed to medication effects. Sleep deprivation, human immunodeficiency virus infection, and chronic sleep fragmentation can increase scored delta sleep. Medications that increase delta sleep at therapeutic doses include baclofen, old and new antipsychotics, and lithium. 5HT-2c antagonism increases delta sleep.*

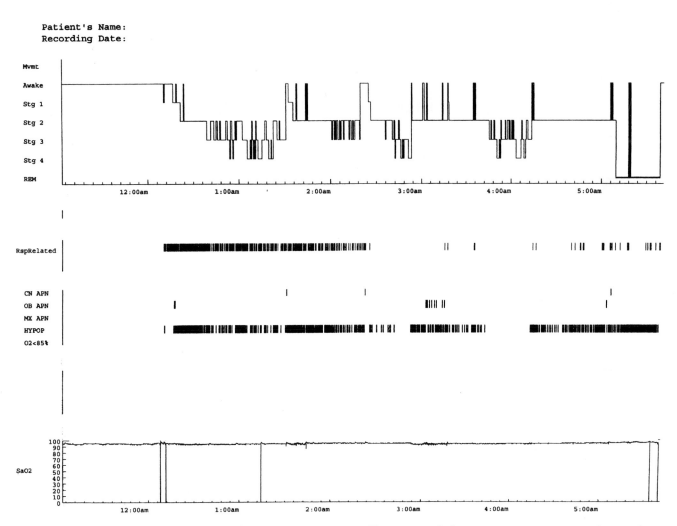

FIGURE 5–6. *Prolonged REM latency, increased delta sleep. A 54-year-old presents with depressive symptoms, snoring, daytime sleepiness, and unrefreshing sleep. Delta sleep is markedly increased for age and may reflect a build up of sleep debt from chronic sleep fragmentation. Prolonged REM latency may reflect increased delta sleep pressure.*

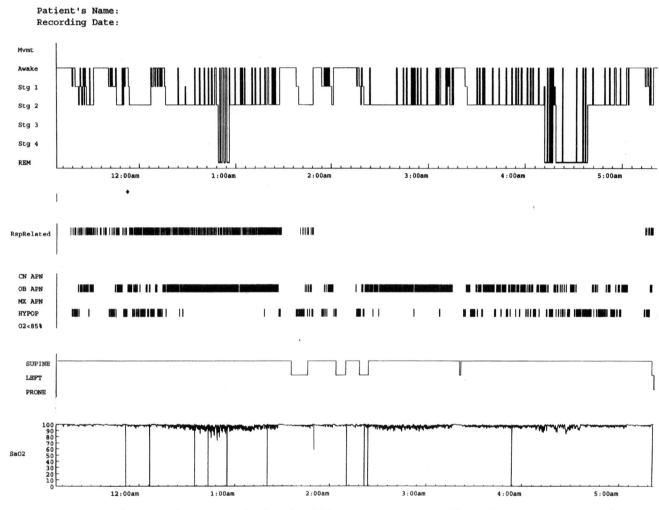

FIGURE 5–7. *Severe obstructive sleep apnea with relatively mild desaturation. A 50-year-old non-obese woman presents with snoring, excessive daytime sleepiness, and unrefreshing sleep. Periodic leg movements in sleep (PLMS) are seen in the first third of the night, but the patient had no clinical restless legs. The observed symmetric fluctuations on the oxymetry trace raised the possibility of underlying periodic breathing, but response to CPAP was complete.*

SLEEP STUDY REPORT

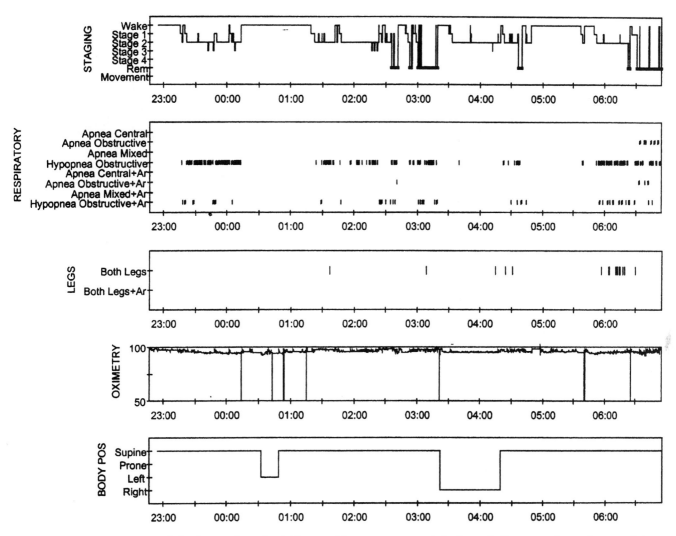

FIGURE 5–8. *Fragmentation of the sleep-wake cycle. A 72-year-old man presents with Parkinson's disease, moderate degrees of sleep-disordered breathing, and severe daytime sleepiness. He takes multiple naps during the day. Severe sleepiness and a narcolepsy-type PSG phenotype are increasingly being recognized in patients with this disorder, and it may be aggravated by treatment with D2/D3 agonists. The distribution of sleep stages shows a clear "separation" of individual sleep cycles by periods of wake. Patients may transiently have this pattern following intensive care unit admissions; it can be seen in elderly institutionalized individuals.*

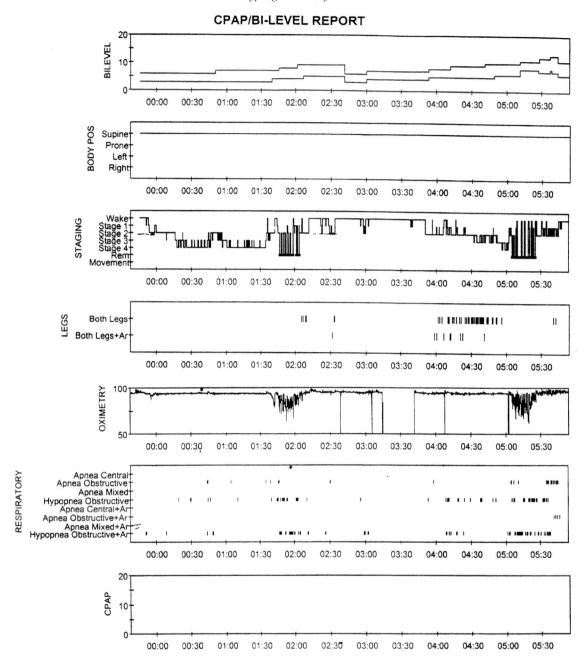

FIGURE 5–9. *REM-hypoventilation unresponsive to BiPAP. A 73-year-old obese diabetic had severe obstructive sleep-disordered breathing with oxygen desaturation to 62% during the diagnostic study. CPAP was not tolerated and did not control oxygen saturation in NREM or REM sleep. Bilevel PAP at tolerable settings controlled oxygen desaturation in NREM sleep, but not in REM sleep. Residual obstructive events were inadequate to explain the oxygenation abnormality. Increased inspiratory positive airway pressure (IPAP) may improve oxygenation further, but this patient required supplemental oxygen (3 L/minute).*

Patient Name :　　　　　**Study Date :**　　　　　**Subject Code :**
D.O.B. :　　　　　　　　**Height :**　　　　　　　　**Ref. Physician :**
Sex :　　　　　　　　　　**Weight :**　　　　　　　　**Scorer :**

SLEEP STUDY REPORT

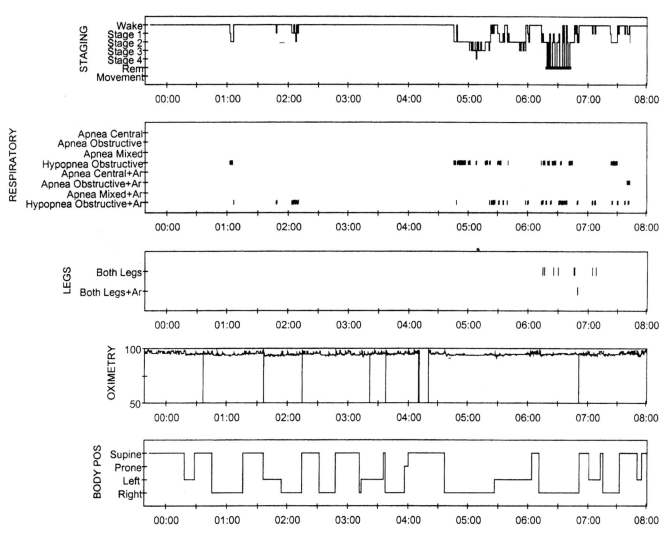

FIGURE 5–10. *Severe first night effect. A 32-year-old woman presented with excessive daytime fatigue and unrefreshing sleep. Normal sleep is from 10 PM to 7 AM, and the recorded pattern was not typical of an average night. Sleep efficiency is markedly reduced. A similar pattern may be seen in severe delayed sleep phase syndrome. A repeat sleep study was recommended to better establish severity of sleep-disordered breathing.*

Patient Name :
D.O.B. :
Sex :

Study Date :
Height :
Weight :

Subject Code :
Ref. Physician :
Scorer :

SLEEP STUDY REPORT

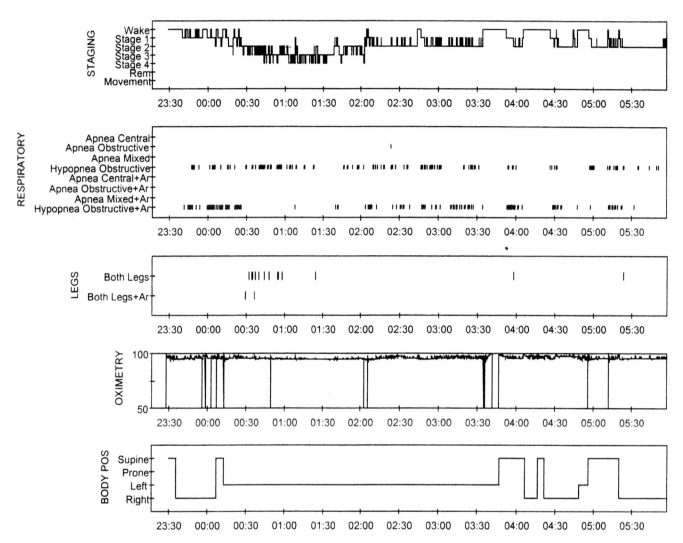

FIGURE 5–11. *Absence of REM sleep-medication effect. A 44-year-old presented to the sleep clinic for the evaluation of severe daytime fatigue in the setting of treatment-resistant depression. Medications included fluoxetine, methylphenidate, and clonazepam. No REM sleep is seen on this night. Non-hypoxic sleep-disordered breathing was also seen.*

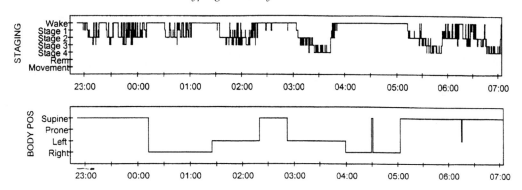

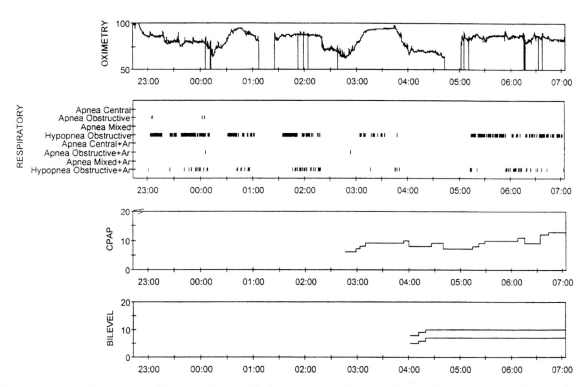

FIGURE 5–12. *Severe sleep hypoventilation. A 70-year-old obese woman with severe chronic obstructive airway disease who uses 24-hour, 5 L/minute of transtracheal oxygen, has severe hypoventilation during sleep. Periods scored wake were prolonged sleep-wake transition periods with unstable breathing and microsleep episodes. CPAP improved oxygenation, even though the obstructions were relatively mild. The patient did not tolerate BiPAP.*

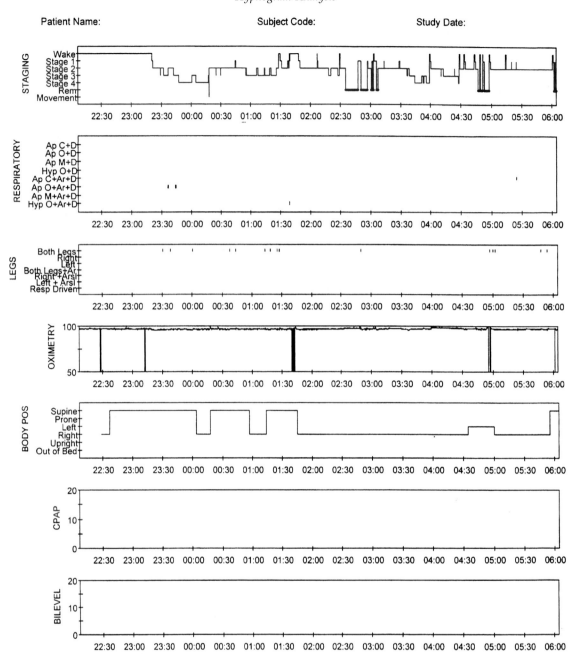

FIGURE 5–13. *Normal sleep. A 34-year-old healthy volunteer for a research study. The subject "skipped" the first REM period, which may be a first night effect.*

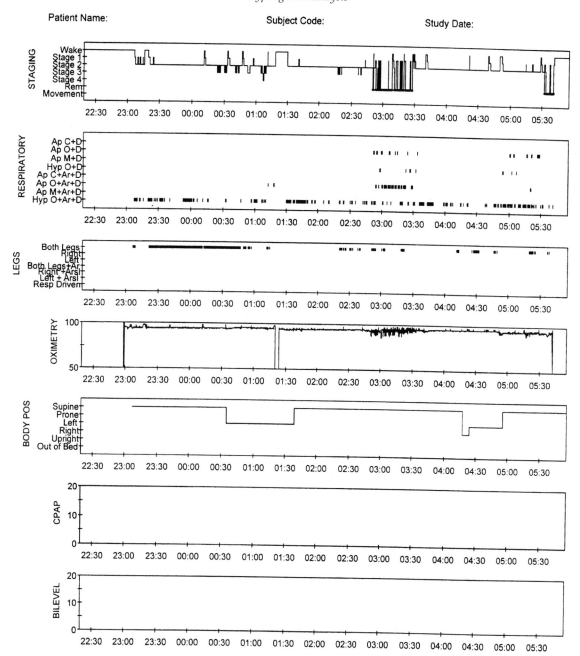

FIGURE 5–14. *Restless legs–related PLMS, REM-dominant sleep-disordered breathing. A 41-year old man presented for the evaluation of sleep-disordered breathing (snoring, daytime fatigue, witnessed apneas). Moderate severity of restless legs was noted, but the patient had no interest in its treatment. Disordered breathing was seen throughout sleep, dominant in REM sleep. PLMS were seen especially in the first third of the night, but did not seem to cause arousals.*

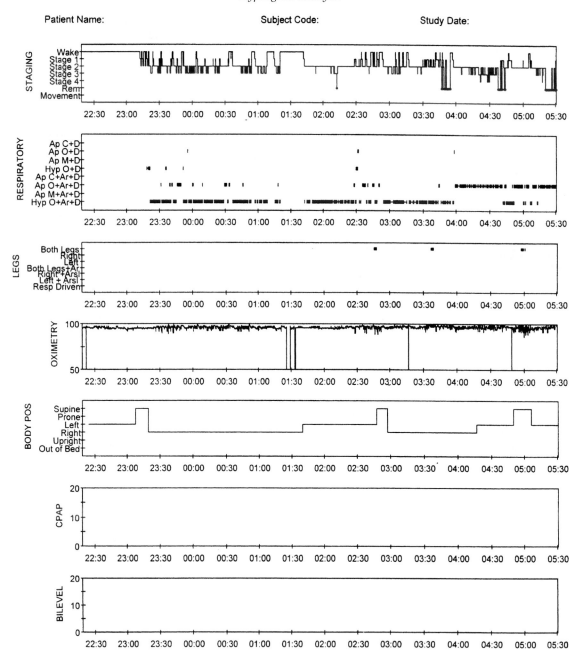

FIGURE 5–15. *Time-of-night effects in sleep-disordered breathing. A 56-year-old man presents with lifelong symptoms suggestive of attention deficit hyperactivity disorder. Daytime sleepiness is denied, but there is a marked mid-afternoon dip in perceived cognitive capabilities. There is a gradual evolution (increasing severity) of the purely obstructive disorder across the night. The last third of the sleep study exhibited repetitive apneas, irrespective of sleep type, sleep depth, or body position.*

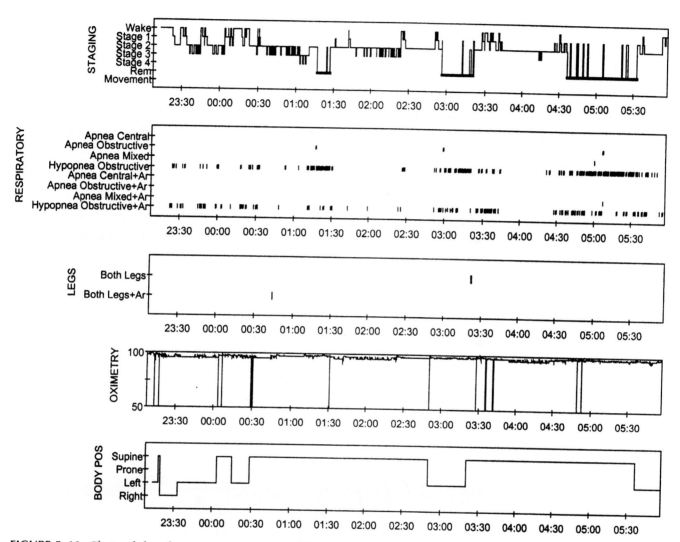

FIGURE 5–16. *Clustered sleep-fragmentation. A 42-year-old man with a diagnosis of attention deficit hyperactivity disorder presents for evaluation of sleep-disordered breathing as a cause of suboptimal response to stimulants. Sleep-disordered breathing was severe during REM sleep. During NREM sleep, periods of non-CAP were perfectly normal (irrespective of simultaneously scored delta sleep), while cyclic alternating pattern demonstrated abnormality of intermediate severity.*

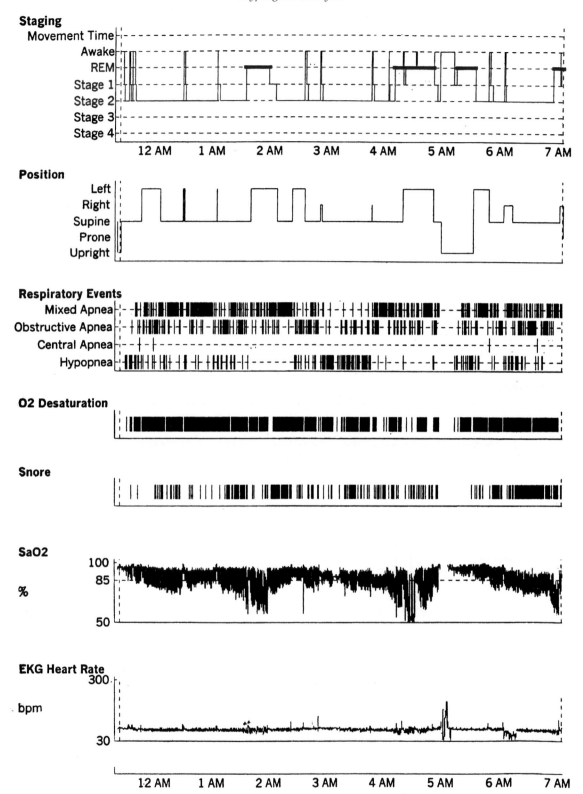

FIGURE 5–17. *Severe upper airway obstructive sleep apnea syndrome. A 38-year-old man presented with a history of loud snoring, choking during sleep, excessive daytime sleepiness (Epworth Sleepiness Scale score of 17) and disturbed night sleep. Hypnogram shows absent slow-wave sleep, recurrent episodes of obstructive and mixed apneas and hypopneas with an apnea-hypopnea index of 110.6, severe oxygen desaturation (for 21 minutes the level fell below 70 percent), and snoring. Following CPAP titration with an optimum titration pressure of 20 centimeters of water, the apneas and hypopneas were largely eliminated (the index fell to 5.8) and oxygen saturation remained above 90 percent.*

6

Cardiac Arrhythmias

ROBERT J. THOMAS, SUDHANSU CHOKROVERTY, MEETA BHATT, AND TAMMY GOLDHAMMER

The polysomnogram (PSG) provides a good opportunity to evaluate cardiac rhythms. Although medically threatening abnormalities are seen less frequently today than in the past, sleep specialists and technicians must be able to recognize the basic abnormalities. The following 10 PSG segments show some of the cardiac arrhythmias seen during overnight PSG recording.

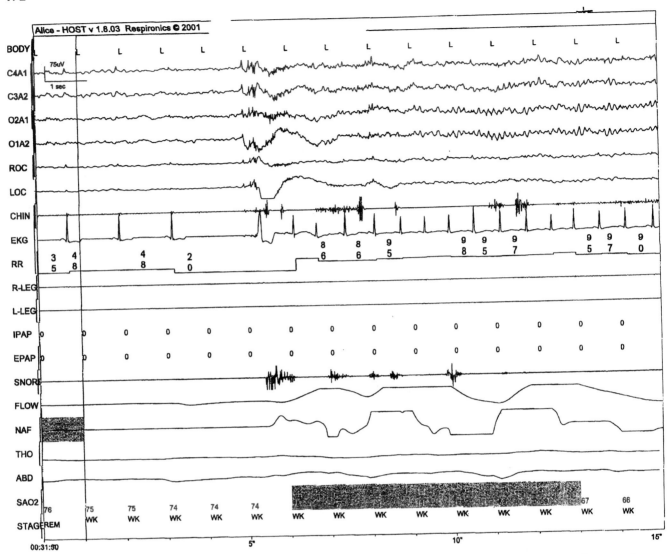

FIGURE 6–1. *Severe disease-related bradyarrhythmia in rapid eye movement (REM) sleep. A 56-year-old man with severe daytime sleepiness. The left side of the snapshot shows a heart rate less than 50, the termination of an apnea, and severe hypoxia (saturation in the mid-70s). Just prior to the arousal, there is a 4-second period with no electrocardiographic (EKG) rhythm (possible sinus arrest or sinoatrial exit block), followed by a ventricular escape, and post-arousal tachycardia, with a near doubling of heart rate. The EKG R wave amplitude also shows fluctuations that track respiratory effort: This EKG-derived respiration signal is secondary to changes in the cardiac axis generated by positional variation of the heart in the thoracic cavity associated with respiration.*

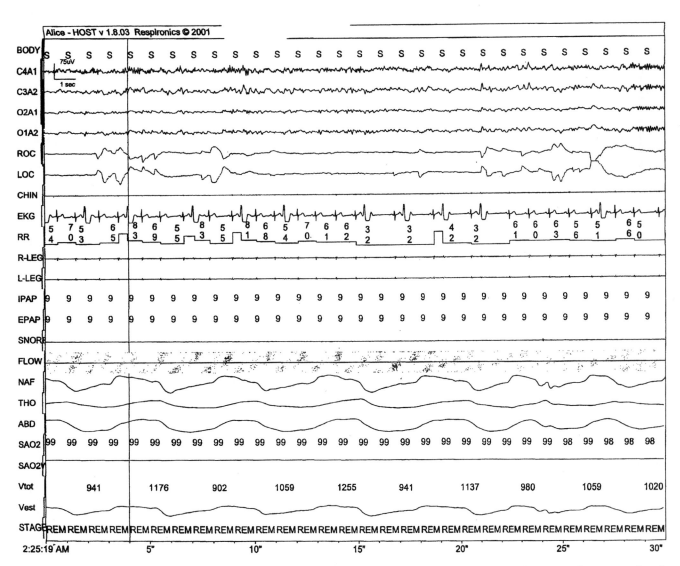

FIGURE 6–2. *Ventricular ectopy in REM sleep. Bigeminy and trigeminy is noted in this 26-year-old woman who presented with nonhypoxic obstructive sleep-disordered breathing. This finding was not seen in non-REM (NREM) sleep. There was excessive use of caffeine (four to five large cups of strong coffee across the day). The patient has no palpitations during the day or night.*

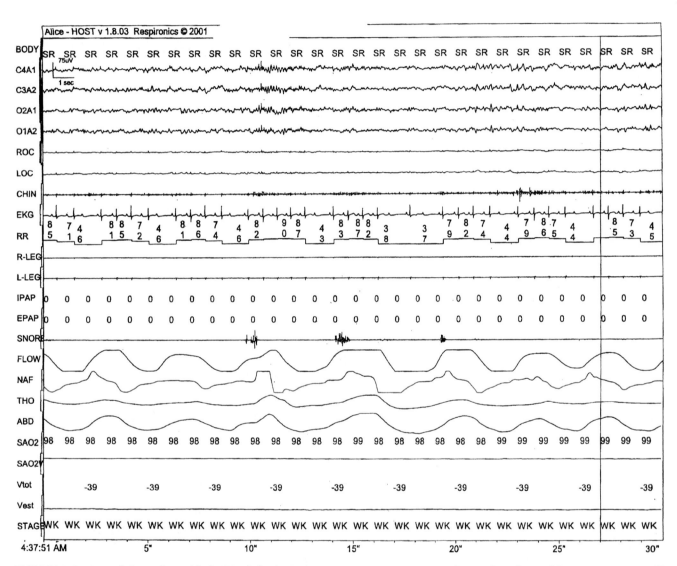

FIGURE 6–3. *Second-degree heart block, Wenckebach. Progressive increase in PR interval preceding dropped beats in a 48-year-old patient with delayed sleep phase syndrome, seen unchanged during wake and sleep. This is an innocent arrhythmia and requires no treatment.*

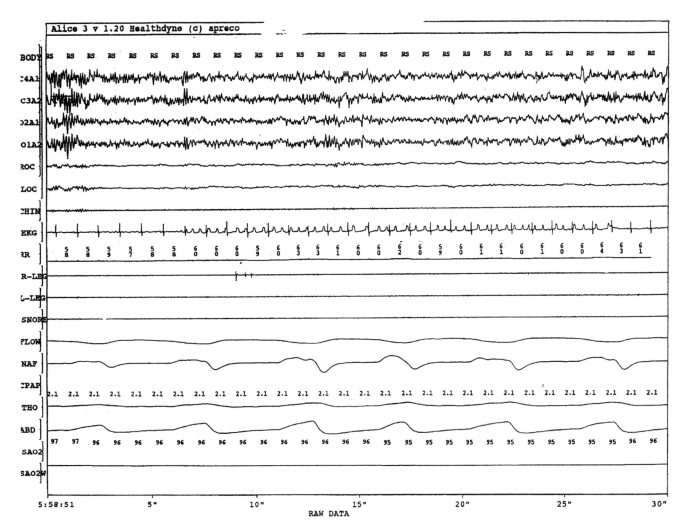

FIGURE 6–4. *Supraventricular tachycardia. Atrial tachycardia with varying block or a run of atrial flutter with varying block. The abrupt change in P wave morphology is not associated with any change in QRS morphology. The ability of a single EKG channel in precisely determining the origin of rhythms can be limited. This patient was not on any medication such as digitalis.*

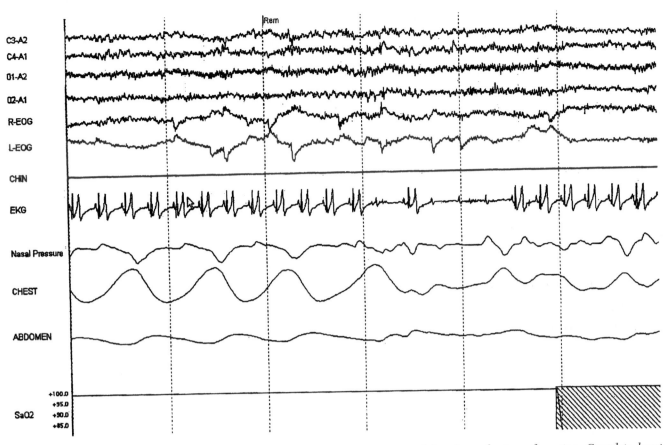

FIGURE 6–5. *REM-bradyarrhythmia. A 26-year-old asymptomatic man presented for the evaluation of snoring. Complete heart block.*

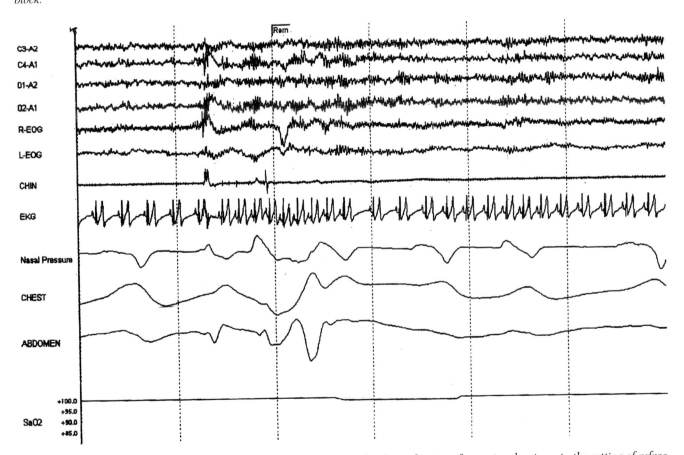

FIGURE 6–6. *Postarousal tachycardia. A 36-year-old woman presents for the evaluation of excessive sleepiness in the setting of refractory depression. This pattern of postarousal bursts of heart rate increase was noted throughout the study. Such cyclic variations in heart rate have been used to develop EKG-based screening tools for sleep-disordered breathing. One disadvantage of such tools is that severity information cannot be assessed from the degree of heart rate change, and some patients with the worst disease (e.g., heart failure) may show very little RR variability.*

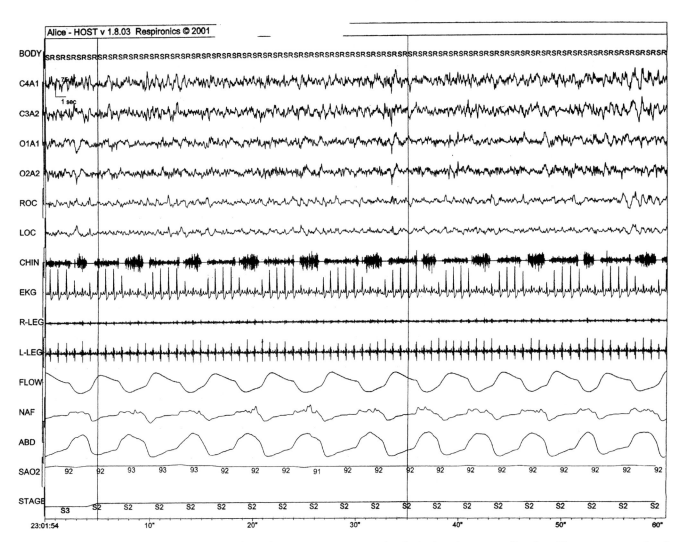

FIGURE 6–7. *EKG-derived respiration signal. Cyclic variation in RR amplitude (rather than interval) induced by respiratory-related fluctuations in cardiac positions. This signal has also been evaluated as a noninvasive EKG-derived method to assess sleep respiration. The disadvantages are similar to RR variability—it is rarely as prominent as in this sample.*

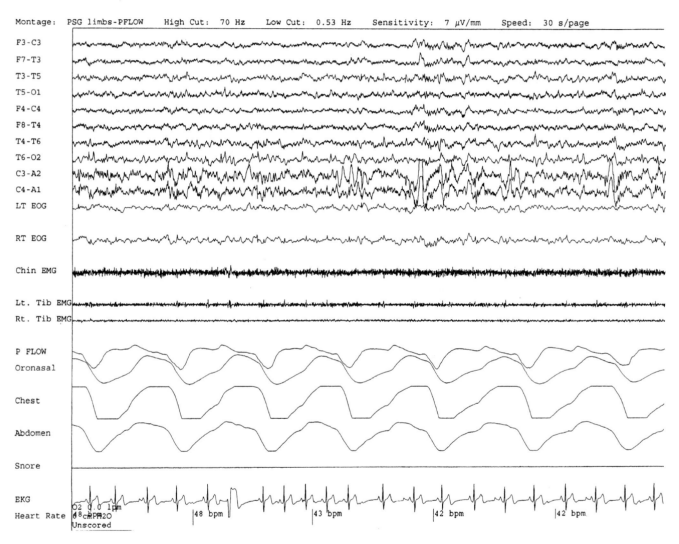

Montage: PSG limbs-PFLOW   High Cut: 70 Hz   Low Cut: 0.53 Hz   Sensitivity: 7 µV/mm   Speed: 30 s/page

FIGURE 6–8. *Ventricular premature contractions. A 30-second epoch from an overnight PSG study of a 40-year-old woman with a history of restless legs syndrome reveals the presence of ventricular ectopic beats. The patient reported occasional palpitations. This phenomenon may be rate dependent, and a faster heart rate may not be associated with the ventricular ectopic beats. Sinus arrhythmia is also noted.*

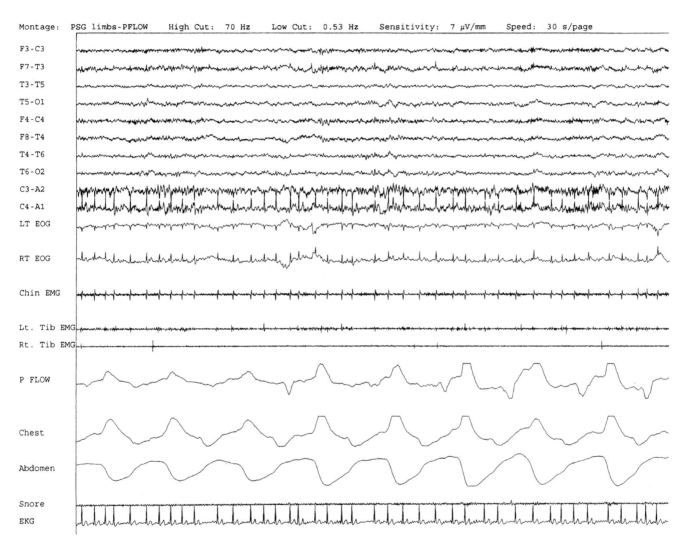

Montage: PSG limbs-PFLOW   High Cut: 70 Hz   Low Cut: 0.53 Hz   Sensitivity: 7 μV/mm   Speed: 30 s/page

FIGURE 6–9. *Atrial fibrillation. A 47-year-old man with a history of atrial fibrillation was referred for evaluation of sleep apnea. A 30-second epoch of REM sleep from an overnight PSG demonstrates the presence of atrial fibrillation. The association of sleep apnea and recurrence/triggering of atrial fibrillation has been reported.*

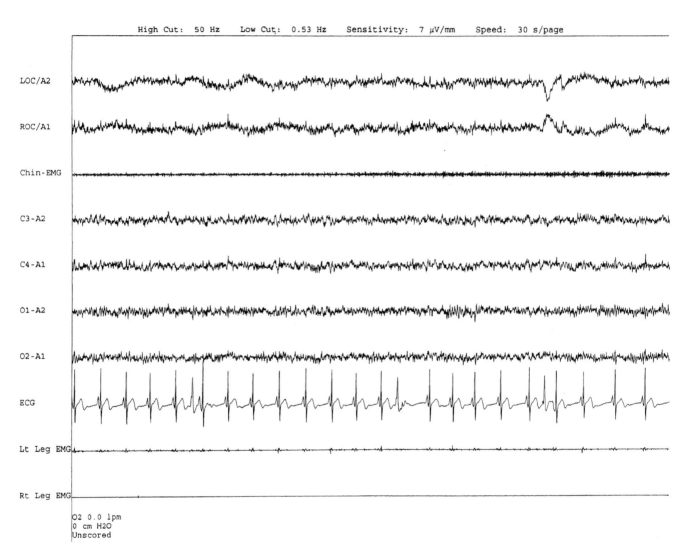

High Cut: 50 Hz   Low Cut: 0.53 Hz   Sensitivity: 7 µV/mm   Speed: 30 s/page

FIGURE 6–10. *Aberrant conduction. A 51-year-old woman was referred for the evaluation of sleep apnea. A 30-second epoch from the PSG shows premature ventricular complexes with slight widening of the QRS but maintained axis. This may be an aberrant beat secondary to a junctional ectopic.*

7

Uncommon and Atypical PSG Patterns

Sudhansu Chokroverty, Meeta Bhatt, and
Tammy Goldhammer

A case of rhythmic leg movements with blinking in wakefulness.

Montage: SLEEP   High Cut: 70 Hz   Low Cut: 1.00 Hz   Sensitivity: 7 μV/mm   Speed: 30 s/page

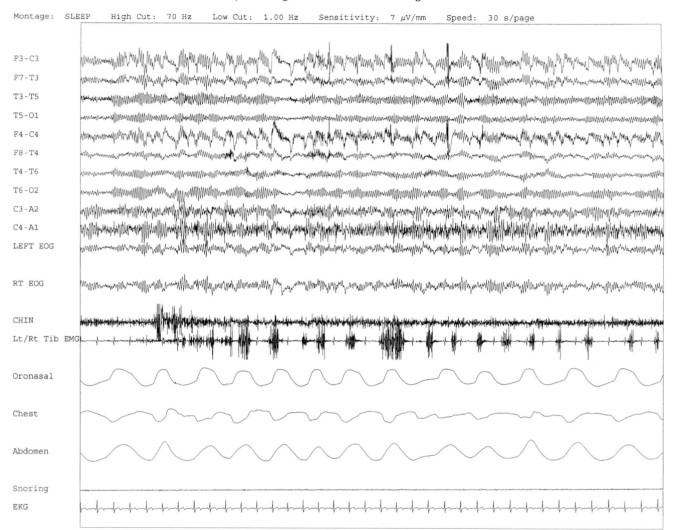

FIGURE 7–1. *A 70-year-old woman with history of insomnia and early morning awakenings. Normal neurological examination with no evidence of Parkinson's disease or other neurodegenerative disorders. Nocturnal polysomnography (PSG) revealed mild obstructive sleep apnea. An unusual pattern of episodes of rhythmic leg movements at approximately 0.5 to 1.5 hertz and/or rapid blinking is noted repeatedly during periods of wakefulness but not during sleep. The significance of these events limited to wakefulness remains uncertain. One such 30-second epoch is demonstrated. EEG, Top 10 channels; Lt. and Rt. EOG, left and right electrooculograms; electromyography of chin; Lt./Rt. Tib. EMG, left and right tibialis anterior EMG; oronasal thermistor; chest and abdomen effort channels; snore monitor; EKG, electrocardiography.*

A case of rhythmic leg movements in sleep associated with arousals

Montage: PSG limbs   High Cut: 70 Hz   Low Cut: 1.00 Hz   Sensitivity: 7 µV/mm   Speed: 30 s/page

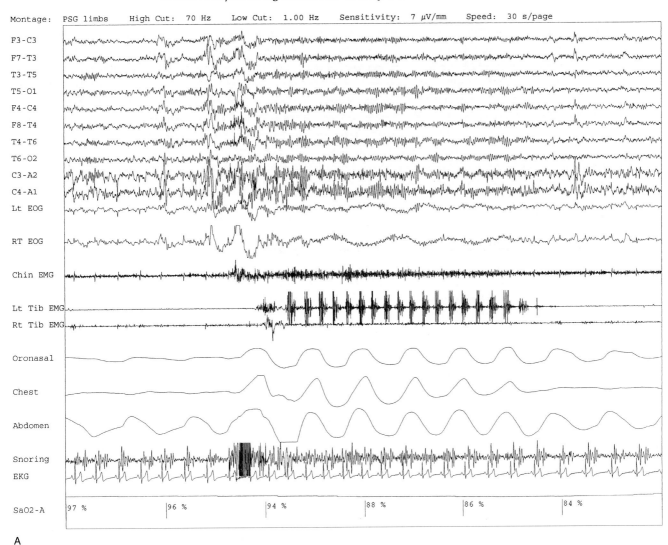

A

FIGURE 7–2. *A 40-year-old man with chief complaint of loud snoring, "fighting for breath," and excessive daytime drowsiness is diagnosed with severe obstructive sleep apnea on nocturnal PSG. A 30-second excerpt (**A**) from stage II non–rapid eye movement (NREM) sleep shows the presence of obstructive respiratory apnea associated with rhythmic foot and leg movements during arousal from the respiratory events. The rhythmic movements are noted in either or both legs at approximately 1.4 hertz.*

Montage: PSG limbs   High Cut: 70 Hz   Low Cut: 1.00 Hz   Sensitivity: 7 µV/mm   Speed: 120 s/page

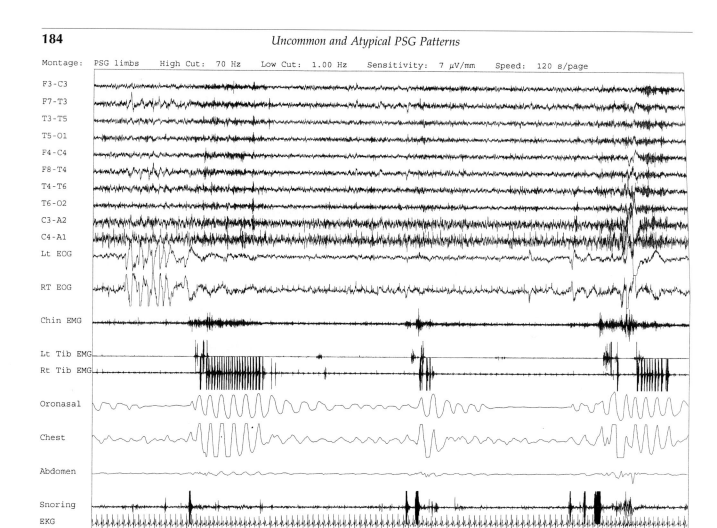

B

FIGURE 7–2, cont'd *A 120-second excerpt* (**B**) *from REM sleep shows three episodes of similar rhythmic leg movements recorded in both tibialis anterior EMG channels following obstructive hypopneic and apneic events.* EEG, *Top 10 channels;* Lt. and Rt. EOG, *left and right electrooculograms;* chin EMG, *EMG of chin;* Lt. and Rt. Tib. EMG, *left and right tibialis anterior EMG;* oronasal thermistor; chest and abdomen effort channels; snore monitor; EKG, *electrocardiography;* SaO2, *oxygen saturation by finger oxymetry.*

A case of rhythmic leg movements in wakefulness and sleep unrelated to respiratory events or periodic leg movements in sleep (PLMS)

Montage: SLEEP   High Cut: 70 Hz   Low Cut: 1.00 Hz   Sensitivity: 7 μV/mm   Speed: 30 s/page

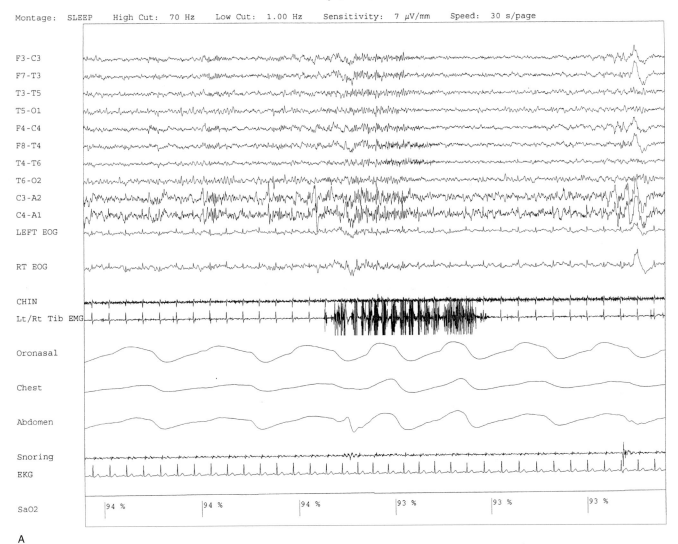

A

FIGURE 7–3. *A 50-year-old man with history of loud snoring, choking in sleep, and intermittent leg jerking at night. Nocturnal PSG shows the presence of mild sleep apnea with an apnea-hypopnea index of 12.3. Three 30-second excerpts from nocturnal polysomnography show bursts of rhythmic foot and leg movements on the left/right tibialis anterior muscle recording channel during stage II NREM sleep (**A**), REM sleep (**B**), and wakefulness (**C**). The movement is not associated with respiratory events, oxygen desaturation, or arousal from sleep. EEG, Top 10 channels;* Lt. *and* Rt. EOG, *left and right electrooculograms;* chin EMG, *EMG of chin;* Lt./Rt. Tib. EMG, *left/right tibialis anterior EMG;* oronasal thermistor; chest and abdomen effort channels; snore monitor; EKG, *electrocardiography;* SaO₂, *oxygen saturation by finger oxymetry.*

Montage: SLEEP   High Cut: 70 Hz   Low Cut: 1.00 Hz   Sensitivity: 7 μV/mm   Speed: 30 s/page

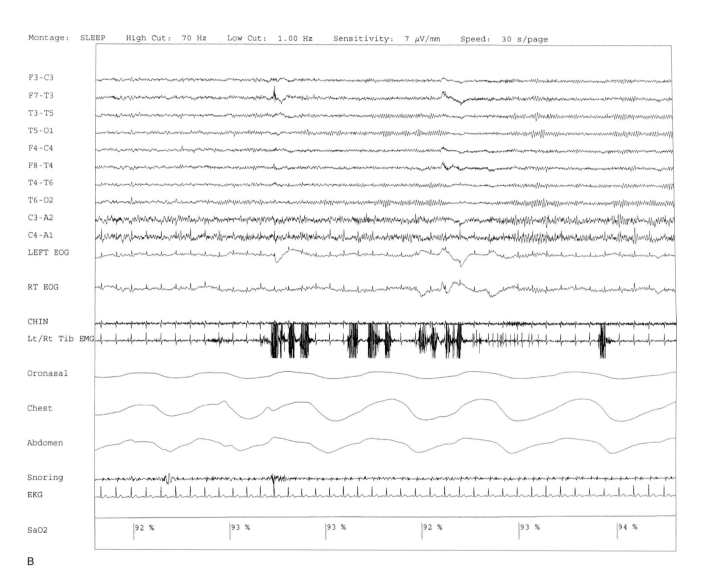

B

FIGURE 7–3, cont'd.

Montage: SLEEP   High Cut: 70 Hz   Low Cut: 1.00 Hz   Sensitivity: 7 µV/mm   Speed: 30 s/page

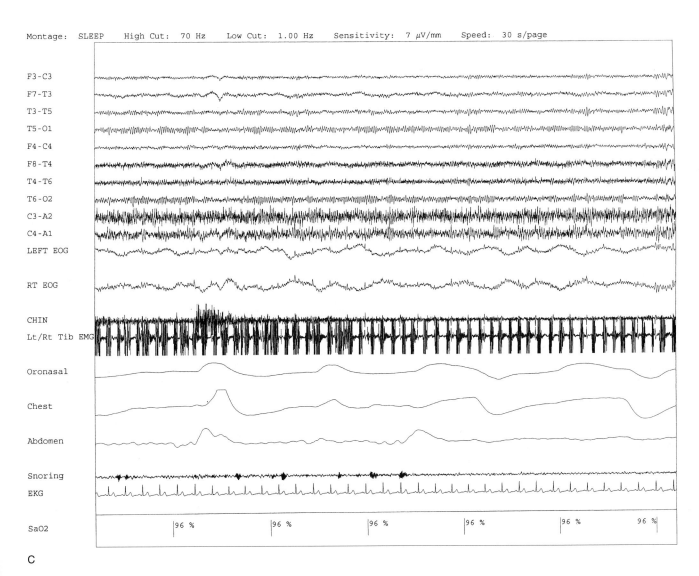

C

FIGURE 7–3, cont'd.

A case of excessive fragmentary myoclonus (EFM)

Montage:	SLEEP	High Cut:	70 Hz	Low Cut:	1.00 Hz	Sensitivity:	7 μV/mm	Speed:	30 s/page

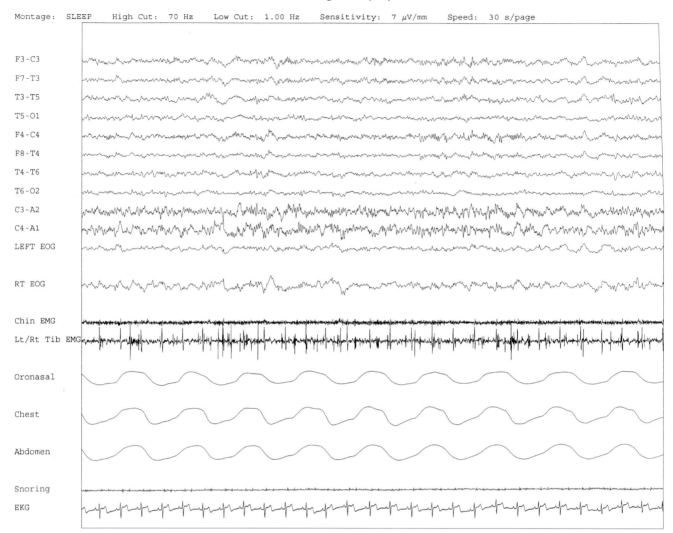

FIGURE 7–4. *A 73-year-old man with history of snoring, gasping, and fighting for breath in sleep for many years. Overnight PSG did not show evidence of apnea or periodic limb movement disorder. An increased amount of myoclonic jerks are noted, characterized by brief (less than 150 milliseconds) sharp EMG potentials in the left and right tibialis anterior EMG recording during NREM sleep suggesting presence of EFM. EFM has been noted in association with several primary sleep disorders but its pathological relationship to them and especially to excessive daytime sleepiness remains uncertain. EEG, Top 10 channels; Lt. and Rt. EOG, left and right electrooculograms; chin EMG, EMG of chin; Lt./Rt. Tib. EMG, left and right tibialis anterior EMG; oronasal thermistor; chest and abdomen effort channels; snore monitor; EKG, electrocardiography.*

A case of Bruxism associated with arousals following respiratory dysrhythmia.

Montage: SLEEP   High Cut: 70 Hz   Low Cut: 1.00 Hz   Sensitivity: 7 μV/mm   Speed: 120 s/page

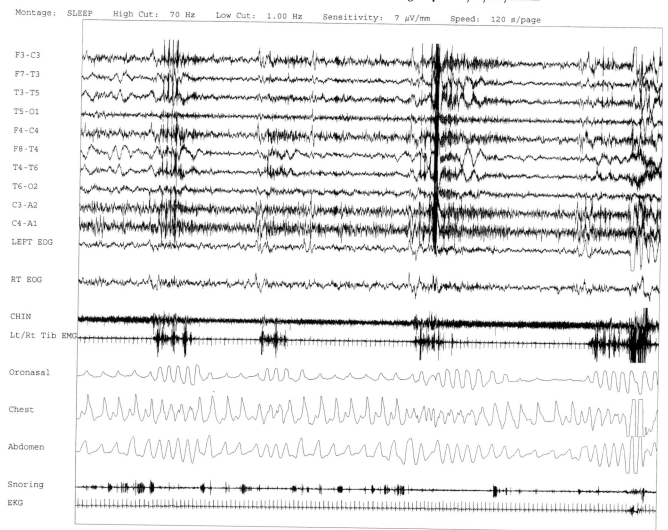

FIGURE 7–5. *A 120-second excerpt from PSG recording reveals sleep bruxism in a 70-year-old woman with a history of insomnia, early morning awakenings, and excessive daytime sleepiness. Overnight PSG revealed the presence of mild-moderate obstructive sleep apnea with an apnea-hypopnea index of 21.5. Episodes of bruxism are recorded repeatedly as part of the arousal response following respiratory events accompanied by tooth grinding on simultaneous audio-video recording. Respiratory related limb movements are recorded on tibialis anterior channel in association with the arousal response. PSG sleep bruxism is characterized by a series of teeth grinding associated with rhythmic EMG artifacts with a frequency of approximately 0.5 to 1.0 hertz in stage I NREM sleep.* EEG, *Top 10 channels;* Lt. and Rt. EOG, *left and right electrooculograms;* chin EMG, *EMG of chin;* Lt./Rt. Tib. EMG, *left/right tibialis anterior EMG;* oronasal thermistor; chest and abdomen effort channels; snore monitor; EKG, *electrocardiography.*

A case of alpha-delta sleep

Montage: SLEEP   High Cut: 70 Hz   Low Cut: 1.00 Hz   Sensitivity: 7 µV/mm   Speed: 10 s/page

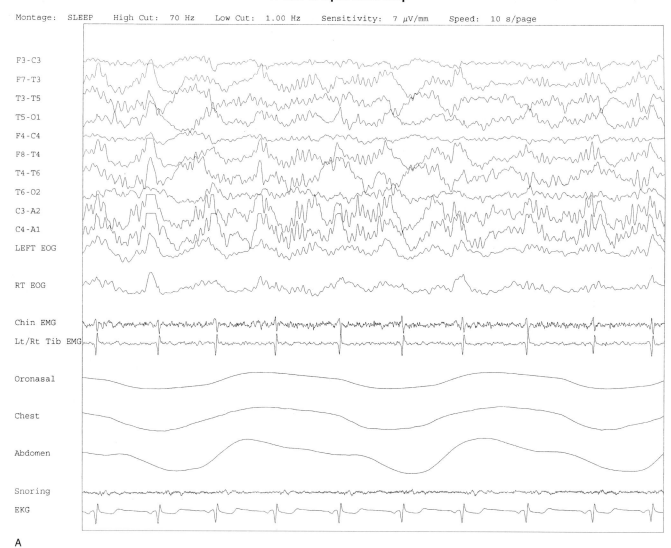

A

FIGURE 7–6. *Ten- and 30-second excerpts from a nocturnal PSG showing alpha-delta sleep in a 30-year-old man with history of snoring for many years. He denied any history of joint or muscle aches and pains. The alpha frequency is intermixed with and superimposed on underlying delta activity. Alpha-delta sleep denotes a nonspecific sleep architectural change noted in many patients with complaints of muscle aches and fibromyalgia. It is also seen in other conditions and many normal individuals. EEG, Top 10 channels; Lt. and Rt. EOG, left and right electrooculograms; chin EMG, EMG of chin; Lt./Rt. Tib. EMG, left/right tibialis anterior EMG; oronasal thermistor; chest and abdomen effort channels; snore monitor; EKG, electrocardiography.*

Montage: SLEEP   High Cut: 70 Hz   Low Cut: 1.00 Hz   Sensitivity: 7 μV/mm   Speed: 30 s/page

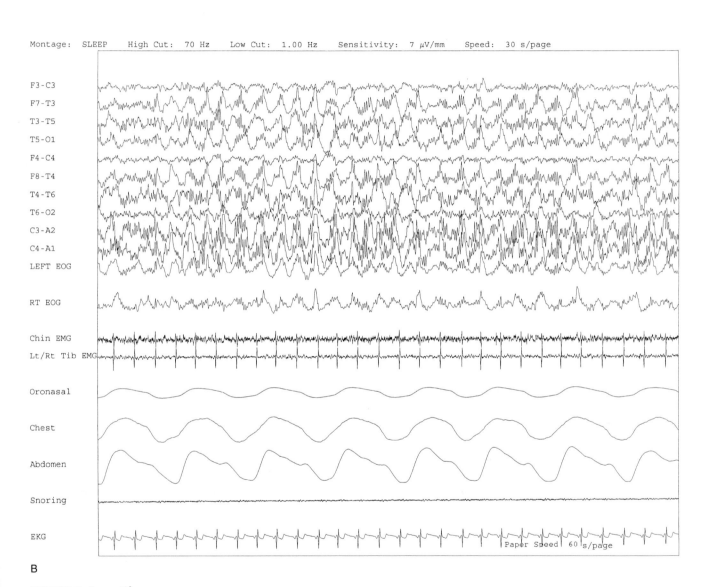

B

FIGURE 7–6, cont'd.

A case of Narcolepsy with obstructive sleep apnea syndrome without REM atonia without features of REM behavior disorder (RBD)

Montage: PSG limbs-PFLOW   High Cut: 70 Hz   Low Cut: 0.53 Hz   Sensitivity: 7 µV/mm   Speed: 30 s/page

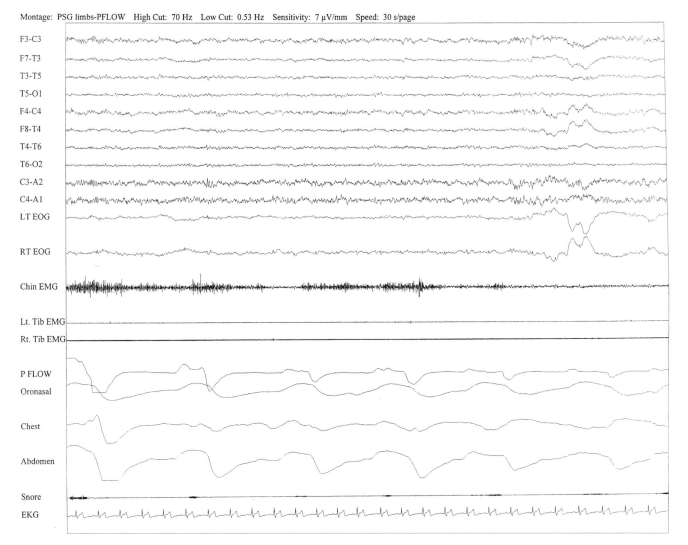

FIGURE 7–7. *A 63-year-old man with episodes of frequent, brief sleep spells during routine daytime activities, for example, relaxing, sitting, or even singing, since early college days with worsening in the last 3 to 4 years. The spells last approximately 5 to 10 minutes and are refreshing on awakening. He denies any history of cataplexy. He experienced sleep paralysis many years ago but there is no clear history of hypnagogic hallucinations. However, more recently there is a complaint of really frightening dreams at night, which are not accompanied by any motor or behavioral disorder. His medical history is significant for adult-onset diabetes mellitus for several years. The neurological examination is significant for evidence suggestive of mild peripheral neuropathy in the legs bilaterally likely related to diabetes mellitus. Of note, there is no suggestion of a movement disorder on neurologic examination. Initial overnight PSG was significant for some nonspecific sleep architectural changes but did not show any evidence of sleep apnea or PLMS. Multiple sleep latency test revealed a mean sleep latency of 2.5 minutes consistent with pathologic sleepiness. Also, two sleep onset rapid eye movements (SOREMs) suggestive of narcolepsy were recorded. He was started on stimulant treatment and responded well until recently when he started complaining of excessive daytime sleepiness and increased snoring. A repeat PSG showed recurrent episodes of apneas and hypopneas during NREM and REM sleep with a moderately severe apnea-hypopnea index of 33, accompanied by mild oxygen desaturation, snoring, and increased arousal index suggestive of sleep apnea syndrome in conjunction with narcolepsy. Interestingly, the PSG showed frequent periods of phasic muscle bursts and intermittent loss of muscle atonia on chin EMG channel during REM sleep. One such 30-second epoch in REM sleep is shown in this figure. Accompanying motor or behavioral abnormalities were not recorded on simultaneous video monitoring and patient denied any specific dream recollections. An association between narcolepsy and sleep apnea and that between narcolepsy and RBD have been described and close follow-up is indicated to decide if the isolated finding of REM sleep without muscle atonia is a precursor sign of emerging RBD or not. EEG, Top 10 channels; Lt. and Rt. EOG, left and right electrooculograms; chin EMG, EMG of chin; Lt. and Rt. Tib. EMG, left and right tibialis anterior EMG; P flow, peak flow; oronasal thermistor; chest and abdomen effort channels; snore monitor; EKG, electrocardiography.*

A case of sleep spindles in REM sleep

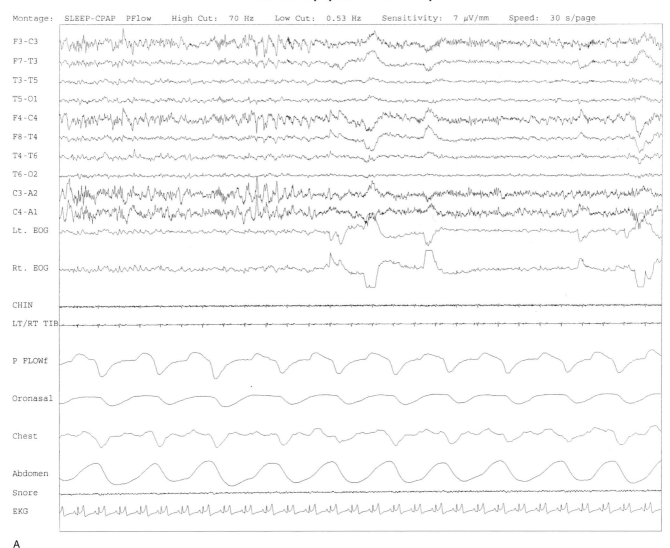

A

FIGURE 7–8. *A 67-year-old man with difficulty sleeping, loud snoring, and excessive daytime sleepiness for 5 years. Medical history is significant for high blood pressure and coronary artery disease. Nocturnal PSG showed the presence of moderate sleep apnea with an apnea-hypopnea index of 29.5. Figures are 30-second excerpts from nocturnal PSG showing the presence of frequent sleep spindles throughout both the epochs of REM sleep. Prominent sawtooth waves of REM sleep in C3- and C4-derived EEG channels, prominent phasic eye movements of REM sleep on electrooculogram channels, and decreased chin muscle tone characteristic of REM atonia are seen in* **A***.*

Montage: SLEEP-CPAP PFlow   High Cut: 70 Hz   Low Cut: 0.53 Hz   Sensitivity: 7 µV/mm   Speed: 30 s/page

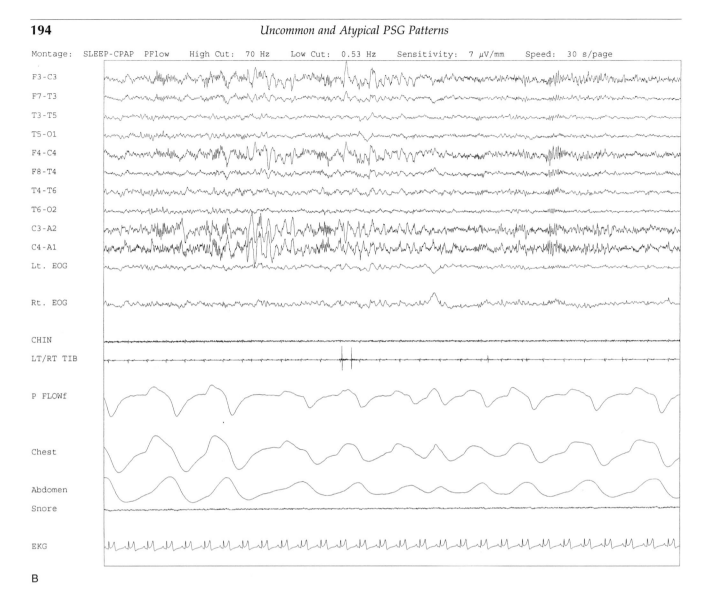

B

FIGURE 7–8, cont'd B *similarly shows prominent sawtooth waves of REM sleep in C3- and C4-derived EEG channels, single phasic eye movement of REM sleep around the middle of the epoch on the electrooculogram channels, decreased chin muscle tone characteristic of REM atonia, and two brief myoclonic bursts representing phasic muscle bursts of REM sleep.*

8

Motor Disorders During Sleep

PASQUALE MONTAGNA, MARCO ZUCCONI, SUDHANSU CHOKROVERTY

Sleep represents a state of relative mental and physical inactivity. Indeed physiologists confirm that sleep is attended by motor inhibition, and consider that motor disfacilitation is itself one of the defining features of sleep. Several types of peculiar sleep-related movements become evident, however, when we examine the sleeping animal more closely and in some unfortunate individuals, sleep becomes a time of motor agitation and turmoil. By virtue of widespread availability of video-polysomnographic (PSG) techniques, the last few decades have witnessed a truly bewildering expansion in the varieties of sleep-related motor disorders, most of them previously unsuspected. In many of the motor disorders, old and new, most of our knowledge is still only of a descriptive kind and we lack an in-depth understanding of the basic physiopathological mechanisms involved.

In the newly developed International Classification of Sleep Disorders (ICSD, 2nd edition), a separate section is devoted to sleep-related movement disorder. This category includes restless legs syndrome (RLS), periodic limb movements in sleep (PLMS) disorder, sleep-related leg cramps, sleep-related bruxism, sleep-related rhythmic movement disorders, and other sleep-related movement disorders due to a known physiologic condition or a substance abuse and those not due to a substance or known physiologic condition (e.g., other psychiatric or behavioral sleep-related movement disorder). Most of the nosologic entities characterized by prominent motor abnormalities are, however, included in the category of parasomnias (e.g., undesirable motor events and behavior occurring during sleep that do not necessarily disturb sleep architecture and that are not due to abnormalities intrinsic to basic sleep mechanisms). Parasomnias include disorders of arousals (e.g., confusional arousals, sleepwalking, sleep terrors arising out of NREM sleep), those associated with REM sleep (e.g., REM behavior disorder, parasomnia overlap disorder, status dissociatus, nightmares, and recurrent isolated sleep paralysis), and other parasomnias (e.g., nocturnal dissociative disorder, catathrenia or nocturnal groaning, exploding head syndrome, sleep-related eating disorders). While we await a deeper understanding of the pathophysiological mechanisms, however, description remains the first step in the knowledge of a phenomenon. Video recordings and polygraphic pictures go a long way in helping clinicians to recognize and characterize the various movement abnormalities encountered in the everyday practice of sleep medicine. Therefore, an atlas of the PSG features characteristic of the different motor disorders arising during sleep provides a good guide in the interpretation of the tracings and helps technicians and physicians alike in recognizing patterns useful in the differential diagnosis.

Text continued on p. 204

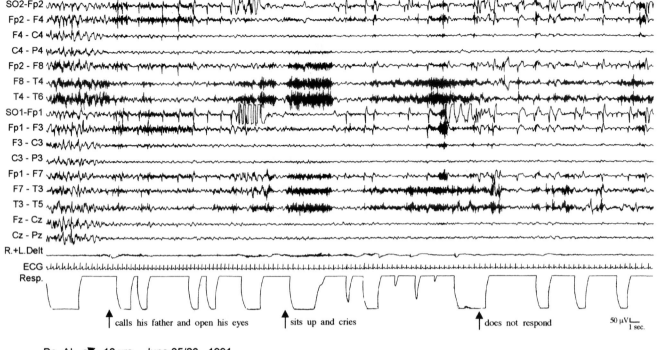

A

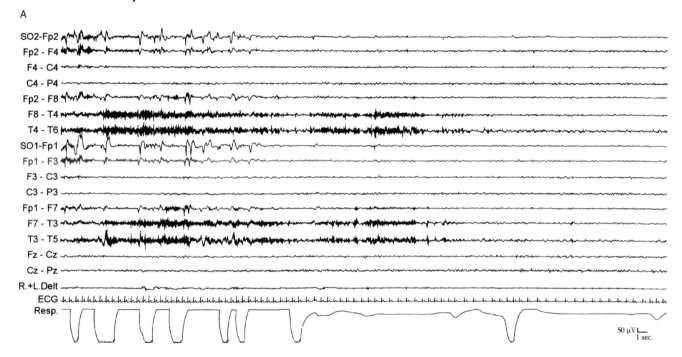

B

FIGURE 8–1. *Sleep terror. A 10-year-old boy presented with a 6-year history of sudden awakenings usually within 2 hours after sleep onset. During the episodes the patient sat up with a fearful expression and glassy eyes, vocalized and screamed with tachycardia, tachypnea, flushing of the skin, and mydriasis. The patient was confused and disoriented if awakened. The PSG recording shows that the episode arises from stage IV of sleep with a diffuse "hypersynchronous" rhythmic delta activity, deep inspiration, and tachycardia. At the beginning of the episode the patient calls his father, open his eyes and cries but electroencephalographic (EEG) background activity remains slow. At the end of the episode, the patient goes back to sleep. SO, Supraorbital electrode; R+L Delt., right and left deltoideus muscle; Resp, thoracoabdominal respiration.*

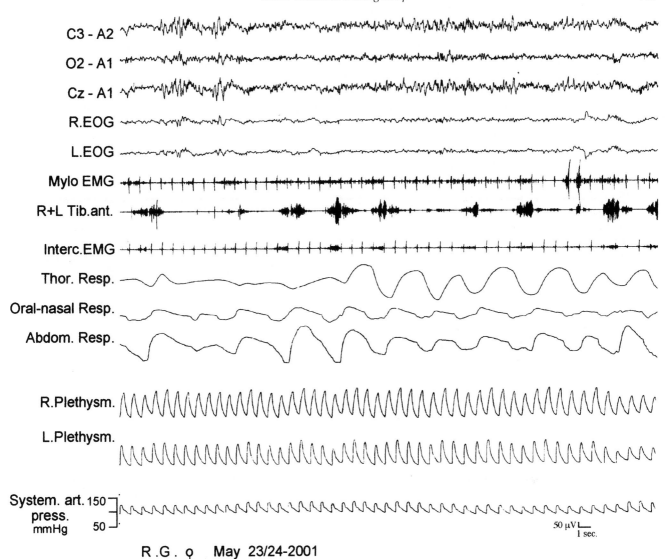

C3 - A2
O2 - A1
Cz - A1
R.EOG
L.EOG
Mylo EMG
R+L Tib.ant.
Interc.EMG
Thor. Resp.
Oral-nasal Resp.
Abdom. Resp.
R.Plethysm.
L.Plethysm.
System. art. press. mmHg 150 50
50 µV
1 sec.

R.G. ♀   May 23/24-2001

FIGURE 8–2. *Status dissociatus. A 66-year-old woman with Harlequin syndrome suffered, approximately one year after right jaw and multiple limb trauma, restless sleep, interrupted by excessive motor and sometimes harmful activities associated with vocalization and a report of dreaming corresponding to the motor manifestations. Hypnagogic hallucinations and sleep paralysis could rarely occur. PSG tracing shows intermingled NREM and REM EEG features. In particular sleep spindles were observed during REM sleep patterns (sawtooth waves, desynchronized high-frequency/low-amplitude activity and REMs). Chin muscle atonia was not complete with brief sudden twitches and tonic electromyographic (EMG) bursts. Respiration shows irregular tracings of REM sleep.* R. EOG, *right electrooculogram;* L. EOG, *left electrooculogram;* Mylo, *mylohyoideus;* R+L Tib ant, *right and left tibialis anterior;* Interc, *intercostalis;* Thor. Resp, *thoracic respiration;* Abdom. Resp, *abdominal respiration;* R. Plethysm, *right plethysmogram;* L. Plethysm, *left plethysmogram;* System. Art. Press, *systemic arterial pressure.*

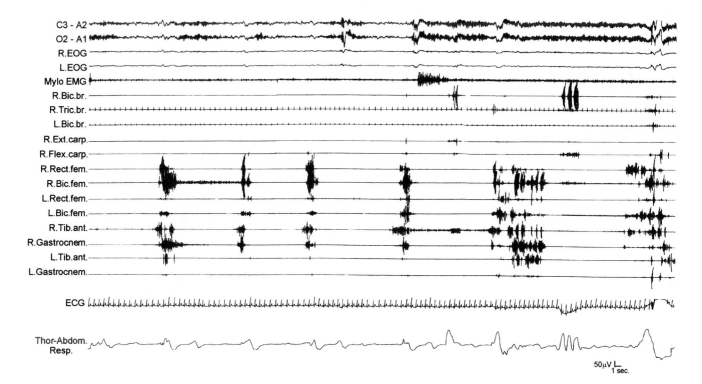

Ro.Li. ♀ 74 yrs July 24/25-2000

FIGURE 8–3. *Periodic limb movements and restless legs syndrome. A 74-year-old man presented with a 4-year history of inability to keep his legs still when trying to fall asleep with an urge to get out of bed and walk around. At the transition from wake to sleep, the PSG recording shows periodic jerks involving the lower limbs. During wakefulness, continuous voluntary and involuntary movements involving upper and lower limbs appear. R, Right; L, left; EOG, electrooculogram; Mylo, mylohyoideus; Bic. Br, biceps brachii; Tric.br, triceps brachii; Ext. carp, extensor carpi; Flex. Carp, flexor carpi; Rect. fem, rectus femori; Bic. fem, biceps femori; Tib. ant, tibialis anterior; Gastrocnem, gastrocnemius; Thor-Abdom. Resp, thoracoabdominal respiration.*

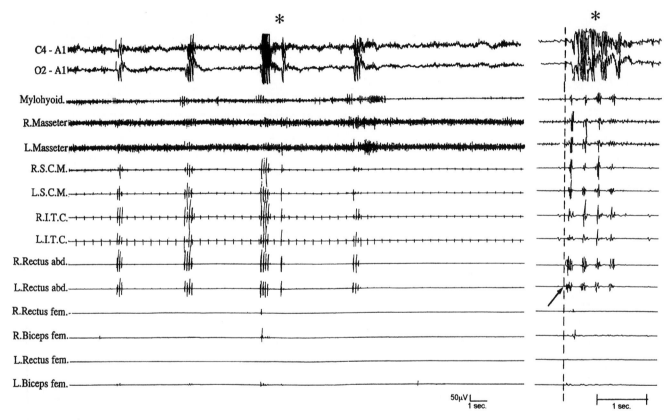

FIGURE 8–4. *Propriospinal myoclonus at the wake-sleep transition. A 40-year-old man presented with a 4-year history of axial jerks during relaxed wakefulness impeding falling asleep. PSG recording shows repetitive myoclonic axial jerks. The EMG activity originates in the left rectus abdominis muscle, thereafter propagating to rostral (sternocleidomastoid, masseter, mylohyoid) and caudal (biceps femoris) muscles. The panel on the left shows jerks at low speed; the right panel shows one of the jerks at high speed. R, Right; L, left; Mylohyoid, mylohyoideus; S.C.M, sternocleidomastoideus; I.T.C, intercostalis; Rectus abd, rectus abdominis; Rect. fem, rectus femoris; Biceps fem, biceps femoris.*

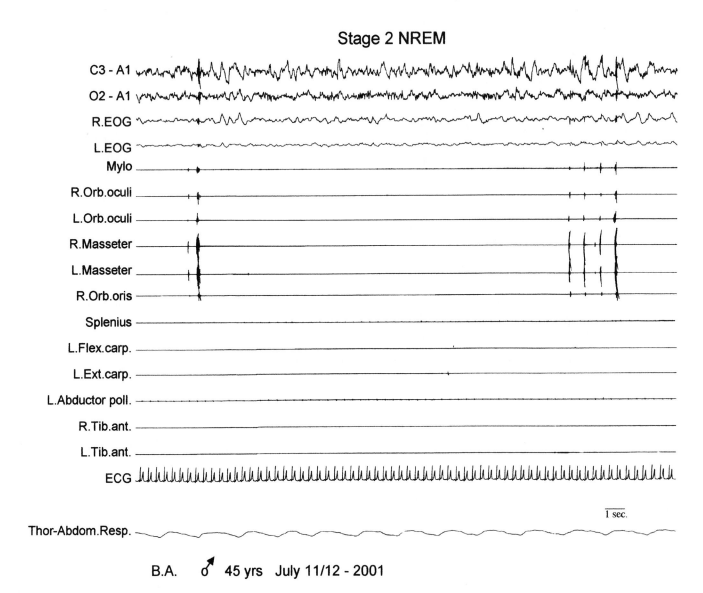

FIGURE 8–5. *Faciomandibular myoclonus. A 45-year-old man presented nocturnal tongue biting and bleeding since age 25 years. Nocturnal PSG recording shows myoclonic EMG activity of orbicularis oculi and oris and masseter muscles during NREM sleep. R, Right; L, left; EOG, electrooculogram; Mylo, mylohyoideus; Orb. Oculi, orbicularis oculi; Orb. Oris, orbicularis oris; Flex. carp, flexor carpi; Ext. carp, extensor carpi; Abductor poll, abductor pollicis; Tib. ant, tibialis anterior; Thor-Abdom. Resp, thoracoabdominal respiration.*

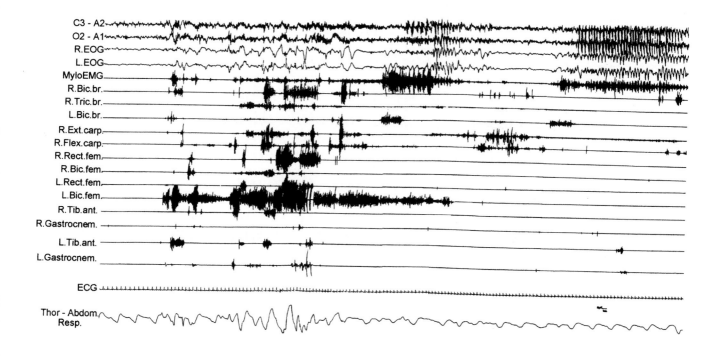

Na.Se. ♂ 43 yrs November 20/21-2000

A

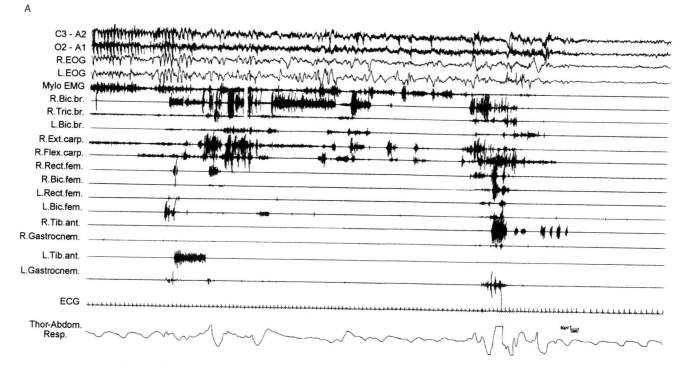

Na.Se. ♂ 43 yrs November 20/21-2000

B

FIGURE 8–6. *Sleep-related eating disorder. A 43-year-old man presented with a history of 20 years of abrupt awakenings from nocturnal sleep associated with compulsive feeding behavior out of control. PSG recording shows an episode of eating behavior arising from sleep (stage II). The patient wakes up and after 40 seconds begins to eat a snack put on a trolley near his bed (observe the artifact of mastication on EEG channels); then he lies down and goes back to sleep. R, Right; L, left; EOG, electrooculogram; Mylo, mylohyoideus; Bic. Br, biceps brachii; Tric.br, triceps brachii; Ext. carp, extensor carpi; Flex. Carp, flexor carpi; Rect. fem, rectus femori; Bic. fem, biceps femori; Tib. ant, tibialis anterior; Gastrocnem, gastrocnemius; Thor-Abdom. Resp, thoracoabdominal respiration.*

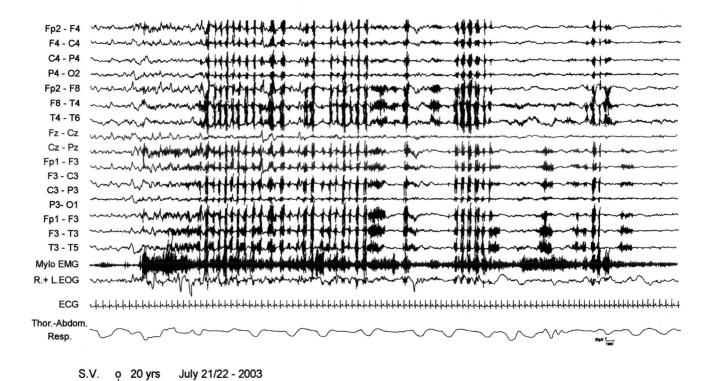

S.V.   ♀ 20 yrs   July 21/22 - 2003

FIGURE 8–7. *A 20-year-old woman referred for sudden nocturnal awakenings with vocalization and sleepwalking. PSG shows an arousal from NREM stage IV sleep with subsequent rhythmic masticatory muscles activation and teeth gnashing (EMG artifacts on EEG channels) typical of sleep bruxism.*

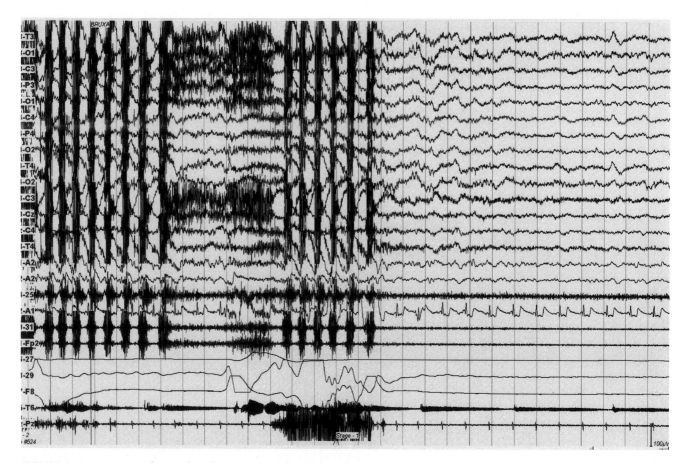

FIGURE 8–8. *Bruxism with episodes of nocturnal groaning (a rare REM-parasomnia but sometimes with NREM-related episodes too, with a noisy "lament" in expiration) in a 31-year-old man with a history of bruxism for more than 10 years (orthodontic surgery at that time). For 2 years he gives a history of a nocturnal noise during sleep (obtained from the wife). Figure 8–10 shows an episode of bruxism in NREM sleep (arousal related) followed by a groaning episode (on the PSG a prolonged central apnea in expiration is noted associated with noise).*

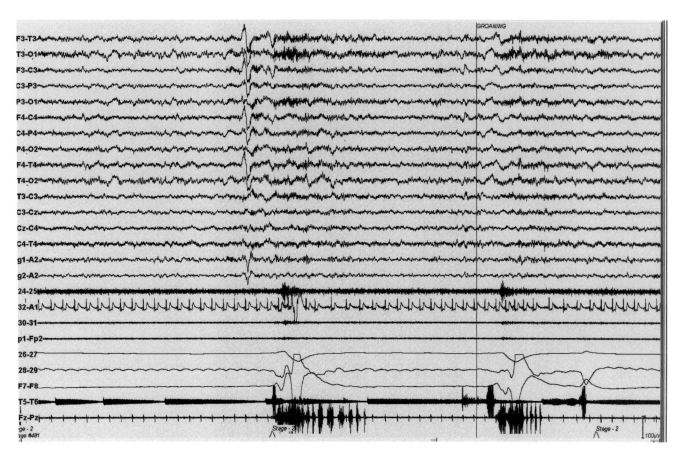

FIGURE 8–9. *Two episodes of groaning in NREM (stage II) that ended with arousals associated with atypical myoclonic jerks (PLMS), polyclonic at the end and of prolonged duration (> 5 seconds).*

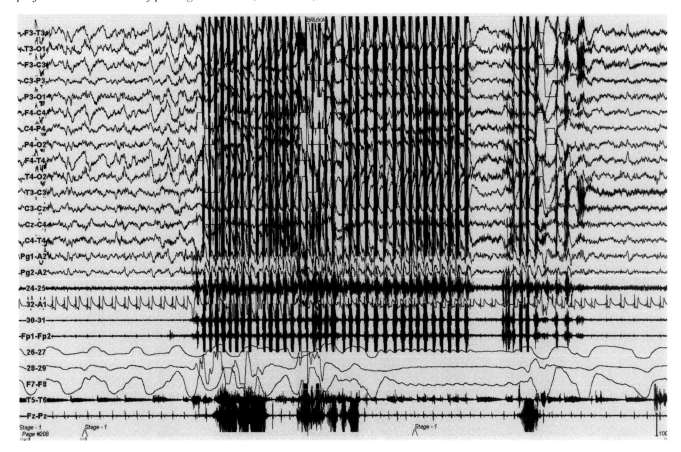

FIGURE 8–10. *An intense and prolonged bruxism episode emerging from stable NREM sleep, during arousal, and a brief groaning episode. The montage is EEG, ROC (Pg1-A2), LOC (Pg2-A2), submental EMG (24-25), EKG (32-A1), EMG m.masseter (30-31 and Fp1-Fp2), oronasal, thoracic and abdominal respiration, microphone (T5-T6), and EMG of anterior tibialis muscles from right and left side (commonly referred to one single channel, Fz-Pz). Epoch is 30 seconds.*

BIBLIOGRAPHY

1. Chokroverty S. Sleep Disorders Medicine: Basic Science, Technical Considerations, and Clinical Aspects. Boston: Butterworth/Elsevier, 1999.
2. Chokroverty S, Hening WA, Walters AS. Sleep and Movement Disorders. Boston: Butterworth/Elsevier, 2003.
3. Culebras A. Sleep Disorders and Neurological Disease. New York: Marcel Dekker, 2000.
4. Kryger M, Roth T, Dement W. Principles and Practice of Sleep Medicine. Boston: Butterworth/Elsevier, 2001.

9

Sleep and Epilepsy

Marco Zucconi, Pasquale Montagna, and Sudhansu Chokroverty

Epilepsy is a condition of recurrent unprovoked seizures, whereas a seizure is a paroxysmal event as a result of sudden excessive discharge of cerebral cortical neurons. There is a reciprocal relationship between sleep and epilepsy: Sleep triggers seizures and seizures disrupt sleep architecture. The estimated frequency of nocturnal seizures varies between 7.5 percent and 45 percent reflecting the heterogeneity of such seizures. Some types of epileptiform syndromes are prone to recur exclusively or frequently during sleep. Examples of predominantly sleep (nocturnal) seizures include the following: benign partial epilepsy of childhood with centrotemporal spikes or occipital paroxysms; nocturnal frontal lobe epilepsy (this includes nocturnal paroxysmal dystonia, paroxysmal arousals and episodic nocturnal wanderings); autosomal dominant nocturnal frontal lobe epilepsy; juvenile myoclonic epilepsy; generalized tonic-clonic seizures on awakening; nocturnal temporal lobe epilepsy (a subgroup of partial complex seizure of temporal lobe origin); tonic seizure (as a component of Lennox-Gastaut syndrome);

epilepsy with continuous spike and waves during non–rapid eye movement (NREM) sleep (CSWS); and Landau-Kleffner syndrome, probably a variant of CSWS.

Most interictal epileptiform discharges are triggered during NREM stages I and II but occasionally in stages III and IV sleep. In epileptic patients, NREM sleep acts as a convulsant causing excessive synchronization and activation of seizure in an already hyperexcitable cortex. In contrast, REM sleep generally behaves like an anticonvulsant because of inhibition of thalamocortical synchronizing mechanism and tonic reduction of interhemispheric impulse transmission through the corpus callosum. Overnight polysomnography (PSG) using multiple channels of electroencephalography (EEG) recording combined with simultaneous video recording is the single most important test for evaluating nocturnal seizure. For recognition of epileptiform patterns in the EEG, the readers are referred to Chapter 2. In this section of the atlas we provide several case vignettes along with overnight EEG and PSG segments showing characteristic patterns.

Text continued on p. 220

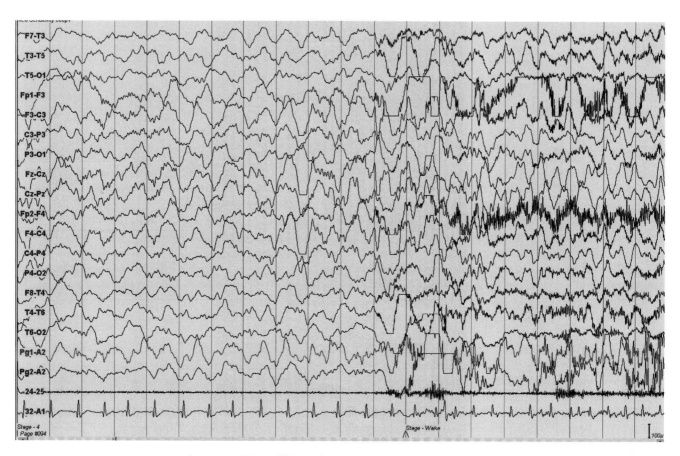

FIGURE 9–1–9–3. *PSG sequence of a nocturnal frontal lobe epilepsy (NFLE) seizure in a 10-year-old boy with onset of episodes, during sleep at the age of 6½ years and characterized by arousal with sudden elevation of head and trunk, sitting , fearful expression, sometimes jumping ahead or ambulating, and rare similar episodes during wakefulness. Wake EEG is normal, and sleep EEG shows rare sharp waves on Fz-Cz channel. Duration, less than 15 to 20 seconds, sometimes 30 seconds for prolonged episodes; frequency, 7 to 10 per night, with similar morphology and stereotypical features; good response to carbamazepine. The montage of PSG is EEG (top 16 channels), ROC (Pg 1-A2), LOC (Pg 2-A2), submental EMG (24-25), and EKG (32-A1). Epoch is 20 seconds.*

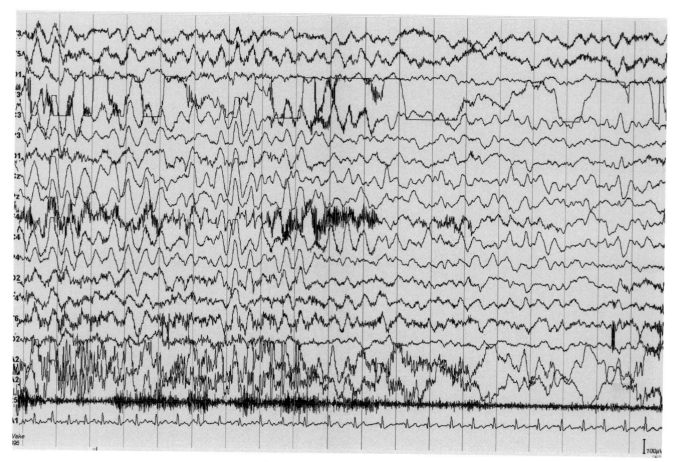

FIGURE 9–2.

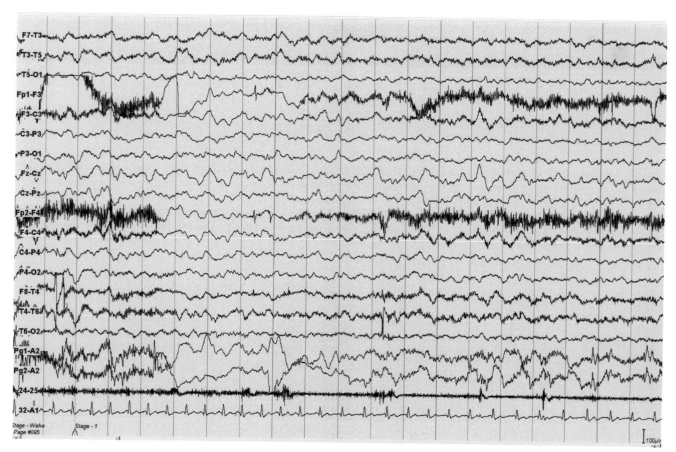

FIGURE 9–3.

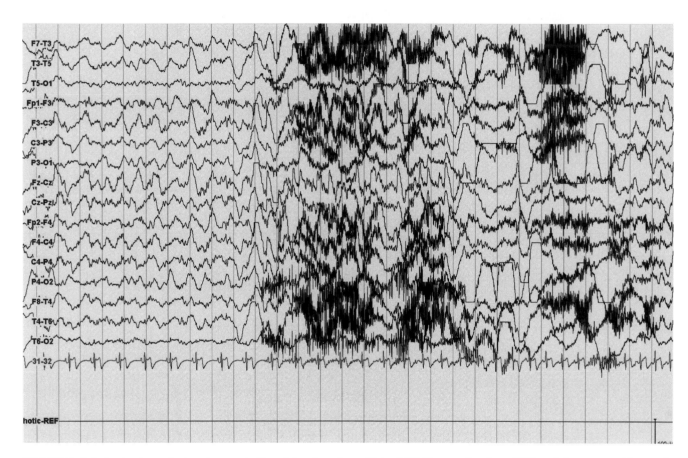

FIGURE 9–4–9–6. *A seizure during sleep probably arising from frontal lobe (NFLE) emerging from SWS and characterized by awakening followed by choking sensation. We recorded two episodes in that night. PSG shows an awakening from SWS followed after 10 seconds by an epileptiform discharge probably starting from frontotemporal leads (right), spreading bilaterally in the EEG. The patient's episodes had been misdiagnosed as panic attack in the past. He is a 23-year-old man whose episodes started at 12 to 13 years of age. There is no family history of epilepsy. The montage is only EEG + EKG and we recorded the episode during a morning video-PSG after sleep deprivation the night before.*

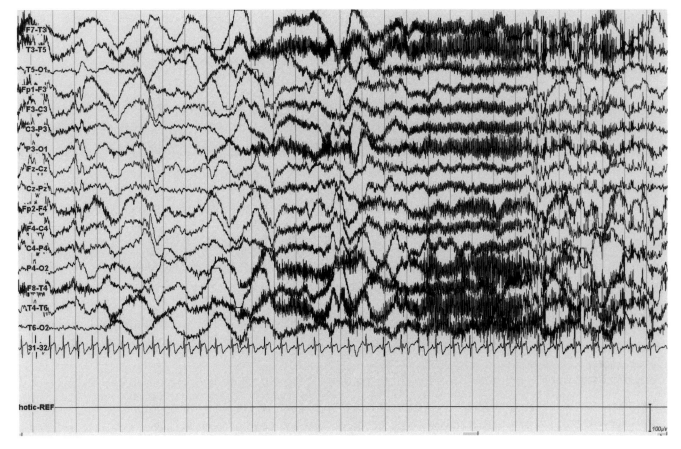

FIGURE 9–5.

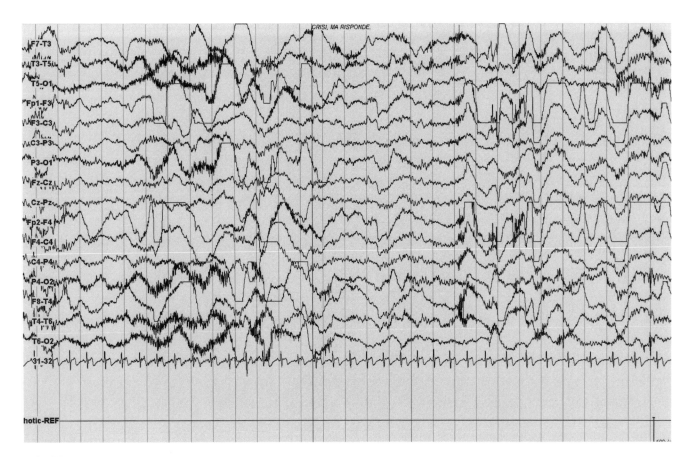

FIGURE 9–6.

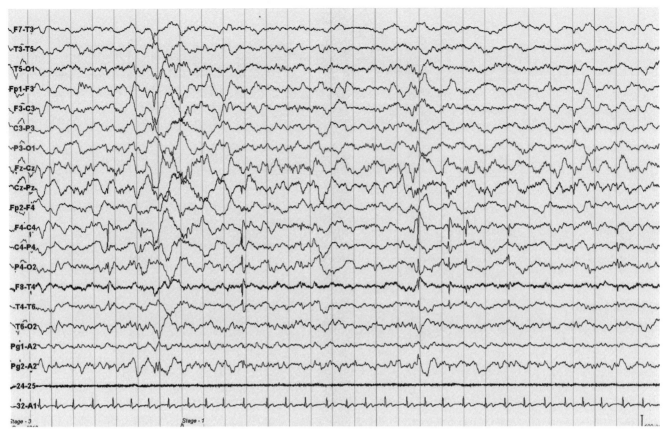

FIGURE 9–7. *Interictal epileptic paroxysms originating from right frontal region in a 9½-year-old boy with episodes of parasomnia-like behavior during sleep, starting at age 6, and clinically characterized by eyes opening, but without contact, sometimes crying or sleep talking (stereotyped, frequency of two per week), and rare episode of sudden arising in the bed, screaming, and pavor-like behavior (two to three episodes). He has a family history of parasomnia-like episodes. The montage is similar to that in Case 1 (Figures 9–1 through 9–3). Note interictal spikes at C4 and T4.*

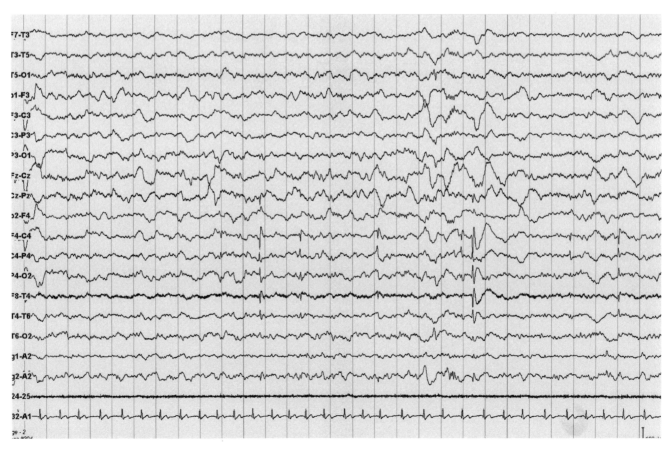

FIGURE 9–8. *Same as in Figure 9–7.*

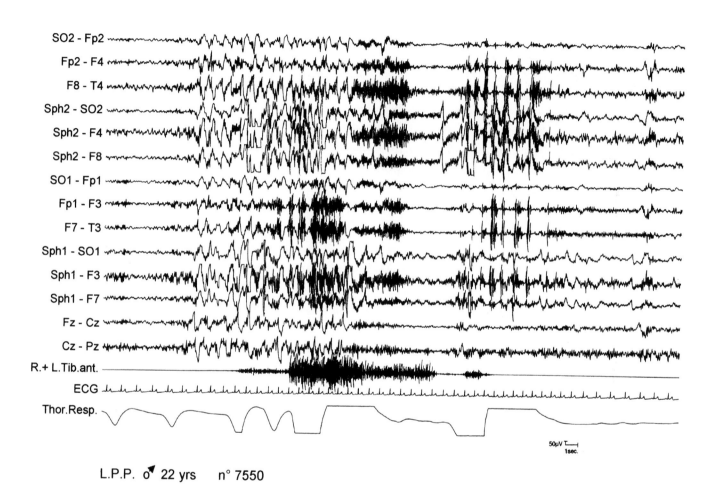

SO2 - Fp2

Fp2 - F4

F8 - T4

Sph2 - SO2

Sph2 - F4

Sph2 - F8

SO1 - Fp1

Fp1 - F3

F7 - T3

Sph1 - SO1

Sph1 - F3

Sph1 - F7

Fz - Cz

Cz - Pz

R.+ L.Tib.ant.

ECG

Thor.Resp.

50μV
1sec.

L.P.P. ♂ 22 yrs   n° 7550

FIGURE 9–9. *Paroxysmal arousals in NFLE. A 22-year-old woman presented with epileptic seizures only during nocturnal sleep or a few minutes after waking up. Motor manifestation consisted of raising her arms and stretching her legs with jerks and dystonic postures of the four limbs. Seizures recurred one to two times per night. PSG recordings show a paroxysmal arousal arising from stage II of sleep during which the patient presents a sudden abduction and extension of lower limbs with an abduction of upper limbs, tachycardia, and modification of respiration. Ictal EEG is characterized by a paroxysmal activity of diffuse slow waves. SO, Supraorbital electrode; Sph, sphenoidal electrode; R+L Tib ant, right and left tibialis anterior; Thor. Resp, thoracic respiration.*

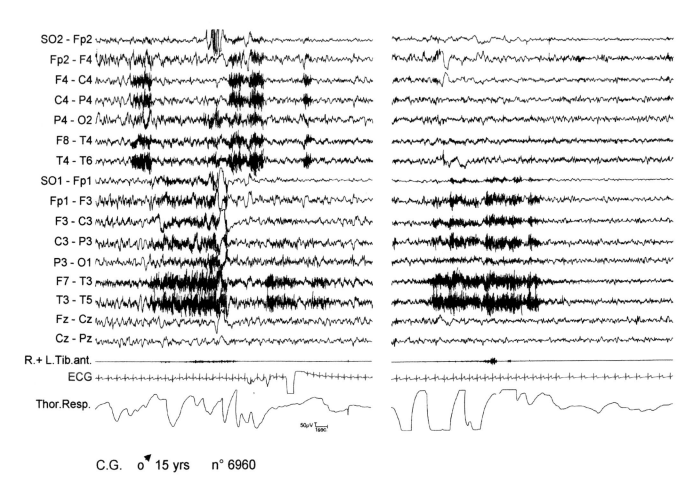

C.G.   o⚲ 15 yrs   n° 6960

FIGURE 9–10. *Two paroxysmal arousals in NFLE. A 15-year-old boy presented with nocturnal seizures since age 13, during which he suddenly opened his eyes and stretched his four limbs with a twist of upper limbs and oral automatisms. Sometimes he jumped out of bed and walked around with repetitive gestural automatisms. More than one seizure appeared nightly, almost every night. The figure shows the polygraphic recording of two different arousals in the same night arising from NREM sleep. Note the absence of clear-cut EEG abnormalities. During both episodes, tachycardia and modification of respiration are evident. SO, Supraorbital electrode; R+L Tib ant, right and left tibialis anterior; Thor. Resp, thoracic respiration.*

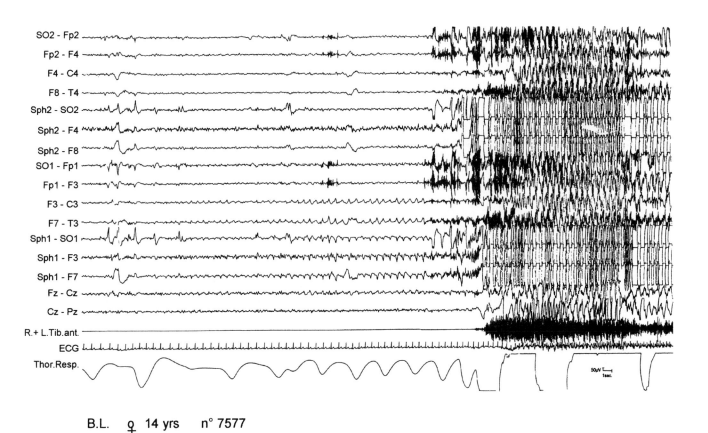

SO2 - Fp2
Fp2 - F4
F4 - C4
F8 - T4
Sph2 - SO2
Sph2 - F4
Sph2 - F8
SO1 - Fp1
Fp1 - F3
F3 - C3
F7 - T3
Sph1 - SO1
Sph1 - F3
Sph1 - F7
Fz - Cz
Cz - Pz
R.+ L.Tib.ant.
ECG
Thor.Resp.

50μV
1sec.

B.L. ♀ 14 yrs   n° 7577

A

FIGURE 9–11. *Nocturnal paroxysmal dystonia in NFLE. A 14-year-old girl presented with nocturnal episodes since age 12, characterized by head rising and complex motor automatism involving both legs, arms, and trunk with dystonic postures. Seizures recurred several times a night, two to three times per month. Video-PSG recordings showed that at the beginning of the seizure the patient opens her eyes, presents a deep inspiration while raising her head, then abducts her hyperextended upper limbs and presents rhythmic movements of limbs and trunk with back arching. Polygraphic tracing shows this seizure arising from sleep stage II. The motor manifestation is preceded for 10 to 15 seconds by repetitive sharp waves on left anterior EEG channels; then paroxysmal EEG activity is almost completely masked by muscle artifacts. During the seizure, tachycardia and modification of respiration occur. SO, Supraorbital electrode; Sph, sphenoidal electrode; R+L Tib ant, right and left tibialis anterior; Thor. Resp, thoracic respiration.*

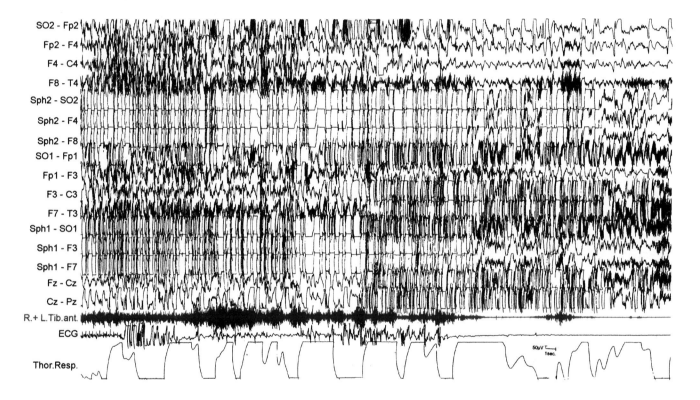

SO2 - Fp2
Fp2 - F4
F4 - C4
F8 - T4
Sph2 - SO2
Sph2 - F4
Sph2 - F8
SO1 - Fp1
Fp1 - F3
F3 - C3
F7 - T3
Sph1 - SO1
Sph1 - F3
Sph1 - F7
Fz - Cz
Cz - Pz
R.+ L.Tib.ant.
ECG
Thor.Resp.

50μV
1sec.

B.L.   ♀ 14 yrs   n° 7577

B

FIGURE 9–11, cont'd.

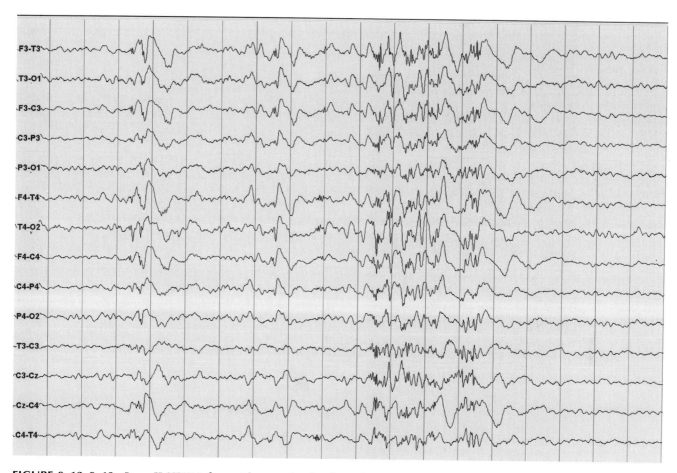

FIGURE 9–12–9–13. *Stage II NREM sleep with generalized spike and waves and multiple spike and wave bursts during a 24-hour ambulatory EEG recording. This is a 24-year-old woman with a drug-resistant partial idiopathic epilepsy, with psychomotor seizures (alteration of consciousness and flexion of the head with automatisms and sometimes secondary generalization). The seizures appear in cluster. EEG during wake shows rare generalized paroxysms (slow spike and wave) with left hemispheric prevalence. EEG during sleep shows activation of generalized epileptiform discharges as described above, both during stage II NREM (Figure 9–12) and stage III-IV NREM (Figure 9–13).*

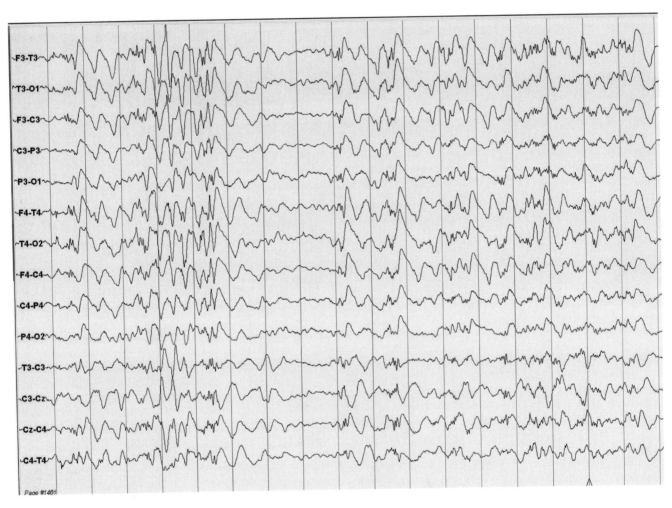

Page #1461

FIGURE 9–13.

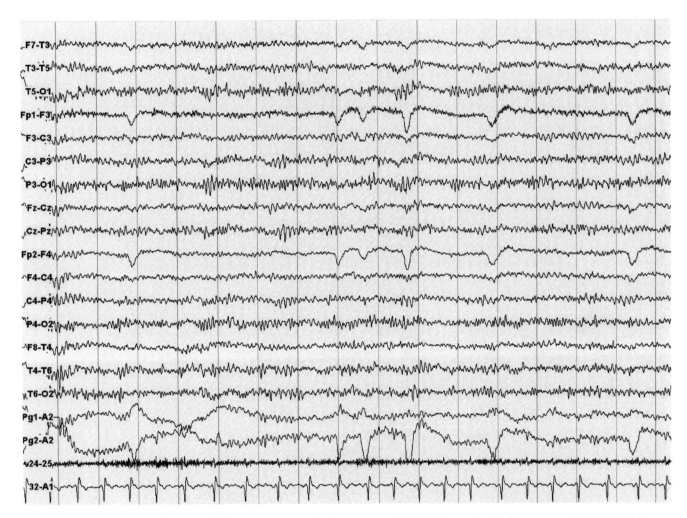

FIGURE 9–14–9–17. *EEG during wakefulness (Figure 9–14), during stage II NREM (Figure 9–15), during stage III-IV NREM (Figure 9–16), and during REM (Figure 9–17) sleep. An 11-year-old girl with a history of rare episodes of "absence" during wake and no other seizures, but with a mild psychomotor retardation. During wake (Figure 9–14), 10 to 11 hertz posteriorly dominant alpha activity is noted without epileptiform discharges. Sleep-activated generalized paroxysms (spikes and spike-wave complexes) both during stage III-IV NREM (Figure 9–16) and stage II NREM (Figure 9–15). During REM sleep (Figure 9–17), epileptiform discharges decreased and there are some isolated spikes in the posterior regions. Montage: EEG (top 16 channels), ROC (Pg1-A2), LOC (Pg2-A2), submental EMG (24-25), and EKG (32-A1) in all the figures.*

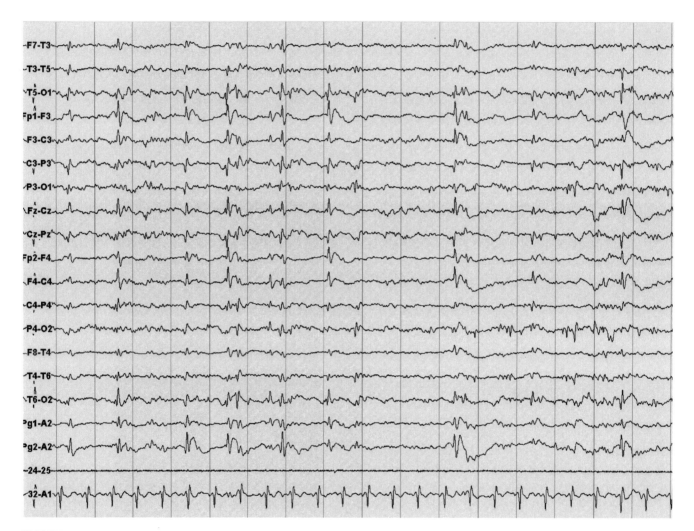

FIGURE 9–15.

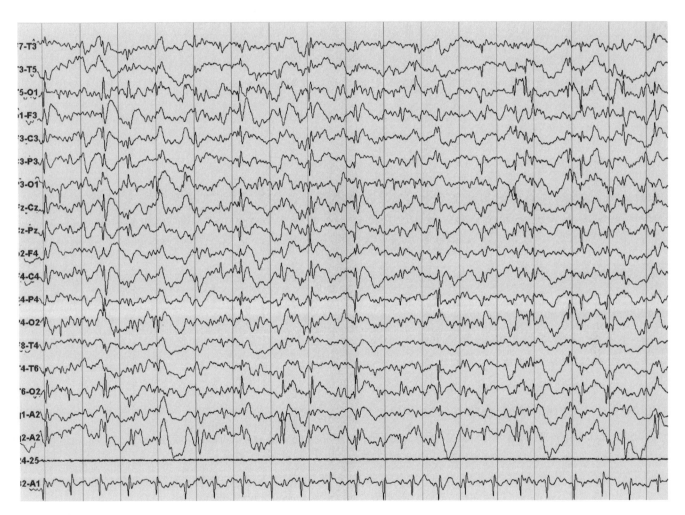

FIGURE 9–16.

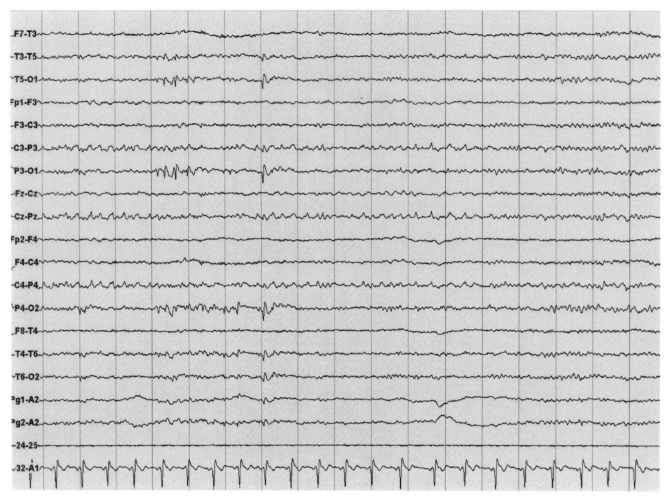

FIGURE 9–17.

BIBLIOGRAPHY

1. Chokroverty S, Quinto C. Sleep and epilepsy. In Chokroverty S, ed. *Sleep Disorders Medicine: Basic Science, Technical Considerations and Clinical Aspects,* 2nd ed. Boston: Butterworth/Elsevier, 1999:697–727.

2. Bazil C, Malow B, Sammaritano M. *Sleep and Epilepsy: The Clinical Spectrum.* Amsterdam, The Netherlands: Elsevier Science B.V., 2002.

3. Dinner DS, Luders HO. Relationship of epilepsy and sleep: An overview. In Dinner DS, Luders HO, eds. *Epilepsy and Sleep. Physiological and Clinical Relationships.* San Diego: Academic Press, 2001:2–18.

4. Malow B. Paroxysmal events in sleep. *J Clin Neurophysiol* 2002;19:522–534.

5. Provini F, Plazzi G, Tinuper P, et al. Nocturnal frontal lobe epilepsy. A clinical and polygraphic overview of 100 consecutive cases. *Brain* 1999;122:1017–1031.

6. Scheffer IE, Bhatia KP, Lopes-Cendes I, et al. Autosomal dominant nocturnal frontal lobe epilepsy: A distinctive clinical disorder. *Brain* 1995;118:61–73.

10

Miscellaneous Neurological Disorders and Sleep-Disordered Breathing

Sudhansu Chokroverty, Meeta Bhatt,
and Tammy Goldhammer

Neuroanatomical substrates responsible for controlling sleep-wakefulness and respiration are all located within the central nervous system. It is therefore logical to have sleep-disordered breathing (SDB) in patients with a variety of neurological disorders as a result of direct or indirect involvement of those structures. Neuroanatomical substrates for wakefulness include the ascending reticular activating system terminating in the thalamus and extrathalamic regions and thalamocortical projections to widespread areas of the cerebral cortex. The major neurotransmitter pathways include cholinergic neurons in the laterodorsal and pedunculopontine tegmental nuclei, noradrenergic neurons in the locus ceruleus, serotonergic neurons in the raphe region, and posterior hypothalamic histaminergic neurons. In addition, recently described hypocretin (orexin) in the lateral hypothalamic and perifornical region with its widespread ascending and descending projections throughout the entire central nervous system plays a significant role in the maintenance of wakefulness. Neuroanatomical substrates for non–rapid eye movement (NREM) sleep are located primarily in the ventrolateral preoptic region of the anterior hypothalamus and also in the region of the nucleus tractus solitarius in the medulla. The rapid eye movement (REM)–generating neurons are located in the pons.

The central respiratory neurons controlling respiration during sleep and wakefulness (metabolic or automatic system) are located in the medulla in the region of nucleus tractus solitarius, nucleus ambiguus, and nucleus retroambigualis. The voluntary respiratory system is located in the cerebral cortex and projects partly to the metabolic system in the medulla but mostly descends to the upper cervical spinal cord where the metabolic and the voluntary systems

are integrated. Therefore these anatomical locations make these structures controlling sleep-wakefulness and breathing highly vulnerable to the neurological lesions affecting the cortical and subcortical structures. SDB therefore occurs in many central neurological disorders as well as in peripheral neurological disorders such as polyneuropathies, neuromuscular junction disorders, and muscle diseases by causing weakness of the respiratory muscles. SDB has been described in many neurodegenerative disorders, "strokes," other structural affections of the brainstem and upper cervical spinal cord, as well as in many neuromuscular diseases.

In this section of the atlas we are illustrating a few selected neurological disorders causing a variety of SDB. SDB has been estimated to be present in 33 percent to 53 percent of Alzheimer's disease (AD) patients. Whether the prevalence of sleep apnea in AD patients is related to the advancing age of the patient and whether sleep apnea increases its severity of illness or more rapid progression of the disease remains to be determined. SDB causes cognitive impairment and therefore it is most probable that the presence of SDB will adversely affect these demented patients. SDB (obstructive, central, and mixed apneas) as well as laryngeal stridor may be more common in Parkinson's disease (PD) patients than in age-matched controls. Those PD patients with autonomic dysfunction show increased incidence of SDB. The factors contributing to SDB include impairment of respiratory muscle function owing to rigidity or an impairment of the central control of breathing in addition to other contributing factors such as laryngeal spasms associated with off stage of dystonic episodes, diaphragmatic dyskinesias, and upper airway dysfunction. Multiple system atrophy (MSA), another degen-

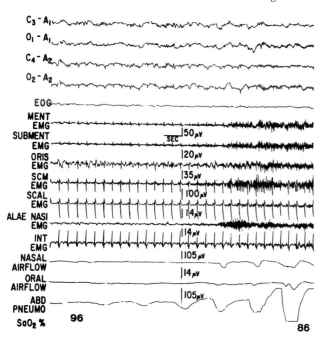

FIGURE 10–1. *A case of Alzheimer's dementia and SDB. Polysomnographic (PSG) recording in a 68-year-old man in an advanced stage of Alzheimer's disease with profound dementia, excessive daytime sleepiness, and severe nocturnal sleep disturbance. PSG shows a portion of mixed apnea during stage II non-REM sleep accompanied by oxygen desaturation. Top four channels represent electroencephalography (EEG) (Key: international electrode placement system). Electromyograms (EMG) of mentalis (MENT), submental (SUBMENTAL), orbicularis (ORIS), sternocleidomastoid (SCM), scalenus anticus (SCAL), alae nasi, and intercostals (INT) muscles are shown. Also shown are nasal and oral airflow, abdominal pneumogram (ABD PNEUMO), and oxygen saturation (SaO₂%). EOG, Electrooculogram. (From Chokroverty S. Sleep, breathing, and neurological disorders. In Chokroverty S, ed. Sleep Disorders Medicine. Boston: Butterworth-Heinemann, 1999:519, with permission.)*

erative disease of the autonomic and somatic neurons, initially presents with progressive autonomic failure followed by progressive somatic neurologic manifestations affecting multiple systems. The term *Shy-Drager syndrome* is used to describe the condition in which autonomic failure is the predominant feature. The term *strionigral degeneration* thus is used to describe the condition in which the predominant feature is parkinsonism whereas sporadic *olivopontocerebellar atrophy* (OPCA) is used when cerebellar features are the predominant manifestations. A variety of sleep-related respiratory disturbances may occur, which include obstructive, central and mixed apneas and hypopneas, dysrhythmic breathing, Cheyne-Stokes respiration and nocturnal inspiratory stridor. SDB in MSA may result from direct and indirect mechanism such as degeneration

of sleep-wake generating neurons in the brainstem and hypothalamus, degeneration of respiratory neurons or direct involvement of the projections from the hypothalamus and the central nucleus of the amygdala to the respiratory neurons in the nucleus tractus solitarius and nucleus ambiguus, interference with the vagal inputs from peripheral respiratory receptors to central respiratory neurons, as well as an alteration of the neurochemical environment. In addition to the sporadic OPCA, patients with dominant OPCA may also have central, upper airway obstructive, or mixed apneas but these are less frequent and less intense in this condition than in MSA. In several multiple sclerosis patients, SDB abnormalities have been described. SDB in such a condition may result from a demyelinating plaque involving the hypnogenic and respiratory neurons in the brainstem. In Arnold-Chiari malformation, particularly in type I malformation, several patients have been described with central and upper airway obstructive sleep apneas as well as profound sleep hypoventilation.

Sleep, epilepsy, breathing, and sleep apnea are all interrelated but sleep and seizures may adversely affect breathing, and disordered breathing during sleep may in turn adversely affect seizures. Sleep and sleep deprivation may trigger seizures in susceptible individuals. Epileptogenesis depends on cortical hyperexcitability and excessive neuronal synchronization. NREM sleep acts as a convulsant as a result of thalamocortical synchronization and hence predisposes to the activation of seizure in an already hyperexcitable cortex. In contrast, during REM sleep there is inhibition of thalamocortical synchronization as well as a tonic reduction in the interhemispheric impulse traffic through the corpus callosum. As a result, REM sleep generally attenuates epileptiform discharges and lateralizes generalized discharges to a focal area. Generalized seizures as well as seizure discharges in the limbic-hypothalamic system may cause SDB. Reciprocal connections between the central respiratory neurons in the medulla and the limbic, hypothalamic, and other forebrain structures explain why epileptic seizures are triggered during sleep and the discharges in the limbic-hypothalamic region may interfere with the respiratory regulation causing SDB. The association of epilepsy and sleep apnea, once thought to be rare, is increasingly recognized. The true prevalence of sleep apnea or SDB in epilepsy however remains undetermined at present in absence of well-controlled large-scale epidemiological studies. There are scattered case reports of upper airway obstructive, central and mixed apneas in patients with epilepsy and improvement of seizure control with treatment of apneas.

Patients with narcolepsy-cataplexy syndrome may also have sleep apnea, which is present in up to 30 percent of narcoleptic patients. SDB most commonly occurs as a central apnea but patients may also have obstructive and

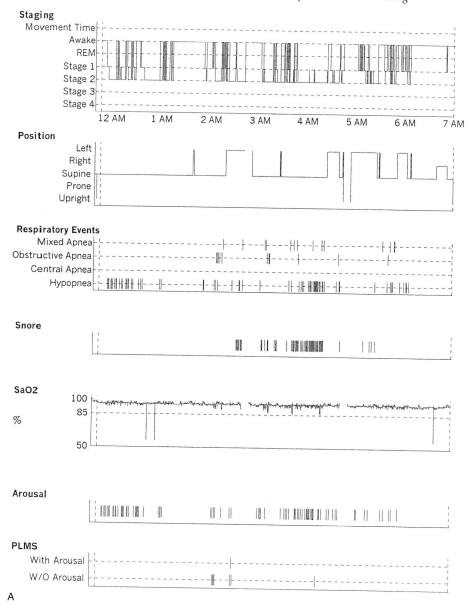

FIGURE 10–2. *A case of Parkinson's disease and SDB. A 67-year-old man with history of loud snoring for several years, mild daytime sleepiness, and light-headedness on standing up in the last 2 to 3 months. His past medical history is significant for Parkinson's disease diagnosed about 2 years ago (currently stage II Hoehn-Yahr scale) and hypertension. A prior sleep study performed approximately 3 years ago had diagnosed him with severe obstructive sleep apnea syndrome. He tried continuous positive airway pressure (CPAP) treatment unsuccessfully and has been using a dental appliance every night for the last 2 years, which has somewhat decreased his daytime sleepiness. Hypnogram in* **A** *shows sleep architectural changes with frequent stage shifts, and awakenings resulting in a decreased sleep efficiency of 54 percent. Slow-wave sleep (SWS) and REM sleep are conspicuously lacking. Frequent respiratory events, particularly hypopneas, are recorded throughout the night associated with mild O_2 desaturation and arousals. The apnea-hypopnea index is moderately increased at 25. The multiple sleep latency test (MSLT) shows a mean sleep latency of 1.75 minutes consistent with pathological sleepiness. Several sleep complaints, commonly sleep maintenance insomnia, hypersomnia, and parasomnias, particularly REM behavior disorder (RBD), are reported in Parkinson's disease patients. Some patients may also have obstructive and central sleep apnea but adequate studies have not been undertaken to see if apneas are part of the intrinsic disease process or related to aging.*

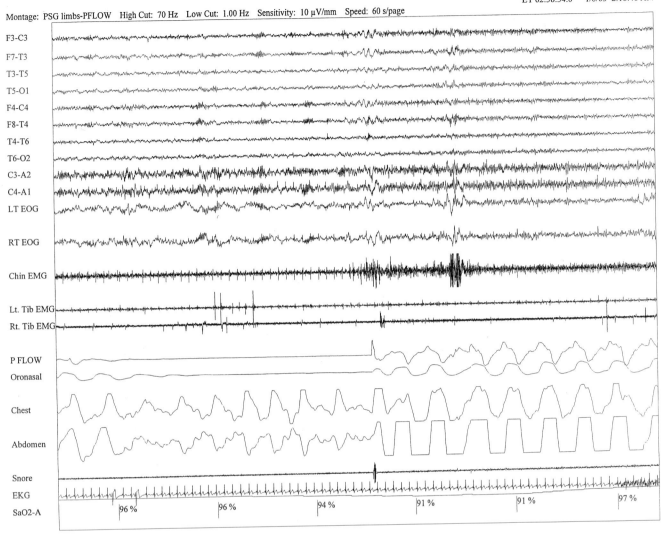

ET 02:36:34.0   1/6/03 2:16:46 AM

B

FIGURE 10–2, cont'd B: *A 60-second excerpt from overnight PSG showing an obstructive sleep apnea in stage II NREM sleep associated with mild O₂ desaturation and followed by an arousal. EEG, Top 10 channels; Lt., left; Rt., right; EOG, electrooculograms; chin EMG, electromyography of chin; Tib. EMG, tibialis anterior electromyography; P Flow, peak flow; oronasal thermistor; chest and abdomen effort channels; snore monitor; EKG, electrocardiography; SaO₂, oxygen saturation by finger oxymetry.*

mixed apneas. Sleep attacks with narcolepsy may be aggravated by such associated sleep apnea and therefore recognition of this is important in these patients as they may require additional treatment with continuous positive airway pressure for relief of apnea and excessive daytime somnolence.

Sleep disturbances in neuromuscular disorders are usually the result of sleep-related respiratory dysrhythmias but in some cases direct dysfunction of the respiratory premotor and motor neurons in the brainstem and spinal cord

are responsible for sleep complaints. Involvement of the respiratory muscles, the phrenic and intercostals nerves, or the neuromuscular junctions of the respiratory and oropharyngeal muscles may cause SDB in neuromuscular disorders causing excessive daytime somnolence, repeated arousals, and sleep fragmentation. SDB has been described in many patients with neuromuscular disorders including myotonic dystrophy and other primary muscle diseases, motor neuron disease or amyotrophic lateral sclerosis, and neuromuscular junctional disorders and

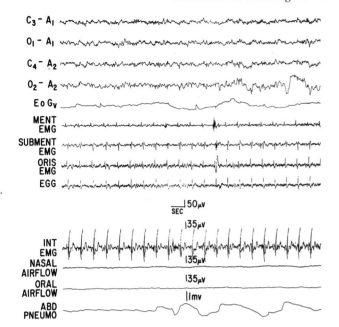

FIGURE 10–3. *A case of multiple systems atrophy (Shy-Drager syndrome) and SDB. PSG recording in a 58-year-old patient with olivopontocerebellar atrophy presenting with ataxic gait, scanning dysarthria, nystagmus, marked finger-nose and heal-knee incoordination, and bilateral extensor plantar responses. Laboratory tests showed evidence of dysautonomia. PSG shows a portion of an episode of mixed apnea during stage II non-REM sleep. EEGs are shown in the top four channels. EOGv, vertical electrooculogram; ment, mentalis; EMG, electromyography; SUBMENT, submentalis; ORIS, orbicularis; INT, intercostals muscles; ABD PNEUMO, abdominal pneumogram; EGG, electroglossogram. (From Chokroverty S, Sachdeo R, Masdeu J. Autonomic dysfunction and sleep apnea in olivopontocerebellar degeneration. Arch Neurol 1984;41:509, with permission.)*

polyneuropathies. Many reports of central, mixed, and upper airway obstructive sleep apneas, and alveolar hypoventilation associated with excessive daytime somnolence have been described in such patients. Respiratory disturbances are generally noted in the advanced stage of such disorders but sometimes SDB may be the presenting complaint in patients with motor neuron disease or with acid maltase deficiency. In amyotrophic lateral sclerosis, SDB may result from weakness of the upper airway and the diaphragmatic and intercostal muscles due to involvement of the bulbar, phrenic, and intercostal motor nuclei. In addition degeneration of central respiratory neurons may occur, causing central and obstructive sleep apneas in this condition.

SDBs causing sleep disturbance are well known in patients during the acute and convalescent stage of poliomyelitis. Sleep disorders, however, in post-polio syndrome are less well known. Patients with post-polio syndrome present with increasing weakness, wasting of previously affected muscles, and additional involvement of the unaffected regions of the body. Patients may present with excessive daytime somnolence and fatigue as a result of sleep-related hypoventilation or apneas.

In summary, it is important to recognize SDB in a variety of neurological conditions as appropriate treatment may improve the quality of life and improve the long-term prognosis of the primary neurological disorder. The clinical clues to SDB in neurological disorders include sleep disturbances at night and presence of excessive daytime sleepiness for which no obvious cause is found.

Text continued on p. 239

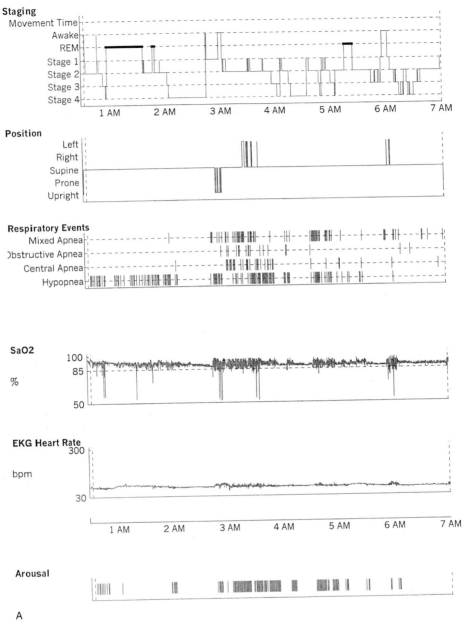

FIGURE 10–4. *A case of multiple sclerosis and SDB. A 51-year-old woman with history of multiple sclerosis diagnosed 7 years ago. Her sleep difficulties started approximately 3 years ago and are described as frequent night awakenings, sleepwalking, and brief episodes consisting of sudden sleepiness or impairment of consciousness resulting in falls and multiple fractures but never accompanied by jerky movements of the limbs, tongue biting, or incontinence, with spontaneous recovery in 5 to 10 minutes without residual confusion. These episodes occur during early morning hours as well as during the day. Her neurological examination is significant for the presence of decreased visual acuity and impaired saccades bilaterally, horizontal nystagmus on looking to the left, intention tremor (left more than right) on finger-to-nose testing, mild ataxia in the lower extremities on heel-to-shin testing, tandem ataxia, and impaired joint and position sense in the toes bilaterally. She was clinically evaluated with a differential diagnosis of SDB related to multiple sclerosis, narcolepsy-cataplexy secondary to multiple sclerosis, and sleepwalking. Unusual nocturnal seizures remained unlikely given the clinical features, the several negative EEGs, and the negative long-term epilepsy monitoring. A: Hypnogram significant for REM sleep distribution abnormality (longest REM in the early part of the night); frequent obstructive, mixed, and central apneas and hypopneas both during NREM and REM sleep; mild-moderate O_2 desaturation; and frequent arousals. Sleep-related respiratory dysrhythmias due to brainstem involvement are a common finding in multiple sclerosis patients.*

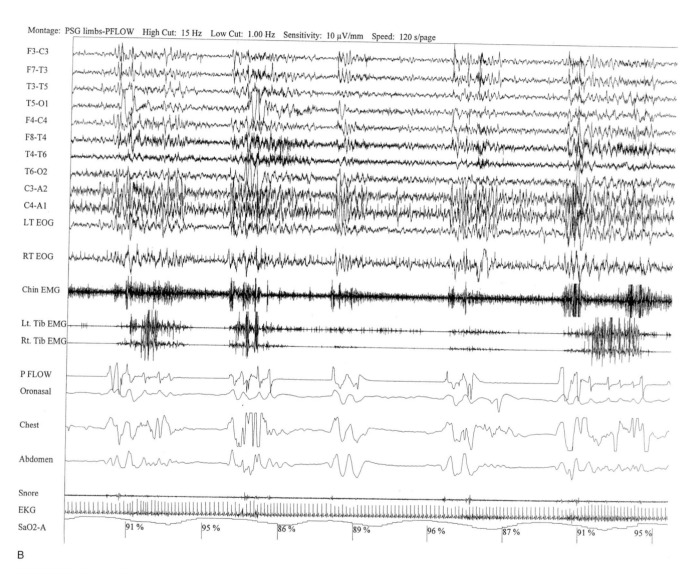

Montage: PSG limbs-PFLOW   High Cut: 15 Hz   Low Cut: 1.00 Hz   Sensitivity: 10 µV/mm   Speed: 120 s/page

B

FIGURE 10–4, cont'd B: *A 120-second excerpt from overnight PSG recording showing repeated central apneas with O₂ desaturation. An increase in muscle tone is noted on chin and tibialis anterior EMG channels following some central events. EEG, Top 10 channels; Lt., left; Rt., right; EOG, electrooculograms; Chin EMG, electromyography of chin; Tib., tibialis anterior muscle; electromyography; P Flow, peak flow; oronasal thermistor; chest and abdomen effort channels; snore monitor; EKG, electrocardiography; SaO₂ oxygen saturation by finger oxymetry.*

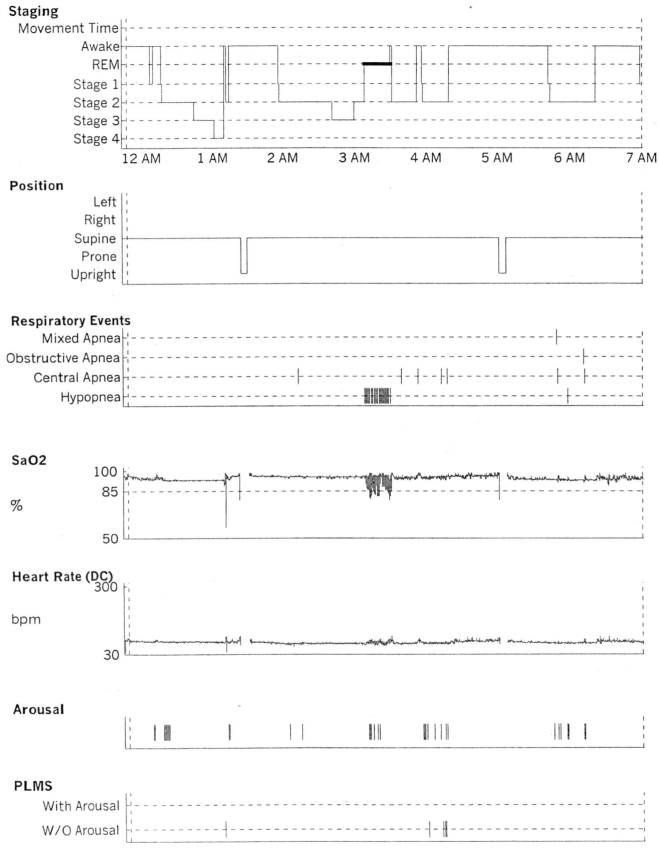

A

For legend see opposite page

FIGURE 10–5. *A case of Arnold-Chiari malformation and SDB. A 52-year-old man with history of tiredness and excessive daytime sleepiness for many years but no cataplexy, sleep paralysis, or hypnagogical hallucinations. At the age of 27 years, he complained of gait problems and magnetic resonance imaging (MRI) examination revealed Arnold-Chiari malformation type 1. His neurological examination is significant for the presence of a coarse horizontal nystagmus, minimal right lower facial weakness, minimal right wrist extensor muscle weakness, minimal to mild ataxia in upper and lower extremities on coordination testing, and presence of ataxia on tandem gait.* **A:** *Hypnogram shows a few periods of apneas and hypopneas accompanied by mild-moderate oxygen desaturation and arousals limited exclusively to a single REM sleep period recorded during the night. A supine posture is maintained throughout the PSG recording. These findings are suggestive of REM sleep-related hypoventilation. Central sleep apnea, obstructive sleep apnea, and hypoventilation have all been described in patients with Arnold-Chiari malformation, likely from brainstem involvement.*

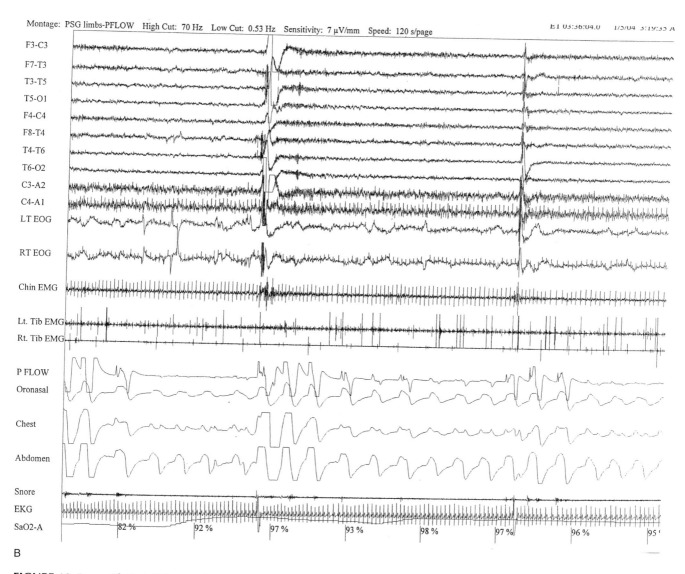

B

FIGURE 10–5, cont'd B: *A 120-second excerpt from REM sleep showing one obstructive apnea followed by two sequential hypopneas. O₂ desaturation of 82 percent, likely from a prior respiratory event, is recorded at the onset of the epoch. The first two events are followed by an arousal response and the epoch does not include the complete recovery phase of the third event. Phasic eye movements of REM sleep are noted on the EOG channels in the early part of the epoch. Phasic muscle twitches of REM sleep are noted on both tibialis anterior EMG channels. Chin EMG channel shows electrocardiography artifact. EEG, Top 10 channels; Lt., left; Rt., right; EOG, electrooculograms; Chin EMG, electromyography of chin; Tib. EMG, tibialis anterior electromyography; P Flow, peak flow; oronasal thermistor; chest and abdomen effort channels; snore monitor; EKG, electrocardiography; SaO₂, oxygen saturation by finger oxymetry.*

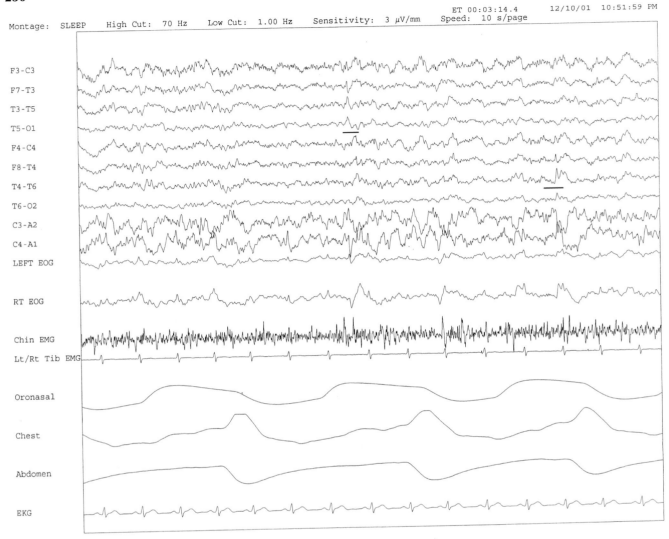

A

FIGURE 10–6. *A case of seizure disorder and SDB. A 53-year-old man with history of frequent night awakenings and excessive daytime sleepiness. Over the last 2 months he reports awakening with choking and "fighting for breath" along with episodes of transient dizziness and unsteadiness during the day. In addition, he reports several episodes of nocturnal tongue biting and two episodes of nocturnal enuresis over the last 20 years. The only significant finding on neurological examination is the presence of postural tremor of outstretched hands bilaterally. Differential diagnostic possibilities of sleep apnea and nocturnal seizures are raised. MRI of the brain revealed no intracranial pathology. Overnight PSG showed the presence of mild sleep apnea with an apnea-hypopnea index of 10.4. The presence of spike and wave activity (as underlined) independently over both temporal regions, left more often than right, was also noted and further confirmed on a prolonged daytime EEG.*

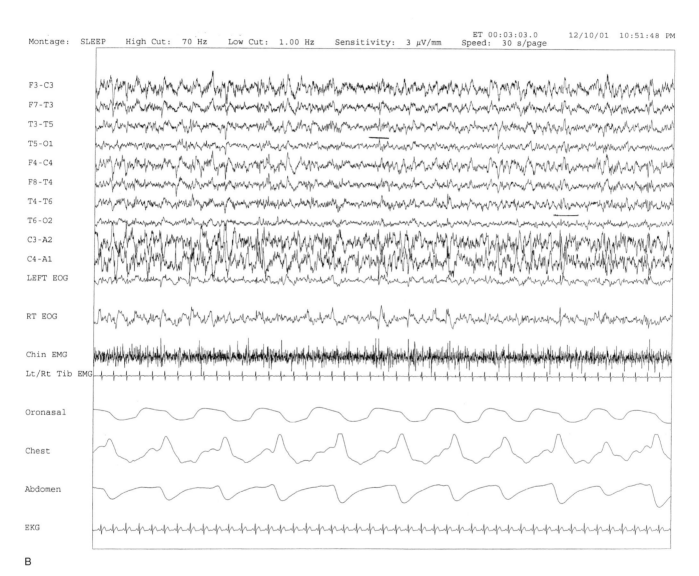

B

FIGURE 10–6, cont'd *A and B: Ten- and 30-second excerpts, respectively, from an overnight PSG recording showing the presence of independent left and right temporal spike and wave discharges (as underlined). EEG, Top 10 channels; Lt., left; Rt., right; EOG, electrooculograms; electromyography of chin, Tib. EMG, tibialis anterior electromyography; P Flow, peak flow; oronasal thermistor; chest and abdomen effort channels; snore monitor; EKG, electrocardiography; SaO₂, oxygen saturation by finger oxymetry.*

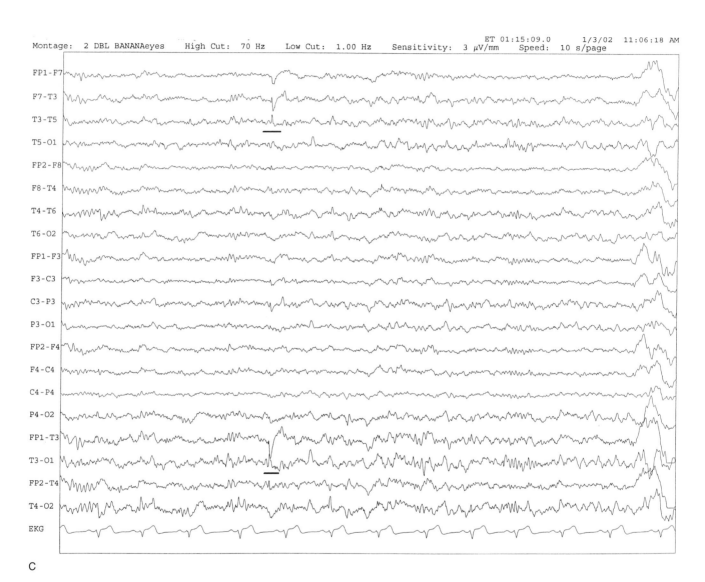

C

FIGURE 10–6, cont'd *C* and *D:* *Ten- and 30-second excerpts, respectively, from an EEG similarly showing the presence of spike and wave discharges in the left temporal region (as underlined). K complex is noted in* *D*.

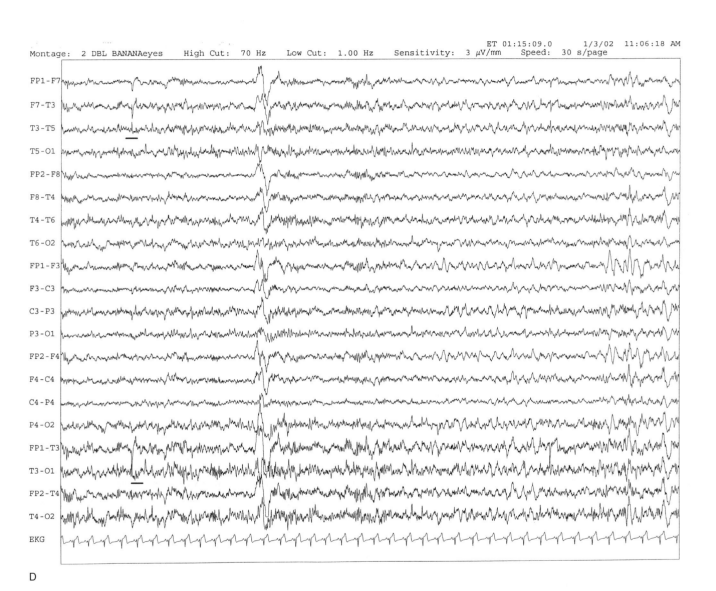

D

FIGURE 10–6, cont'd.

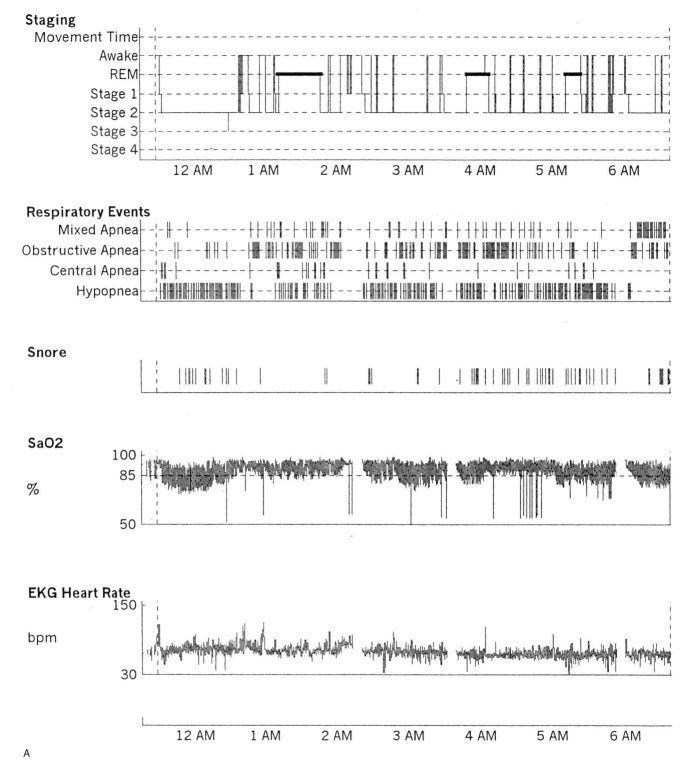

Staging

Movement Time
Awake
REM
Stage 1
Stage 2
Stage 3
Stage 4

12 AM   1 AM   2 AM   3 AM   4 AM   5 AM   6 AM

Respiratory Events

Mixed Apnea
Obstructive Apnea
Central Apnea
Hypopnea

Snore

SaO2

%

100
85

50

EKG Heart Rate

bpm

150

30

12 AM   1 AM   2 AM   3 AM   4 AM   5 AM   6 AM

A

FIGURE 10–7. *A case of narcolepsy and SDB. A 27-year-old man complaining of fatigue and excessive daytime sleepiness with snoring and disturbed sleep at nights for several years. Daytime sleepiness was characterized by feeling sleepy during classes in high school and while driving but there was no history of cataplexy, sleep paralysis, or hypnagogical hallucinations. Evaluation of the throat and neurological examinations were normal. Overnight PSG in 1998 was significant for slightly increased respiratory disturbance index at 8.7 with some nonspecific sleep architectural changes and absence of oxygen desaturation consistent with mild sleep apnea. The mean sleep latency on MSLT was, however, 1.12 minutes consistent with pathological sleepiness and he had two sleep-onset REMs (SOREMs). Given the clinical history and disparity between PSG and MSLT findings, he was diagnosed with narcolepsy and started on stimulant treatment. He responded well and his daytime sleepiness decreased. In 2001 his daytime sleepiness and fatigue returned despite taking the stimulant. He had disturbed sleep with cessation of breathing and frequent awakenings at night. He was also reported to snore loudly in sleep. He reported having put on approximately 20 pounds of weight in the last 6 months. A repeat PSG study in 2001 showed recurrent episodes of obstructive, mixed, and central apneas and hypopneas during NREM and REM sleep accompanied by moderate-severe O_2 desaturation, repeated arousal, snoring, and a severely increased apnea-hypopnea index of 85. The hypnogram is shown in **A**. Thus he was diagnosed to have sleep apnea in conjunction with narcolepsy. Sleep apnea, predominantly central, has been described in patients with narcolepsy.*

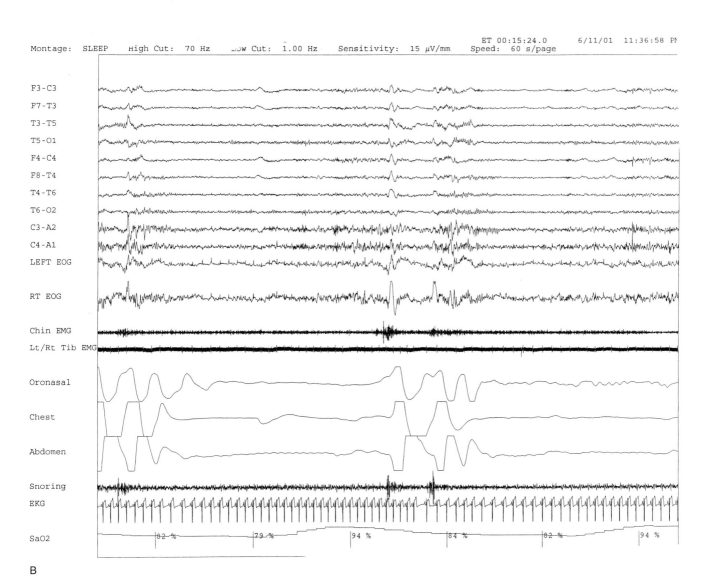

B

FIGURE 10–7, cont'd B: *A 60-second excerpt from overnight PSG showing two central apneas accompanied by mild-moderate O$_2$ desaturation.*

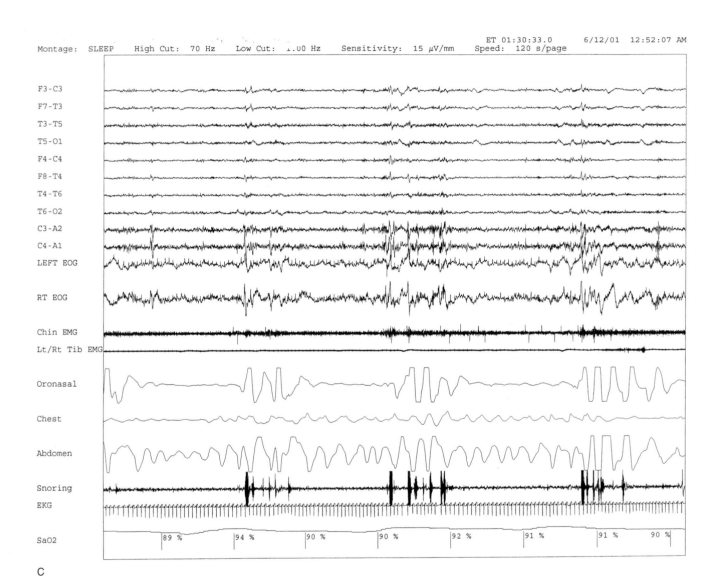

C

FIGURE 10–7, cont'd C: *A 120-second excerpt from overnight PSG showing obstructive apneas with mild O₂ desaturation. EEG,* Top 10 channels; Lt., *left;* Rt., *right;* EOG, *electrooculograms;* Chin EMG, *electromyography of chin;* Tib. EMG, *tibialis anterior electromyography; oronasal thermistor, chest and abdomen effort channels; snore monitor;* EKG, *electrocardiography;* SaO₂, *oxygen saturation by finger oxymetry.*

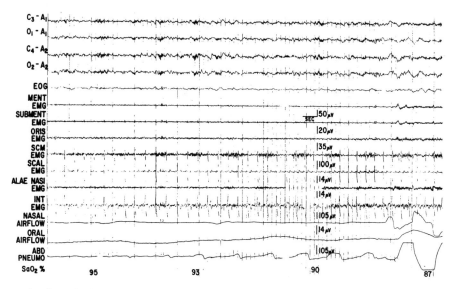

FIGURE 10–8. *Amyotrophic lateral sclerosis (ALS) and SDB. PSG recording in a 50-year-old man with ALS presenting with upper and lower motor neuron signs including bulbar palsy. PSG shows mixed apnea during stage II non-REMG sleep. Top four channels represent EEG (Key: international electrode placement system). Electromyograms (EMG) of mentalis (MENT), submental (SUBMENTAL), orbicularis (ORIS), sternocleidomastoid (SCM), scalenus anticus (SCAL), alae nasi, and intercostals (INT) muscles are shown. Also shown are nasal and oral airflow, abdominal pneumogram (ABD PNEUMO), and oxygen saturation (SaO₂%). EOG, electrooculogram. (From Chokroverty S. Sleep, breathing, and neurological disorders. In Chokroverty S, ed. Sleep Disorders Medicine. Boston: Butterworth-Heinemann, 1999:531.)*

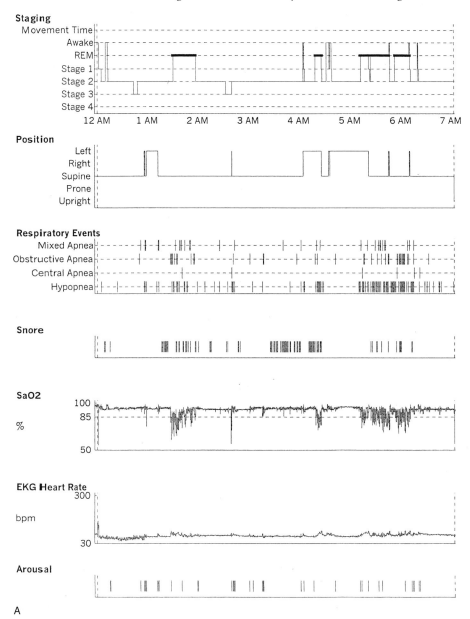

FIGURE 10–9. *A case of post-polio syndrome and SDB. A 56-year-old woman with a 2- to 3-year history of shortness of breath and choking sensation when she lies in bed at night. Past medical history is significant for poliomyelitis at the age of 17 years, which paralyzed her from the neck down. She slowly recovered to a great extent and could eventually walk without aid but continued to have residual weakness in both legs. In the last 2 to 3 years she has noticed weakness in the upper extremities as well and pains all over her body. Her recent complaints are consistent with diagnosis of post-polio syndrome with SRB dysfunction, which is commonly seen in patients with neuromuscular disorders. She also has adult-onset diabetes mellitus, high blood pressure, hypercholesterolemia, and recently diagnosed left breast carcinoma pending mastectomy.* **A:** *Hypnogram is significant for frequent respiratory events particularly hypopneas most marked during REM sleep, which is commonly noted in patients with SDB secondary to neuromuscular disorder. The total apnea-hypopnea index is 30.3 but 86.7 in REM sleep. This is accompanied by moderate-severe oxygen desaturation most marked in REM sleep. A minimum oxygen saturation of 61 percent and a mean of 87 percent during REM sleep are noted. A REM sleep distribution abnormality (with a long REM sleep period recorded in the early part of the night) is also recorded on sleep staging. This can be frequently encountered in patients with disturbed night sleep.*

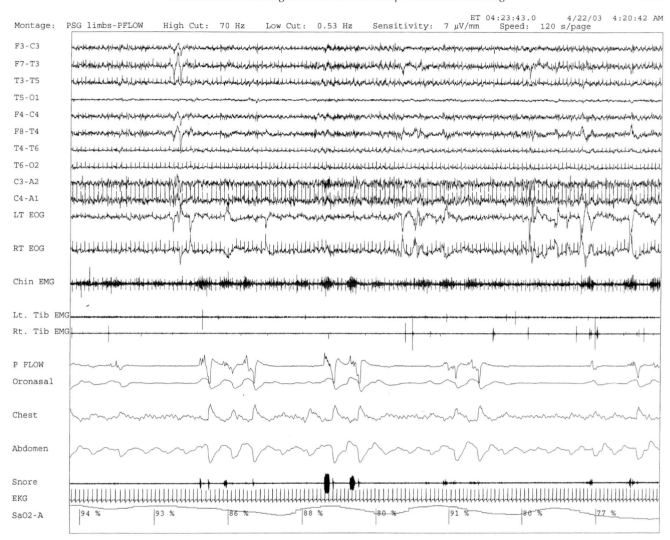

B

FIGURE 10–9, cont'd *B:* *A 120-second excerpt from overnight PSG recording showing repeated obstructive apneas in REM sleep. EEG, Top 10 channels; Lt., left; Rt., right; EOG, electrooculograms; Chin EMG, electromyography of chin; Tib, tibialis anterior muscle; P Flow, peak flow; oronasal thermistor; chest and abdomen effort channels; snore monitor; EKG, electrocardiography; SaO₂, oxygen saturation by finger oxymetry.*

BIBLIOGRAPHY

1. Chokroverty S. Sleep, breathing and neurologic disorders. In: Chokroverty S, ed. *Sleep Disorders Medicine: Basic Science, Technical Considerations, and Clinical Aspects.* 2nd ed. Boston, MA: Butterworth Heinemann; 1999:509–571.
2. Culebras A. *Sleep Disorders and Neurological Disease.* New York: Marcel Dekker, Inc, 2000.
3. Chokroverty S. Sleep and degenerative neurologic disorders. *Neurol Clin* 1996;14(4):807–826.
4. Diederich NJ, Comella CL. Sleep Disturbances in Parkinson's Disease. In Chokroverty S, Hening W, Walters A, eds. *Sleep and Movement Disorders.* Philadelphia, PA: Butterworth-Heinemann, 2003:478–488.
5. Schenck CH, Bundlie SR, Mahowald MW. Delayed emergence of parkinsonian disorder in 38% of 29 older men initially diagnosed with idiopathic rapid eye movement sleep behaviour disorder. *Neurology* 1996;46(2):388–393.
6. Plazzi G, Corsini R, Provini F, et al. REM sleep behavior disorders in multiple system atrophy. *Neurology* 1997;48(4):1094–1097.
7. Chokroverty S, Qunito C. Sleep and epilepsy. In: Chokroverty S, ed. *Sleep Disorders Medicine: Basic Science, Technical Considerations, and Clinical Aspects.* 2nd ed. Boston, MA: Butterworth-Heinemann; 1999:697-727.
8. Gibbs EL, Gibbs FA. Diagnostic and localizing value of electroencephalographic studies in sleep. *Res Publ Assoc Res Nerv Ment Dis* 1947;26:366.

11

Specialized Techniques

Chapter 11A

Multiple Sleep Latency Testing

Sudhansu Chokroverty and Meeta Bhatt

The most common indication for referring a patient for laboratory assessment is excessive daytime sleepiness (EDS), although sleep onset and sleep maintenance insomnia is the most common complaint in the general population. The initial step in assessment of a patient with EDS is detailed sleep and other histories, and physical examination. For assessment of persistent sleepiness, the Epworth Sleepiness Scale (ESS) is often used to assess a general level of sleepiness. This is a subjective propensity to sleepiness assessed by the patient under eight situations on a scale of 0 to 3, with 3 indicating a situation when chances of dozing off are highest. The maximum score is 24 and a score of 10 suggests the presence of EDS. This test has been weakly correlated with multiple sleep latency test (MSLT) scores. The ESS and MSLT, however, test different types of sleepiness. MSLT tests the propensity to sleepiness objectively and ESS tests the general feeling of sleepiness or subjective propensity to sleepiness. The Stanford Sleepiness Scale (SSS) is a 7-point analog scale to measure subjective sleepiness but it does not measure persistent sleepiness. Visual Analog Scale is the other scale used to assess alertness and well-being in which subjects indicate their feelings of alertness at an arbitrary point on a line of 0 to 100 millimeter scale with 100 being the maximum sleepiness and 0 being the most alert.

TECHNIQUE OF MULTIPLE SLEEP LATENCY TEST

The MSLT has been standardized and includes several general and specific procedures. The general procedures before the actual recording include keeping a sleep diary for 1 to 2 weeks before the test, which records the information about bedtime, time of rising, napping, and any drug use. The test is preceded by an overnight polysomnographic (PSG) study and MSLT is scheduled about 2 to 3 hours after the conclusion of the overnight PSG study. The actual test consists of four to five opportunities for napping at 2-hour intervals and each recording session lasts for a maximum of 20 minutes. Between tests subjects must remain awake. The subjects must not smoke for 30 minutes before lights are turned off. Physiologic calibrations (i.e., grit teeth, blink your eyes, look up, look down, look to the right, look to the left, open your eyes and close your eyes) are then performed, and the patient is instructed to relax and fall asleep, and the lights are turned off. The test must be conducted in a quiet, dark room. The specific recording includes two to four channels of electroencephalography (EEG), submental electromyography (EMG), and electrooculography (EOG) recordings. Ideally, four channels of EEG (C3-A2, C4-A1, 01-A1, and 02-A2) are recommended to document alpha activity in relaxed wakefulness in adults and its disappearance at sleep onset.

The measurements include average sleep-onset latency and the presence of sleep-onset rapid eye movements (SOREMs). If no sleep occurs, then the test is concluded 20 minutes after lights are turned off. The test is terminated 15 minutes after the first 30-second epoch of any stage of sleep. If the finding is indefinite, then it is better to continue the test than to end it prematurely. Mean sleep latency is calculated from the sum of the latency to sleep onset for each of the four to five naps. Mean sleep latency of less than 5 minutes is consistent with pathologic sleepiness. A mean sleep latency of 10 to 15 minutes is considered normal; a mean sleep latency of up to 5 to 10 minutes is consistent with mild sleepiness. The occurrence of REM

Montage: MSLT-NEW   High Cut: 70 Hz   Low Cut: 0.53 Hz   Sensitivity: 7 μV/mm   Speed: 30 s/page

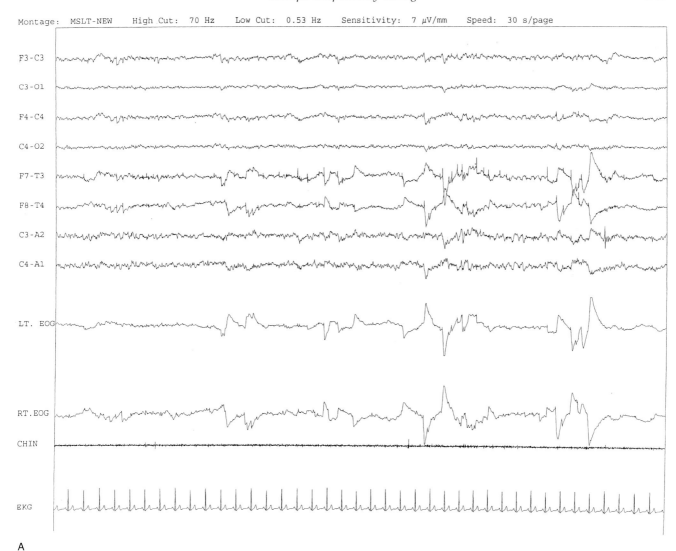

A

FIGURE 11A–1. *A case of narcolepsy. A 60-year-old woman with new onset of intermittent episodes of sudden transient bilateral leg weakness, excessive daytime sleepiness, and intermittent periods of transient confusion. A daytime EEG was normal. Overnight PSG was significant for sleep architecture changes with an immediate sleep onset latency, presence of only one REM cycle, with a decreased REM sleep percentage (7 percent), an increased arousal index of 23 without associated apnea or periodic limb movements, and with excessive fragmentary myoclonus in non-REM and REM sleep. MSLT showed a mean sleep latency of 1.6 minutes consistent with pathologic sleepiness and the presence of 2 (out of 4) sleep-onset REM naps suggestive of REM sleep dysregulation as seen in narcolepsy. **A:** A 30-second epoch from MSLT showing the presence of sleep-onset REM occurring 7 minutes after sleep onset. Prominent REMs are seen in the EOG channels and anterior temporal EEG electrodes.*

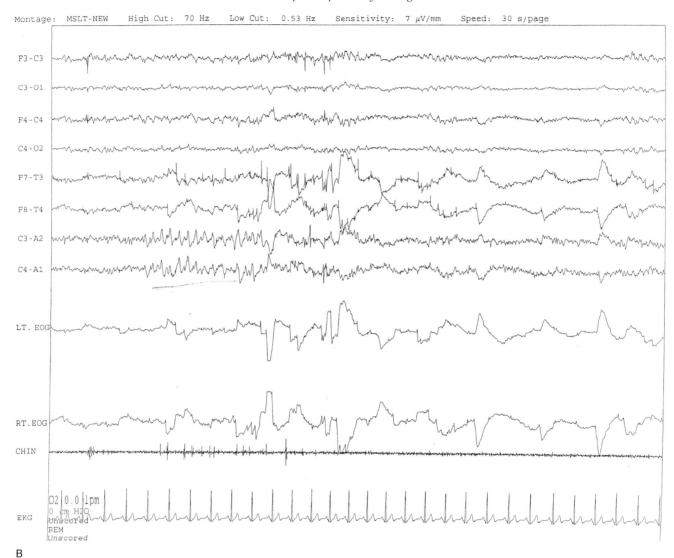

B

FIGURE 11A–1, cont'd B: *A 30-second epoch taken from the same sleep nap as above, showing the presence of prominent sawtooth waves (as underlined) in C3 and C4 electrode channels referenced to contralateral ears. Eye movements characteristic of REM sleep are noted as described above.* EEG, *Top eight channels;* Lt. *and* Rt. EOG, *left and right electrooculograms;* chin, *electromyography of chin;* EKG, *electrocardiography.*

sleep within 15 minutes of sleep onset is defined as SOREMs.

Repeat MSLT is required if the patient is strongly suspected to have narcolepsy but did not show the characteristic findings as may be seen in a certain percentage of narcolepsy patients. MSLT may not be diagnostic in the initial test and the diagnostic yield increases after the second test. The other situation for repeating MSLT is when the findings are ambiguous and the sleep onset or REM sleep cannot be adequately interpreted. Finally, if the MSLT guidelines have not been followed, the test results may be invalid.

INDICATIONS FOR MSLT

The American Academy of Sleep Medicine (AASM) standards of practice committee recommended indications for MSLT. Narcolepsy is the single most important indication for performing the MSLT (Figure 11A–1). A mean sleep latency of less than 5 minutes combined with SOREMs in two or more of the four to five recordings during MSLT is strongly suggestive of narcolepsy, although REM sleep dysregulation and circadian rhythm sleep disorders may also lead to such findings.

In patients with upper airway obstructive sleep apnea syndrome (OSAS), the MSLT is not routinely indicated in the initial evaluation and diagnosis or in assessment of change following treatment with nasal CPAP. However, in those patients previously diagnosed with OSAS or other sleep-related breathing disorder, periodic limb movement disorder, or mood disorders who continue to have excessive sleepiness despite optimal treatment may require evaluation by the MSLT to exclude associated narcolepsy. The coexistence of OSAS and narcolepsy is well known.

An MSLT is indicated in patients suspected of having idiopathic hypersomnia; in this condition the MSLT findings will be consistent with pathologic sleepiness but without SOREMs.

In patients with medical and neurologic disorders (other than narcolepsy), insomnia or circadian rhythm disorders, the MSLT is not routinely indicated for evaluation of sleepiness.

Following are the recommended indications for repeat MSLT: *i.* extraneous circumstances or inappropriate conditions affecting the initial MSLT; *ii.* presence of ambiguous or uninterpretable findings; *iii.* initial MSLT without polygraphic confirmation in a patient suspected to have narcolepsy.

RELIABILITY, VALIDITY, AND LIMITATION OF THE MULTIPLE SLEEP LATENCY TEST

The sensitivity and specificity of the MSLT in detecting sleepiness have not been clearly determined. The test-retest reliability of the MSLT, however, has been documented in both normal subjects and patients with narcolepsy. In subjects with sleepiness caused by circadian rhythm sleep disorders, sleep deprivation, and ingestion of hypnotics and alcohol, pathologic sleepiness has been validated by MSLT. However, there is poor correlation between the MSLT and ESS. The patient's psychological and behavioral state also interferes with the MSLT results. If the patient suffers from severe anxiety or psychological disturbances causing behavioral stimulation, MSLT may not show sleepiness even in a patient complaining of EDS.

MAINTENANCE OF WAKEFULNESS TEST

The maintenance of wakefulness test (MWT) is a variant of the MSLT that measures an individual's ability to stay awake. It should be clearly understood that the MLST and MWT assess separate functions: The MSLT unmasks physiology sleepiness, which depends on both circadian and homeostatic factors; in contrast, the MWT is a reflection of the individual's capability to resist sleep and is influenced by physiologic sleepiness.

TECHNIQUE OF THE MWT

The MWT protocols require 4 trials at two hour intervals to test an individual's ability to stay awake. For total duration of each trial, both 20 and 40 minute protocols have been used. However, based on studies published in the peer-reviewed literature, the Standards of Practice Committee of the American Academy of Sleep Medicine (AASM) recommended the MWT 40 minute protocol. Unlike the MSLT, the MWT does not require prior overnight polysomnography. The test is performed about $1\frac{1}{2}$–3 hours after the individual's usual wake-up time. The recording montage is similar to that used for the MSLT. The patient calibrations prior to each test are similar to those used for the MSLT. Prior to the beginning of the recording, the patients are asked to sit still in bed with a back and headrest, and remain awake as long as possible. Sleep onset is defined as the time between the beginning of the recording and the onset of three consecutive epochs of stage 1 non-REM or one epoch of any other stage of sleep. The test should be terminated after sleep onset or after 40 minutes if no sleep occurs. A mean sleep latency (the arithmetic mean of the 4 trials) of less than 8 minutes is considered abnormal.

INDICATIONS FOR THE MWT

The AASM Standards of Practice Committee recommended the following indications for the MWT:

- Assessment of the individuals employed in occupations involving public transportation or safety for their ability to remain awake;
- Assessment of response to treatment (e.g., response to stimulants in narcolepsy and CPAP titration in OSAS patients).

There is clear need for further research to obtain well-defined normative data, sensitivity and specificity of the MWT to assess ability to stay awake.

BIBLIOGRAPHY

1. Carskadon MA, Dement WC, Mitler M, et al. Guidelines for the multiple sleep latency test MSLT: A standard measure of sleepiness. *Sleep* 1986;9:519–524.
2. Roth T, Roehrs TA, Rosenthal L. Measurement of sleepiness and alertness: Multiple sleep latency tests. In Chokroverty S, ed. *Sleep Disorders Medicine*, Boston: Butterworth-Heinemann, 1999:223–236.
3. Cherbin R. Assessment of sleepiness. In Chokroverty S, Hening WA, Walters AS, eds. *Sleep and Movement Disorders*, Philadelphia: Butterworth/Elsevier, 2003:132–143.
4. Practice parameters for clinical use of the multiple sleep latency tests and the maintenance of wakefulness test. An American Academy of Sleep Medicine report. *Standards of Practice Committee of the American Academy of Sleep Medicine*. Sleep 2005;28:113–121.
5. Arand D, Bonnet M, Hurwitz T, et al. The clinical use of the MSLT and MWT. *Sleep* 2005;28:123–144.
6. Doghramji K, Mitler M, Sangal R, et al. A normative study of the Maintenance of Wakefulness Test (MWT). *Electrocencephal Clin Neurophysiol* 1997;103:554–562.

Chapter 11B

Actigraphy

Sudhansu Chokroverty and Marco Zucconi

An actigraph, also known as an actometer or actimeter, monitors body movements and other activities continuously for days, weeks, or even months. This can be worn on the wrist or alternatively on the ankle for recording arm, leg, and body movements. Actigraph uses piezoelectric sensors which function as accelerometers to record acceleration or deceleration of movements rather than the actual movement. The mechanical movements are converted into electrical signals, which are then sampled every tenth second over a predetermined time or epoch and then retrieved and analyzed in a computer. The principle of analysis is based on the fact that increased movements (as indicated by black bars in the actigraph) are seen during wakefulness in contrast to markedly decreased movements or no movements (as indicated by the white area interrupting the black bars) during sleep, although normal physiological body and limb movements, and postural shifts during sleep will cause interruptions (black bars) of the white background (Figure 11B–1). Several actigraph models are in developing stage to carefully regulate the sampling frequencies and duration, filters, sensitivities, and dynamic range in order to detect and quantify periodic limb movements in sleep (PLMS), but no generally accepted standardized technique of quantifying and identifying PLMS discriminating from other movements (e.g., those resulting from parasomnias, nocturnal seizures, and other dyskinesias) is currently available. Studies have been conducted using actigraph and PSG recordings simultaneously to validate the ability of the actigraph to distinguish sleep from wakefulness. Computer algorithms are available for automatic sleep-wake scoring; however, visual inspection of the raw data is necessary. The reliability and validity of the data are available only for a specific actigraph model but no universally validated data are available. Actigraphs can differentiate indirectly sleep from wakefulness (see Figure 11B–1) but cannot differentiate REM from NREM sleep and cannot identify different NREM sleep stages. Actigraphs and sleep logs are complementary.

INDICATIONS FOR ACTIGRAPH

The AASM Standards of Practice Committee suggested the following recommendations for actigraph:

- Actigraph may be a useful adjunct to history, physical and sleep logs in patients with insomnia including sleep state misperception and inadequate sleep hygiene (Figures 11B–2 through 11B–7), circadian rhythm sleep disorders (Figures 11B–8 through 11B–10), and excessive daytime somnolence (see Figures 11–4 through 11–7).
- Actigraph may be a useful adjunct to detect the rest-activity patterns during modified portable sleep apnea testing.
- Actigraph is useful to document rest-activity patterns over days and weeks when sleep log is not able to provide such data.

Advantages of Actigraph over Polysomnography

These include the following: easy accessibility; inexpensive recording over extended periods for days, weeks, or

Text continued on p. 257

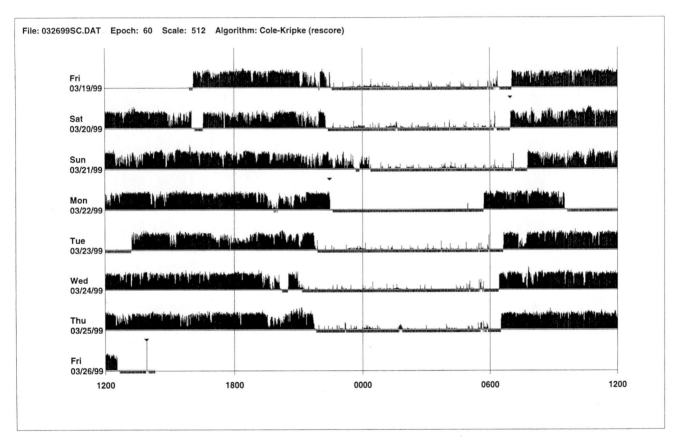

File: 032699SC.DAT   Epoch: 60   Scale: 512   Algorithm: Cole-Kripke (rescore)

Fri 03/19/99
Sat 03/20/99
Sun 03/21/99
Mon 03/22/99
Tue 03/23/99
Wed 03/24/99
Thu 03/25/99
Fri 03/26/99

1200   1800   0000   0600   1200

FIGURE 11B–1. *Normal sleep-wake schedule. This shows a wrist-actigraphic recording from a 55-year-old healthy woman without sleep complaints. This shows a fairly regular sleep-wake schedule except one weekend night (third from the top). She goes to bed between 10:30 PM and 11:00 PM and wakes up around 7:00 AM except on the third day. Physiological body shifts and movements during sleep are indicated by a few black bars in the white areas. The waking period is indicated by black bars.*

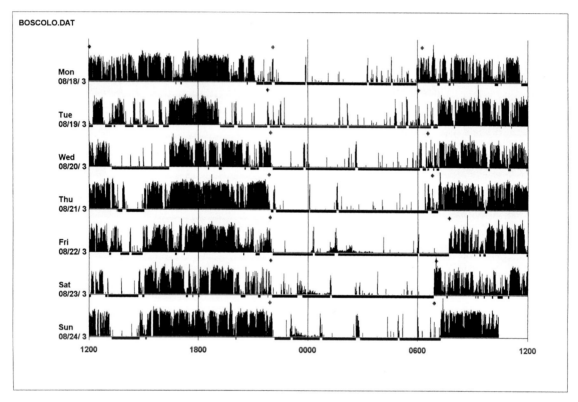

FIGURE 11B–2. *Actigraphy in insomnia (sleep state misperception). A 59-year-old man complaining of insomnia since the age of 12 years. He was diagnosed to have DSM IV Axis 2 personality disorder (dependent personality) and panic attacks in the past, treated with benzodiazepines (clordemetildiazepam 3 mg, flurazepam 30 mg) and zolpidem 10 mg. He denies any symptoms of restless legs syndrome (RLS), excessive daytime sleepiness, or daytime sleep attacks. Subjective sleep duration is 3 to 4 hours per night. In the past he had numerous drugs for sleep amelioration but no clear and stable subjective improvement was noted. An actigraphic monitoring (during drug-reduction, clordemetildiazepam 2 mg, flurazepam 15 mg, and no zolpidem) shows a clear misperception of sleep duration and quality. The recording shows normal nocturnal motor activity and sleep efficiency and duration. Note sleep period during the afternoon. He complained of sleeping not more than 3 hours each night. PSG on the third night: TST, 387 minutes; SE, 73.5; WASO, 122 minutes; number of awakenings, 17; SWS %, 1.3; PLMS index, 1.9. PSG, polysomnography; TST, total sleep time; SE, sleep efficiency; WASO, wake after sleep onset; SWS, slow wake sleep; PLMS, periodic limb movements in sleep.*

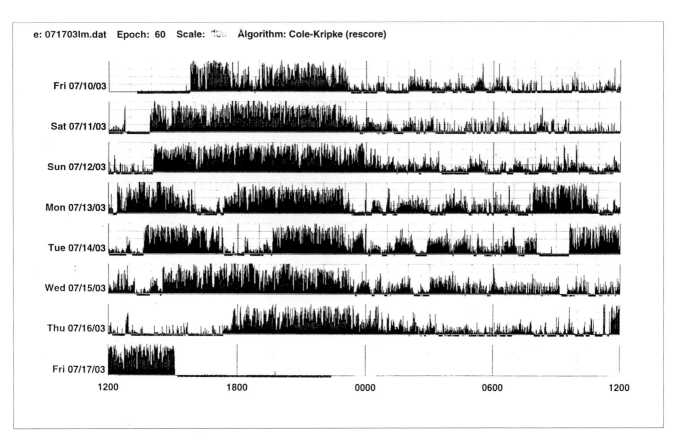

FIGURE 11B–3. *A case of chronic insomnia. This is a wrist actigraph from a 71-year-old woman with complaints of sleep onset and maintenance insomnia for 30 years. She has had many hypnotics over the years with temporary benefits. Despite increasing the doses, the effects wore off over the years. She has had many "street drugs" and now she takes cocaine every night at bedtime. She also complains of excessive daytime somnolence. She is single and has never worked outside the house in her life. She has been living on inherited money. The actigraph shows many periods of wakefulness (intrusion of black bars) during sleep period (white area) and intermittent brief periods of somnolence (intrusion of white areas into the black bars) during daytime wakefulness. This is an example of hypnotic-dependent and stimulant-dependent sleep disorder.*

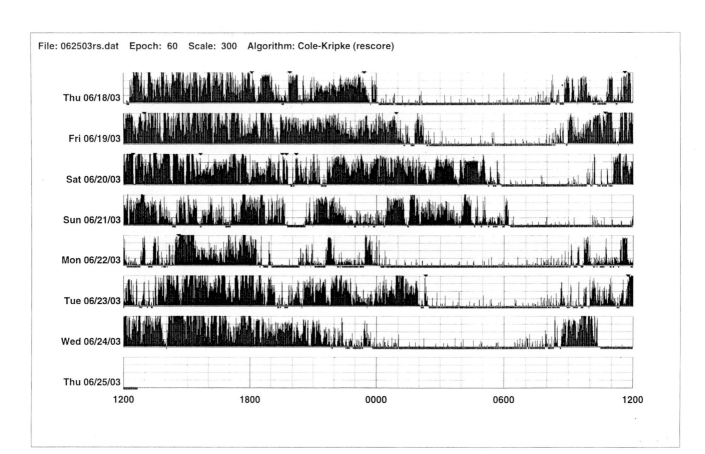

FIGURE 11B–4. *A patient with sleep-onset insomnia and sleep apnea. This wrist actigram is taken from a 31-year-old man who has been complaining of sleep-onset insomnia and excessive daytime sleepiness. The actigram shows irregular sleep onset (delayed) and irregular wake-up time. There are periods of somnolence (intrusion of white areas into black bars) during waking period (black bars). Overnight PSG study showed moderately severe upper airway obstructive sleep apnea (apnea-hypopnea index of 39.8) with oxygen desaturation.*

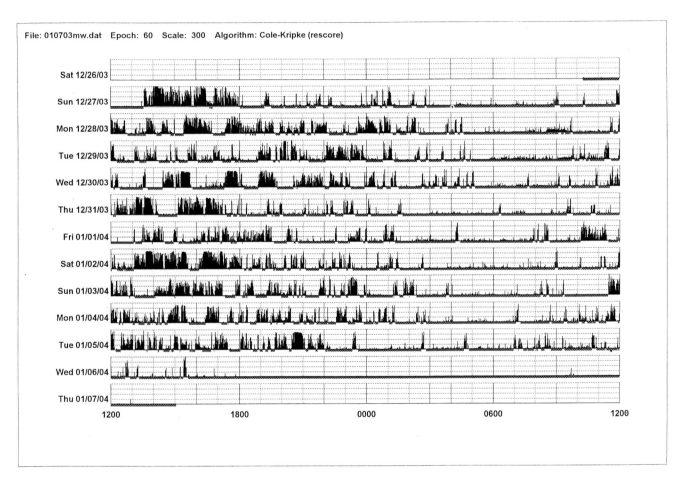

File: 010703mw.dat   Epoch: 60   Scale: 300   Algorithm: Cole-Kripke (rescore)

FIGURE 11B–5. *Parkinson's disease and sleep disorder (see also Chapter 10, Fig. 2). This is an actigraphic recording from the right ankle of a 67-year-old patient with idiopathic Parkinson's disease (Hoehn-Yahr stage 2: mild-moderate). The patient complains of insomnia and daytime hypersomnia. The actigram shows disorganization of sleep-wake schedule with irregular sleep-wake onset and offset, increased activity (black bars in the white area) during nighttime sleep, and many periods of daytime somnolence (intrusions of white areas within the black bars). Overnight PSG shows evidence of upper airway obstructive sleep apnea syndrome (apnea-hypopnea index = 25) and oxygen desaturation.*

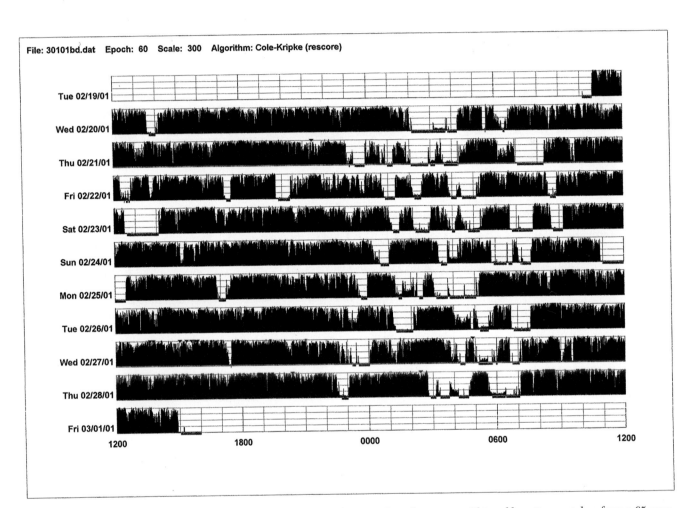

FIGURE 11B–6. *A patient with advanced Parkinson's disease and chronic sleep deprivation. This ankle actigram, taken from a 65-year-old man with advanced Parkinson's disease (Hoehn-Yahr stage 4), shows a complete disorganization of sleep-wake cycling. Between midnight and 7:00 AM (sleep period) there are frequent short episodes of sleepiness (white areas) and wakefulness (black bars). During waking period (7:00 AM to midnight) there are episodes of sleepiness (white areas intruding into black bars).*

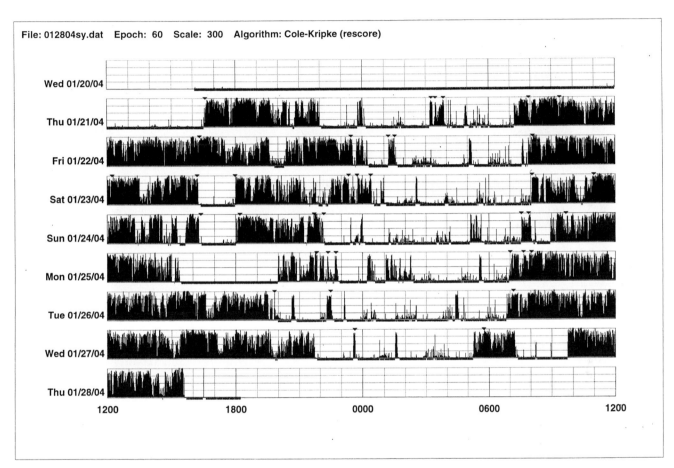

FIGURE 11B–7. *This wrist actigram is taken from a 52-year-old psychologist with type I Arnold-Chiari malformation, who presented with sleep difficulties because of repeated awakenings and excessive daytime somnolence for 15 years (see Chapter 10, Fig. 5). Overnight PSG showed REM hypoventilation. The actigram shows increased activity and periods of wakefulness during nighttime sleep (intrusions of white areas into black bars), irregular sleep onset at approximately 10:00 PM (day 1), midnight (day 2), 1:00 AM (day 3), 10:00 PM (day 4), 11:00 PM (day 5), 8:00 PM (day 6), and 10:00 PM (day 7), and variable wake-up times as indicated by sustained black bars. There are also many brief episodes of daytime somnolence (intrusions of white areas into black bars). On day 5 the actigraph was taken off during part of the waking period as indicated by abrupt onset of white area (no activity).*

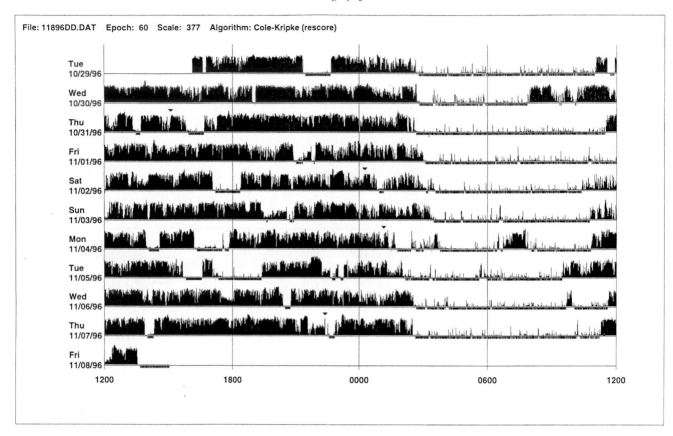

File: 11896DD.DAT   Epoch: 60   Scale: 377   Algorithm: Cole-Kripke (rescore)

FIGURE 11B–8. *Primary delayed sleep phase syndrome. This wrist actigraphic recording is taken from a 29-year-old man with a life-long history of delayed sleep onset and delayed wake-up time. The actigram shows his typical sleep period from 3:00 AM to 4:00 AM to 9:00 AM to noon (white areas). If he has to wake up early in the morning, he feels exhausted and sleepy all day. He feels fine if he is allowed to follow his own schedule. Melatonin at night did not help him. Morning bright light therapy was suggested but the patient declined.*

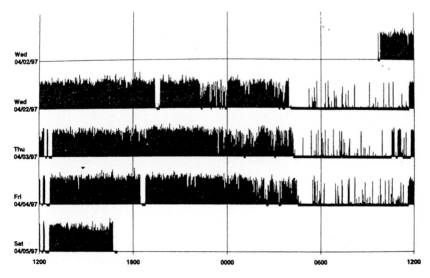

FIGURE 11B–9. *Posttraumatic delayed sleep phase syndrome. A 48-year-old man presented with sleep onset insomnia, cognitive difficulty, and chronic headache for 4 years following a car accident that resulted in multiple injuries including cerebral contusions and coma. The patient was very active before the accident, had no difficulty falling asleep at bedtime, and slept uninterrupted for 6 hours every night. The wrist actigram shows delayed sleep onset around 4:00 AM and wake-up time around noon. Chronotherapy was unsuccessful and the patient declined phototherapy.*

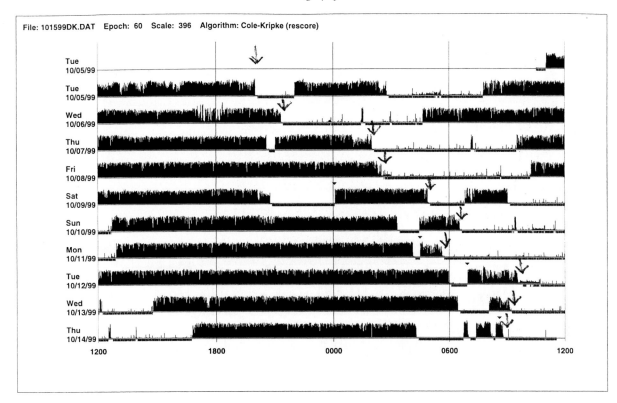

File: 101599DK.DAT   Epoch: 60   Scale: 396   Algorithm: Cole-Kripke (rescore)

FIGURE 11B–10. *Sleep-wake schedule disorder in a patient with acquired immunodeficiency syndrome (AIDS). This wrist actigram is taken from a 46-year-old man with AIDS. The patient presented with sleep difficulty due to inability to fall asleep and wake at desired bedtime and wake-up time. This 10-day recording shows disorganization of the sleep-wake schedule. There is a suggestion of non–24-hour (hypernychthemeral) syndrome with progressive delay of sleep onset (arrows) from day 1 to day 6, and again delayed sleep onset (arrows) from day 7 to day 10.*

even months; recording of 24-hour activities at all sites (home, work, or laboratories); usefulness in uncooperative and demented patients when laboratory PSG study is not possible; ability to conduct longitudinal studies during therapeutic intervention (behavioral or pharmacological treatment) in patients with insomnia; usefulness in sleep state misperception (see Figure 11B–2); ability to document delayed (see Figs. 11B–8 and 11B–9) or advanced sleep phase syndrome or non–24-hour circadian rhythm disorders (see Fig. 11B–10), although sleep logs may suggest such diagnosis; and documentation of excessive daytime sleepiness and repeated episodes of sleepiness (lasting more than a few minutes). Although not adequately standardized, actigraph may have a role in patients with restless legs syndrome and PLMS (Figures 11B–11 through 11B–14).

Disadvantages and Limitations of Actigraph Recordings

These include inability to diagnose sleep apnea, and to clarify the etiology of insomnia, overestimation of sleep when some insomniacs may lie down in bed for prolonged periods without moving; and inability to identify subjects who are feigning sleep problem and to discriminate types of movements such as PLMS from other body movements and provide any information about other physiological characteristics (e.g., EEG, EOG, respiration).

Lack of standardization of placement of the actigraph may be viewed as a pitfall. Most commonly the actigraph is placed on the nondominant side. Activity is somewhat different between the two sides with more activities being recorded from the dominant than the nondominant limbs. However, overall agreement for sleep period between the two sides is not significantly different when compared with the PSG data.

In conclusion, the actigraph is an inexpensive useful method for longitudinal assessment of sleep-wake pattern, can differentiate individuals with normal sleep pattern from those with disturbed sleep due to insomnia or sleep-disordered breathing, and can differentiate normal sleep from sleep-wake schedule disturbances by recording over prolonged period and longitudinal monitoring.

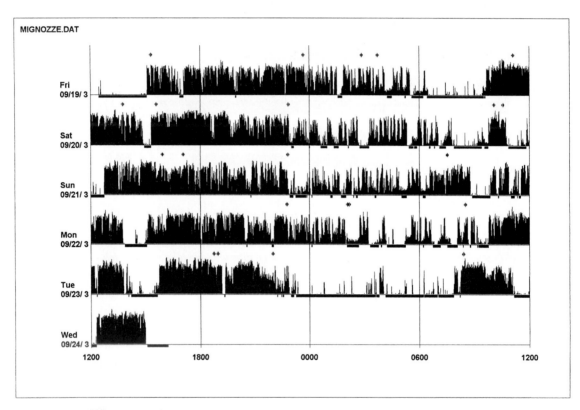

FIGURE 11B–11. *Actigraphy in RLS. A 50-year-old woman with a 2-year history of RLS and a recent increase in severity (International restless legs syndrome study group [IRLSSG] score of 32), of symptoms, and of difficulty in falling asleep (mean 2 hours). Her father and brother are both affected and she is unresponsive to benzodiazepines (lorazepam, clonazepam) and zolpidem. Five-nights monitoring with actigraphy at the calf, 4 days without treatment, and the fifth with dopamine agonist (pramipexole 0.125 mg 2 hours before bedtime). Actigraph shows an increase in nocturnal leg activity during the night (probably PLM) and an increase in number of awakenings in 4 nights. The last night shows very clear increase in sleep duration and quality with a decrease in nocturnal motor activity. PSG on the fourth night: total sleep time (TST), 356 minutes; sleep efficiency (SE), 56.1; wake after sleep onset (WASO), 224; 19 awakenings; PLMS index, 82.2.*

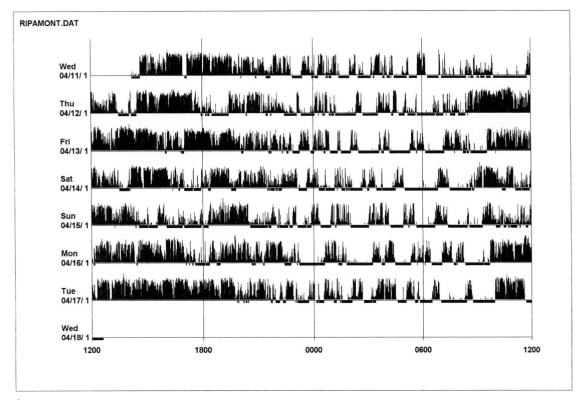

A

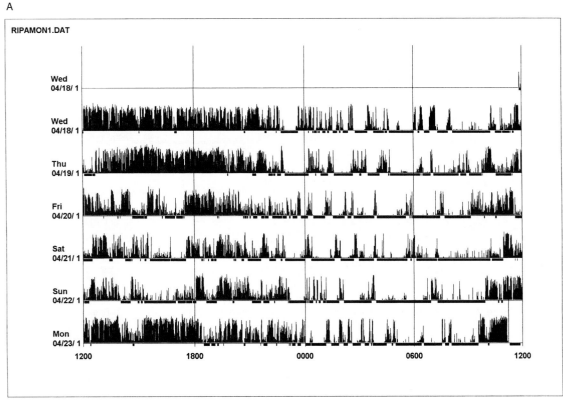

B

FIGURE 11B–12. *Actigraphy at the calf in RLS. A 62-year-old man with an insomnia associated with delayed sleep rhythm with depressive traits (dysthymia). For 6 years he has typical RLS symptoms with leg jerks during sleep (PLMS) and consequent awakenings, sometimes accompanied by nocturnal eating behaviors. Actigraphy monitoring for 3 weeks: 1st week baseline (**A**) (note an increase in number of awakenings with long awake and nocturnal motor activity); 2nd week (**B**) after a week of cabergoline (a long half-life dopamine agonist) 2 hours before bedtime, with an amelioration of motor activity (reduced) and a decrease in the number and duration of awakenings (sleep better after 6 AM); 3rd week (**C**) during the last week of cabergoline treatment with a clear reduction of nocturnal motor activity and an increase in estimated duration and sleep efficiency.*

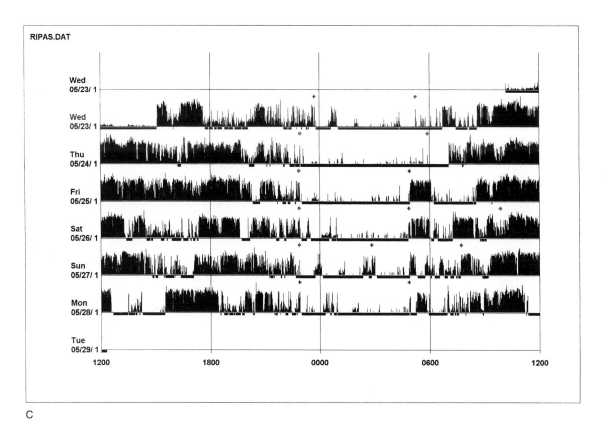

C

FIGURE 11B–12, cont'd.

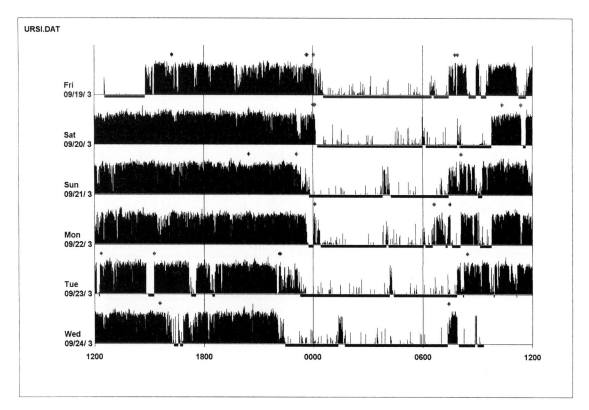

FIGURE 11B–13. *Actigraphy at the calf in RLS. A 59-year-old woman with a 9-year history of mild to moderate RLS (IRLSSG score of 22), positive familiar history for RLS, treated with lorazepam 1 mg for several years. One week of actigraphic monitoring at the calf with an increase in nocturnal motor activity in 4 out of 6 nights and reduced sleep efficiency in the same nights. PSG on the 4th night: TST, 345 minutes; SE, 92.7; WASO, 24 minutes; number of awakenings, 7; PLMS index, 4.9. Compare these findings with those in Figure 11B–11 (severe form of RLS).*

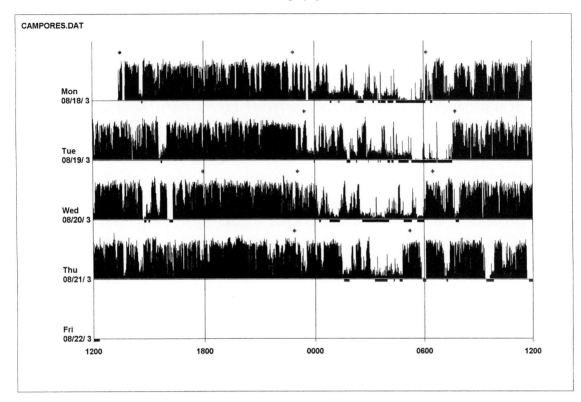

FIGURE 11B–14. *Actigraphy of severe RLS. A 60-year-old woman with familial idiopathic RLS since the age of 30 years but increased in severity for the past 6 years. Symptoms are prominent between 8 PM and 11 PM. Sometimes RLS also occurs during the day. Treatment with ropinirole (slight effect), L-dopa (augmentation after 2 months), and pramipexole as add-on to L-dopa for 2 months. Now RLS during the day and night with 3 to 4 hours (maximum) of sleep per night. IRLSSG score of 35. PSG (the 2nd night of actigraphic monitoring, during L-dopa 250 mg and pramipexole 0.50 mg treatment). TST, 421 minutes; SE, 81.3; WASO, 96 minutes; number of awakenings, 19; PLMS index, 108.*

BIBLIOGRAPHY

1. Sadeh A, Hauri PJ, Kripke DF, et al. The role of actigraphy in the evaluation of sleep disorders. *Sleep* 1995;18:288–302.
2. Standards of Practice Committee. An American Sleep Disorders Association report: Practice parameters for the use of actigraphy in the clinical assessment of sleep disorders. *Sleep* 1995;18:285–287.
3. Tyron WW. *Activity Measurement in Psychology and Medicine*. New York, NY: Plenum Press, 1991.

Chapter 11C

Recommendations for Practical Use of Pulse Transit Time as a Tool for Respiratory Effort Measurements and Microarousal Recognition

JEAN-LOUIS PÉPIN, DEBORAH DALE, JÉRÔME ARGOD,
AND PATRICK LÉVY

The identification and quantification of events characteristic of obstructive sleep apnea and related conditions is a task both laborious and time consuming. The standard polysomnography (PSG) provides the easy detection of events, such as apneas, using basic respiratory effort measurements (thoracic and abdominal movements) although the correct identification of hypopneas and upper airway resistance episodes (UAREs) requires sensitive and quantitative measures of inspiratory effort and airflow. For respiratory effort, methods such as esophageal pressure manometry (Pes) are expensive, cumbersome, invasive and require the investigations to be performed in a sleep laboratory. Thus the inadequacy of current equipment for the characterization of sleep-disordered breathing has led to the use of the promising new technique of pulse transit time (PTT) for measuring respiratory effort and detecting microarousals (MAs).

There is great uncertainty in the level of arousal from sleep sufficient enough to cause sleep fragmentation. Sforza *et al.* have demonstrated the existence of a hierarchical arousal response from autonomic arousals to bursts of delta activity and finally to alpha activity. Thus a predefined arousal stimulus produces, or not, a visible cortical arousal. It is possible that, in certain circumstances, only the first step of the hierarchical arousal response is identifiable, that is, autonomic bursts. Thus, one can choose to detect MAs only by using autonomic markers such as blood pressure (BP) rises, heart rate variations, or transient dips in PTT. It has been demonstrated that autonomic MAs are as sensitive as EEG for detecting sleep disruption.

In summary, the recording of PTT has provided us with a noninvasive method both specific and sensitive in the analysis of variations in sleep fragmentation and respiratory effort during the four stages of sleep. The signal used is not only commercially available, relatively economic to buy, and portable, but also produces a trace, which can be swiftly and efficiently analyzed. The purpose of this review is to describe in a very practical way the interpretation of the signal in clinical practice.

DEFINITION

The "true" PTT value is the time taken for the pulse wave to travel from the aortic valve to the periphery. The speed of this wave is directly proportional to the inverse of the systolic blood pressure. Thus a slight increase in blood pressure causes an increase in vascular tone, which in turn stiffens the arterial wall causing the PTT to shorten (a transient dip in the baseline of the PTT trace). Therefore, PTT is a sensitive tool for measuring transient changes in autonomic tone.

For practical reasons the opening of the aortic valve is assimilated to the R-wave on the electrocardiogram (ECG) (Figure 11C–1). There is a slight delay between the opening of the aortic valve and the R-wave, corresponding to the isometric contraction time (ICT) of the left

Grants: Clinical research funding: PHRC 1997, Ministère de la recherche (249/97). TYCO Healthcare ®

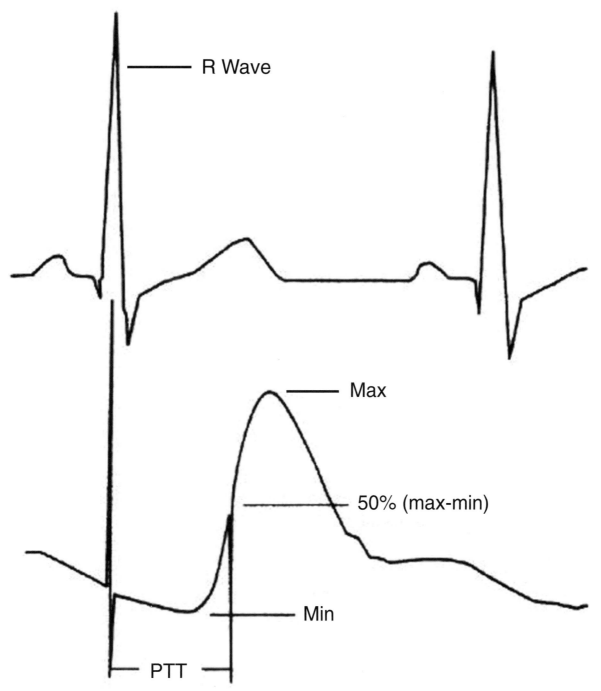

FIGURE 11C–1. *Schematic diagram demonstrating the calculation of PTT using the ECG R-wave as the starting point reference and the arterial pulse wave as the end point (Modified from Smith R, Argod J, Pépin J-L, Lévy P. Pulse transit time: An appraisal of potential clinical applications. Thorax 1999;54:452–457.)*

ventricle. Inspiratory effort causes a prolongation of ICT, which in turn amplifies the PTT signal.

METHOD OF MEASUREMENT

Measuring PTT needs to incorporate ECG leads for the recognition of the R-wave and oximetric photoplethysmography (usually a finger probe) to assess the arrival of the pulse wave in the periphery.

PTT is measured as the interval between the ECG R-wave and the subsequent arrival of the pulse wave at the finger or ear lobe (usually the point on the pulse waveform that is 50% the height of the maximum value). PTT is approximately 200 to 300 ms when using the finger probe and is measured to an accuracy of 2 ms. PTT values are available with every heartbeat and are typically oversampled at 5 hertz to ensure no values are neglected.

MICROAROUSAL RECOGNITION USING PULSE TRANSIT TIME
(Figures 11C–2 and 11C–3)

As PTT is inversely correlated with BP, a PTT MA is defined as a transient dip from the baseline.

PTT is able to assess sleep fragmentation due to non-respiratory causes, whether the cause be immediately obvious, as in the case of PLM (see Figure 11C–2) or not so obvious (see Figure 11C–3). The PTT arousal dip from baseline (ΔPTT) usually ranges from 8 to 15 ms (see Figure 11C–3A) in stage I-II and from 6 to 8 ms during stage III-IV, although there is no clear threshold from one patient to another. Therefore the exact measurement of ΔPTT (number of ms) is less important than the visual aspect, that is, an obvious transient dip from the baseline (see Figure 11C–3). A PTT arousal can be confirmed using corroborative signals such as ECG (increase in heart rate) or BP measurements when available (Figure 11C–4A) (surges in BP) such as "Finapres."

In order to accurately define a PTT arousal it should be noted that the shape of the area above the curve of the PTT is precisely related to the time course evolution of BP. For example, a pointed increase in BP (as seen using a Finapres) is associated with an abrupt transient dip in PTT and a rapid return to baseline presented as a relatively linear PTT trace under the curve (see Figure 11C–4B). In contrast, a more progressive increase in BP is related to a different pattern on the PTT (see Figure 11C–4C).

However, at present, when analyzing the trace, the amplitude of the dip should be the only tool used to define a PTT microarousal (i.e., between 8 ms and 15 ms

during stage II sleep). The area of the trace (this corresponds to the mirror picture of BP evolution during and after MAs) and the length of the dips are probably of importance but their significance remains unknown for the time being.

During REM sleep, variations in sympathetic activity are spontaneously very high and therefore the PTT baseline is highly variable. Thus, the recognition of true MAs during REM sleep is a lot less specific than in other sleep stages (Figure 11C–5).

RESPIRATORY EFFORT (Figures 11C–4, 11C–6, and 11C–7)

Esophageal pressure (Pes) is the "gold standard" measurement used to analyze changes in intrathoracic pressure and, due to the esophagus being anatomically situated in the thorax, it is highly effective at reflecting and quantifying variations in intrathoracic pressure. However this method of analysis is both invasive and frequently unaccepted by the patient.

PTT can be used to analyze respiratory effort and moreover is specific when defining certain respiratory events (hypopneas, UAREs and central events). The heart and large vessels are also located in the thoracic cavity and are thus affected by variations in thoracic volume and pressure. During inspiration, the volume of thoracic cavity increases, reducing thoracic pressure, which in turn reduces the compression of the heart and large vessels (vena cava and aorta), decreasing BP and slowing PTT (PTT dips from the baseline). The opposite is true for expiration. As the thoracic pressure increases, the heart is compressed and BP increases and PTT quickens.

Obstructive Events or Upper Airway Resistance Episodes (see Figure 11C–4)

Obstructive events or upper airway resistance episodes may be recorded on the demonstration of a steady increase in ΔPTT terminated by an MA and then the normalization of the trace (see Figure 11C–4, α1, α2, α3). This is observed simultaneously to a steady increase in Pes to a more negative value (or abdominal thoracic movements with or without a modification of the phase angle or paradoxical movements) terminated by an MA and the normalization of the trace (β1, β2, β3). The increases in ΔPTT are proportional to the increases in Pes. α1 and β1 demonstrate a smaller increase than α2 and β2, which demonstrate a smaller increase than α3 and β3. It is for this reason that PTT has a good specificity, sensitivity, and negative predictive value at differentiating obstructive from central apneas and hypopneas.

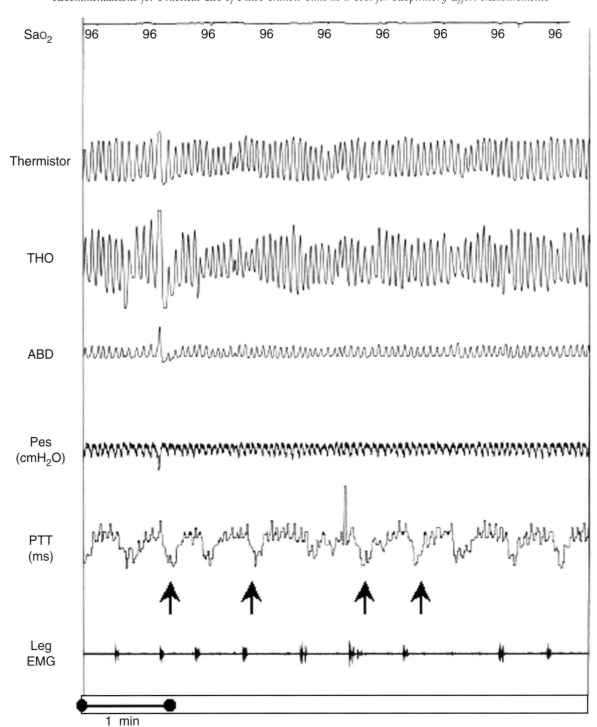

FIGURE 11C–2. *PLMs and associated nonrespiratory MAs. Arrows indicate the typical pattern associated with MAs occurring immediately after the leg movement. The leg movement induces an MA, which is associated with a rise in BP, which in turn induces a transient dip in PTT. The leg movement is probably underestimated by EMG but suspected by the concurrent MAs. Note that no significant respiratory events occur. Pes decreases slightly concurrently with MAs. This figure demonstrates oxygen saturation (SaO₂), thorax (THO), and abdominal (ABD) inductance plethysmography, esophageal pressure (Pes), pulse transit time (PTT), and leg electromyography (EMG).*

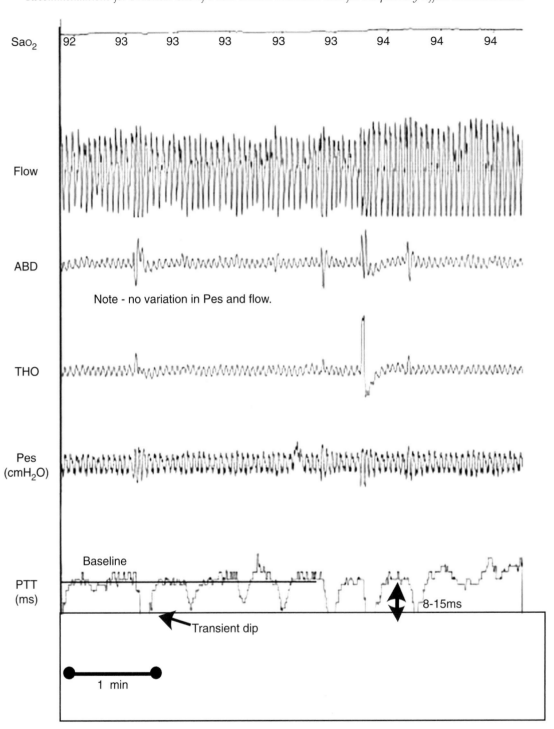

FIGURE 11C–3. *Nonrespiratory arousals detected by PTT. MAs were demonstrated by transient dips from the baseline of 8 to 15 ms during stage II despite no significant variations in Pes or flow. This patient exhibited pain-related MAs owing to rheumatoid arthritis. This figure demonstrates oxygen saturation (SaO₂), thorax (THO) and abdominal (ABD) inductance plethysmography, esophageal pressure (Pes), and pulse transit time (PTT).*

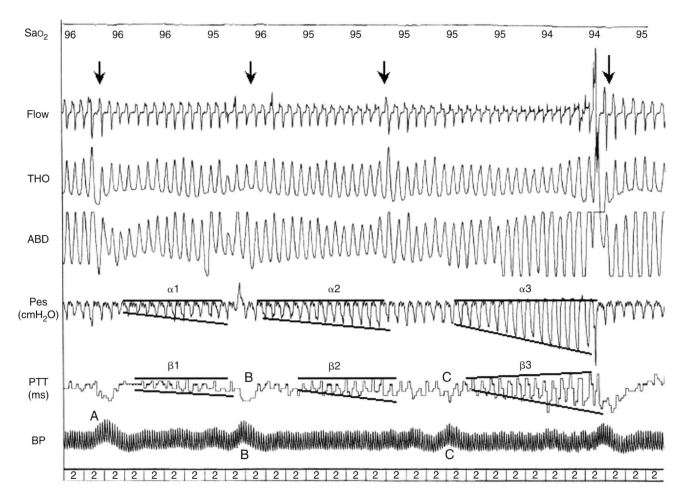

FIGURE 11C–4. *Classic obstructive hypopneas terminated by an MA. The increases in ΔPTT are proportional to the increases in Pes. α1 and β1 demonstrate a smaller increase than α2 and β2, which demonstrate a smaller increase than α3 and β3. The corroborative signal of BP measurements by Finapres (**A**) help confirm an arousal as the time course evolution of BP is precisely related to the shape of the area under the PTT curve. Note a pointed increase in BP (**B**) is associated with an abrupt transient dip in PTT and a rapid return to baseline presented as a relatively linear PTT trace under the curve. In contrast, a more progressive increase in BP (**C**) is related to a different pattern on the PTT. Arrows indicate the disappearance of inspiratory flow limitation occurring concurrently with the MA. This figure demonstrates oxygen saturation (SaO$_2$), thorax (THO) and abdominal (ABD) inductance plethysmography, esophageal pressure (Pes), pulse transit time (PTT), and blood pressure using a Finapres (BP). (From Pépin JL, et al. Chest 2005, in press)*

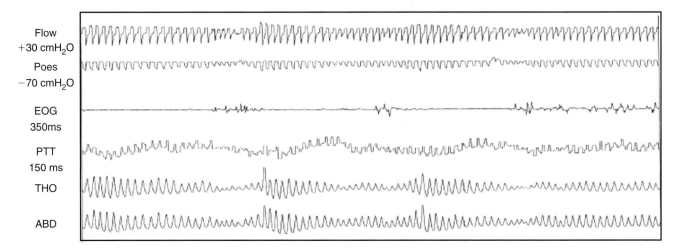

FIGURE 11C–5. *Difficulties of interpretation arising during REM sleep. Note the huge variation in PTT related to physiological fluctuations of autonomic tone during REM sleep. In these conditions, transient dips from the baseline related to MAs are more difficult to identify. REM sleep is associated with marked physiological variations in respiratory effort and airflow so identification of the classic pattern of PTT or Pes changes associated with obstructive respiratory events is more difficult. REM sleep is also associated with marked changes in BP and, as can be clearly seen, this causes the baseline PTT value to fluctuate, compounding further the interpretation difficulties. This figure demonstrates esophageal pressure (Poes), electrooculography (EOG), pulse transit time (PTT), and thorax (THO) and abdominal (ABD) inductance plethysmography. (From Smith R, et al. Thorax 1999;56:452–457)*

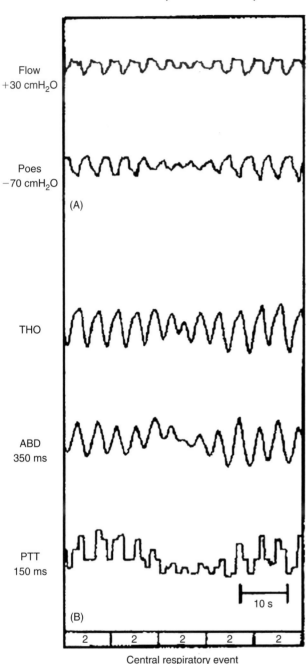

FIGURE 11C–6. *Central respiratory event. The reduction in esophageal pressure (**A**) is similar in fashion to ΔPTT reduction (**B**) during a central respiratory event.*
This figure demonstrates esophageal pressure (Poes), thorax (THO) and abdominal (ABD) inductance plethysmography, and pulse transit time (PTT). (From Argod, et al.)

Central Events (see Figures 11C–6 and 11C–7)

ΔPTT reduces (see Figure 11C–6B) during a central event in a similar fashion to the reduction in esophageal pressure (see Figure 11C–6A). It should be noted that central hypopneas can be judged on the reduction in amplitude of PTT and Pes proportional to the reduction in flow. Except for Pes, PTT is the only tool validated for the recognition of central hypopneas. This pattern of decreasing ΔPTT during a central event terminated by an MA is clearly demonstrated during Cheyne-Stokes respiration (see Figure 11C–7).

LIMITATIONS OF THE TECHNIQUE
(Figure 11C–8)

A drawback with this method of analyzing respiratory effort is that a PTT value is only available every QRS complex. Therefore measurements may fall on either side of the peak or trough of the BP oscillations associated with respiratory effort, which results in a tendency to under-sample. In certain conditions, the minimal value of Pes does not occur concurrently with a QRS complex. This is demonstrated in Figure 11C–8, wherein a given maximum PTT value may (see Figure 11C–8A) or may not (see Figure 11C–8B) correspond to the Pes nadir.

FALSE PULSE TRANSIT TIME VALUES
(Figure 11C–9)

Unfortunately, as the PTT measurements begin with the R-wave on the ECG, false values of PTT occur when the patient suffers from cardiac arrhythmia. Extrasystole produces acute variations in PTT despite the absence of a respiratory event or MA.

MEDICATION

Personal experience has demonstrated that the PTT trace is not generally affected by any cardiac medication such as beta blockers; however, there is no account of this in the literature.

CONCLUSIONS

In conclusion, the measurements of inspiratory swings by PTT can provide quantitative and qualitative information during non-REM sleep in patients suffering from sleep respiratory disorders, thus omitting the necessity for invasive or cumbersome methods of analysis, such as

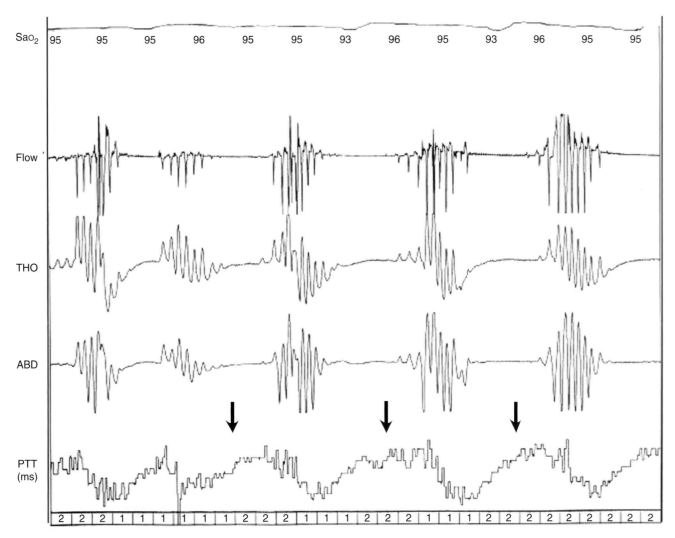

FIGURE 11C–7. *Cheyne-Stokes respiration. During Cheyne-Stokes respiration, a clear increase in ΔPTT may be observed during the crescendo pattern. In contrast, during central apneas (arrows), ΔPTT values are minimal. This figure demonstrates oxygen saturation (SaO₂), thorax (THO) and abdominal (ABD) inductance plethysmography, and pulse transit time (PTT).*

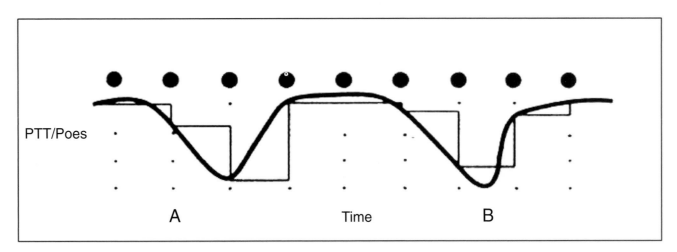

FIGURE 11C–8. *Under sampling error of PTT as reflected by Pes. The points represent each pulse. Breaths corresponding to a selected obstructive respiratory event are represented by a thick sinuous line (Poes) and a thin squared line (PTT). The trace shows two respiratory cycles of obstructive sleep apnea. The nadir of the first cycle happens to coincide with the arterial pulse wave and therefore the PTT amplitude is an accurate representation of the Pes swing (**A**). This second respiratory cycle does not coincide with the pulse wave and consequently the PTT swing underestimates the Pes swing (**B**). (From Smith, et al.)*

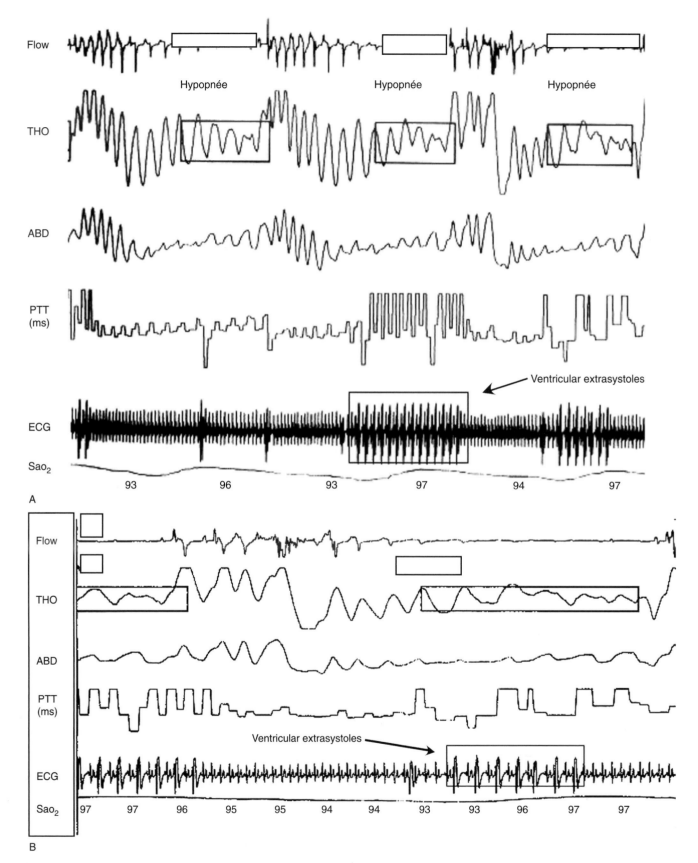

FIGURE 11C–9. *PTT artifacts as a consequence of ventricular extrasystoles. This trace was recorded during a period of frequent hypopneas. Note the false result produced by the PTT simultaneously to a group of extrasystoles occurring close together. This figure demonstrates thorax (THO) and abdominal (ABD) inductance plethysmography, pulse transit time (PTT), electrocardiography (ECG), and oxygen saturation (SAT).*

esophageal pressure. Both respiratory and nonrespiratory MAs can be identified with reasonable sensitivity and specificity using this technique. Care should be taken not to use this portable device on patients with cardiac arrhythmias due to resultant artifacts.

BIBLIOGRAPHY

1. Sforza E, Jouny C, Ibanez V. Cardiac activation during arousal in humans: Further evidence for hierarchy in the arousal response. *Clin Neurophysiol* 2000;111:1611–1619.
2. Pitson D, Stradling JR. Autonomic markers of arousal during sleep in patients undergoing investigation for obstructive sleep apnoea, their relationship to EEG arousals, respiratory events and subjective sleepiness. *J Sleep Res* 1998;7:53–59.
3. Pitson D, Sandell A, van den Hout R, Stradling JR. Use of pulse transit time as a measure of inspiratory effort in patients with obstructive sleep apnoea. *Eur Respir J* 1995;8:1 669–1674.
4. Argod J, Pépin J-L, Lévy P. Differentiating obstructive and central sleep respiratory events through pulse transit time. *Am J Respir Crit Care Med* 1998;158:1778–1783.
5. Argod J, Pépin J-L, Smith RP, Lévy P. Comparison of esophageal pressure with pulse transit time as a measure of respiratory effort for scoring obstructive nonapneic respiratory events. *Am J Respir Crit Care Med* 2000;162:87–93.
6. Smith R, Argod J, Pépin J-L, Lévy P. Pulse transit time: An appraisal of potential clinical applications. *Thorax* 1999;54: 452–457.
7. Pépin J-L, Delavie N, Pin I, Deschaux C, Argod J, Bost M, Lévy P. Pulse transit time improves detection of sleep respiratory events and microarousals in children. *Chest* 2005, in press.
8. Ali N, Davies RJ, Fleetham JA, Stradling JR. Periodic movements of the leg during sleep associated with rises in systemic blood pressure. *Sleep* 1991;14:163–165.

Chapter 11D

The Cyclic Alternating Pattern

Mario Giovanni Terzano, Liborio Parrino, and Arianna Smerieri

PHASIC EVENTS OF NON–RAPID EYE MOVEMENT SLEEP

Sleep staging is based on the application of rules according to which epochs of 20 or 30 seconds are assigned a score that most appropriately characterizes the prevalent pattern occurring during that interval. In the last 35 years, this scoring system has been a methodologic landmark allowing a universal approach to and a standardized training for the analysis of human sleep. There is, however, a huge body of evidence that indicates sleep stages as non-homogeneous states, which contain a mass of neurophysiological phenomena that adjust continuously the restless flow of cerebral activities. Indeed, sleep hosts several phasic events, which play a dynamic role in the structural organization of sleep modulating autonomic and motor correlates (Figures 11D–1 and 11D–2). When these phasic events appear in a periodic manner, the resulting EEG feature is called *cyclic alternating pattern,* or *CAP.*

DEFINITION OF CAP

CAP is a periodic EEG activity of NREM sleep characterized by the repetitive occurrence of phasic events described in Figures 11D–1 and 11D–2. CAP is composed of sequences of CAP cycles. A CAP cycle is composed of a phase A and the following phase B (Figure 11D–3). A CAP sequence begins with a phase A and ends with a phase B. Each phase of CAP is 2 to 60 seconds in duration.

CAP is a global EEG phenomenon involving extensive cortical areas. Under normal conditions, CAP does not occur in REM sleep where the phase A features, consisting mainly of rapid low-amplitude rhythms, are separated by a mean interval of 3 to 4 minutes.

DEFINITION OF NON-CAP

The absence of CAP for more than 60 seconds is scored as non-CAP. An isolated phase A, that is, preceded or followed by another phase A by more than 60 seconds, is classified as non-CAP (Figure 11D–4).

Phase A Subtypes (Figure 11D–5)

Phase A activities can be classified into three subtypes. Subtype classification is based on the reciprocal proportion of high-voltage slow waves (EEG synchrony) and low-amplitude fast rhythms (EEG desynchrony) throughout the entire phase A duration. The three phase A subtypes are as follows:

Subtype A1. EEG synchrony is the predominant activity. If present, EEG desynchrony occupies less than 20 percent of the entire phase A duration. Subtypes A1 include delta bursts, K complex sequences, vertex sharp transients, and polyphasic bursts (clusters of high-voltage delta waves, intermixed with theta, alpha, or beta rhythms) with less than 20 percent of EEG desynchrony.

Subtype A2. The EEG activity is a mixture of slow and fast rhythms with 20 percent to 50 percent of phase A occupied by EEG desynchrony. Subtype A2 specimens include polyphasic bursts with more than 20 percent but less than 50 percent of EEG desynchrony.

Phasic events	**EEG characteristics and neurophysiological significance**
Intermittent alpha rhythm 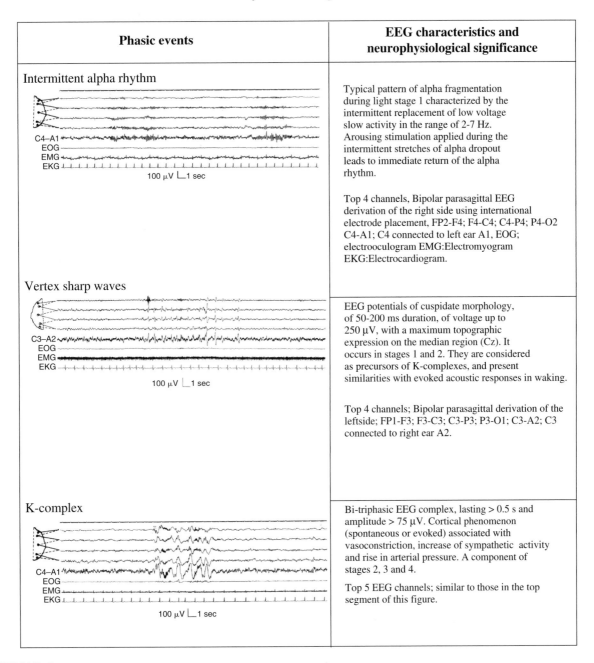	Typical pattern of alpha fragmentation during light stage 1 characterized by the intermittent replacement of low voltage slow activity in the range of 2-7 Hz. Arousing stimulation applied during the intermittent stretches of alpha dropout leads to immediate return of the alpha rhythm. Top 4 channels, Bipolar parasagittal EEG derivation of the right side using international electrode placement, FP2-F4; F4-C4; C4-P4; P4-O2 C4-A1; C4 connected to left ear A1, EOG; electrooculogram EMG:Electromyogram EKG:Electrocardiogram.
Vertex sharp waves	EEG potentials of cuspidate morphology, of 50-200 ms duration, of voltage up to 250 µV, with a maximum topographic expression on the median region (Cz). It occurs in stages 1 and 2. They are considered as precursors of K-complexes, and present similarities with evoked acoustic responses in waking. Top 4 channels; Bipolar parasagittal derivation of the leftside; FP1-F3; F3-C3; C3-P3; P3-O1; C3-A2; C3 connected to right ear A2.
K-complex	Bi-triphasic EEG complex, lasting > 0.5 s and amplitude > 75 µV. Cortical phenomenon (spontaneous or evoked) associated with vasoconstriction, increase of sympathetic activity and rise in arterial pressure. A component of stages 2, 3 and 4. Top 5 EEG channels; similar to those in the top segment of this figure.

FIGURE 11D–1.

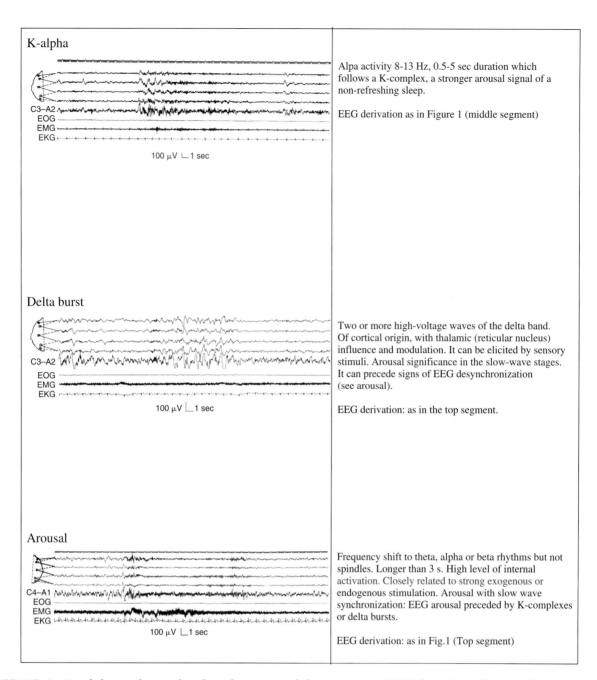

K-alpha

C3–A2
EOG
EMG
EKG

100 μV ⌞1 sec

Alpa activity 8-13 Hz, 0.5-5 sec duration which follows a K-complex, a stronger arousal signal of a non-refreshing sleep.

EEG derivation as in Figure 1 (middle segment)

Delta burst

C3–A2
EOG
EMG
EKG

100 μV ⌞1 sec

Two or more high-voltage waves of the delta band. Of cortical origin, with thalamic (reticular nucleus) influence and modulation. It can be elicited by sensory stimuli. Arousal significance in the slow-wave stages. It can precede signs of EEG desynchronization (see arousal).

EEG derivation: as in the top segment.

Arousal

C4–A1
EOG
EMG
EKG

100 μV ⌞1 sec

Frequency shift to theta, alpha or beta rhythms but not spindles. Longer than 3 s. High level of internal activation. Closely related to strong exogenous or endogenous stimulation. Arousal with slow wave synchronization: EEG arousal preceded by K-complexes or delta bursts.

EEG derivation: as in Fig.1 (Top segment)

FIGURE 11D–2. *Morphology and neurophysiological properties of phasic events in NREM sleep. EOG, Electrooculogram; EMG, electromyogram; EKG, electrocardiogram.*

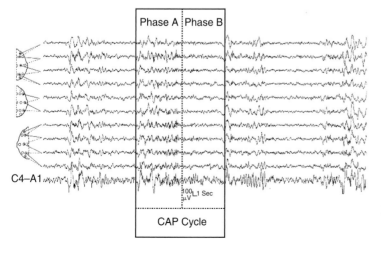

Phase A | Phase B

C4–A1

100 μV⌞1 Sec

CAP Cycle

FIGURE 11D–3. *A CAP sequence in stage II sleep with a highlighted CAP cycle (black box). The CAP cycle is defined by a phase A (aggregate of phasic events) and by a phase B (interval between two successive A phases). Bipolar EEG derivations using international electrode placement; channels 1-6 from top: FP$_2$-F4; F4-C4; C4-P4; P4-O$_2$; F8-T4; T4-T6; Channels 7-11 from top: FP$_1$-F3; F3-C3; C3-P3; P3-O$_1$; C4-A1.*

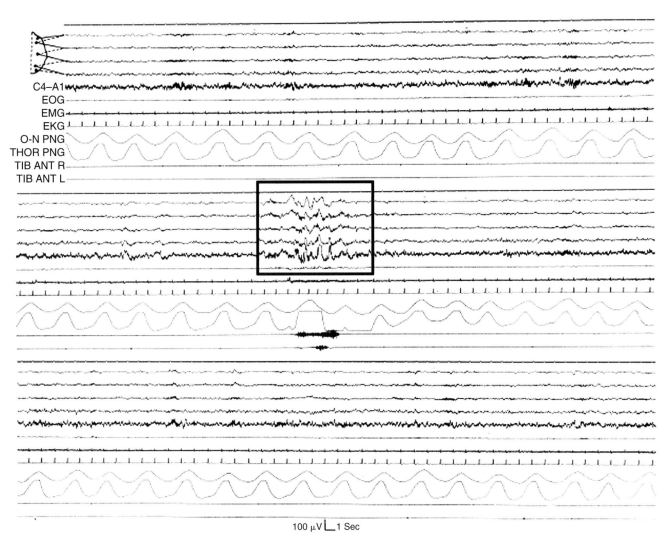

FIGURE 11D–4. *Long stretch of stage II sleep characterized by a stable EEG background (non-CAP) with an isolated phase A* (dotted line box). EOG, *Electrooculogram;* EMG, *electromyogram;* EKG, *electrocardiogram;* O-N PNG, *oronasal airflow;* THOR-PNG, *thoracic pneumogram;* TIB ANT R, *right anterior tibialis muscle;* TIB ANT L, *left anterior tibialis muscle. EEG channel derivations as in Figure 11D–1 (top segment).*

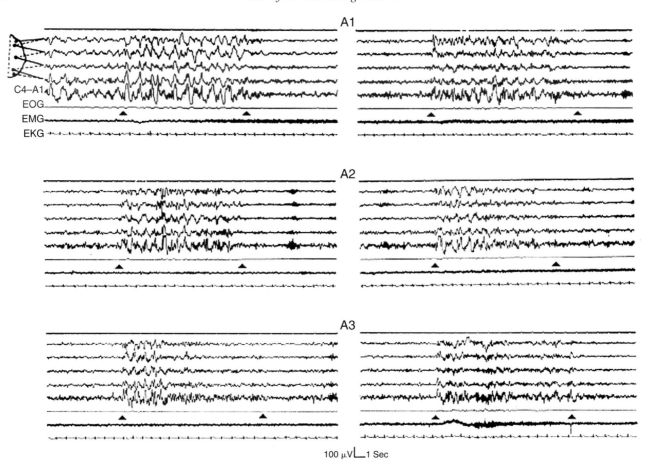

FIGURE 11D–5. *Six specimens of phase A subtypes confined within black triangles. The A1 subtypes (top) are dominated by high-voltage low-frequency EEG frequencies. The A3 subtypes (bottom) contain a prevalent amount of low-voltage high-frequency EEG activities. The A2 subtypes (middle) are characterized by a balanced mixture of EEG synchrony and EEG desynchrony. Notice that in most cases the high-voltage low-frequency EEG activities precede the onset of the fast low-amplitude rhythms. EOG, Electrooculogram; EMG, electromyogram; EKG, electrocardiogram. EEG derivations as in Figure 11D–1 (top segment).*

Subtype A3. The EEG activity is predominantly rapid low-voltage rhythms with more than 50 percent of phase A occupied by EEG desynchrony. Subtype A3 specimens include K-alpha, EEG arousals, and polyphasic bursts with more than 50 percent of EEG desynchrony. A movement artifact within a CAP sequence is also classified as subtype A3.

The majority of EEG arousals occurring in NREM sleep (87 percent) are inserted within the unstable background offered by CAP, where arousals basically coincide with a phase A2 or A3.

The regular oscillations that accompany the transition from light sleep to deep stable sleep are basically expressed by the A1 subtypes (Figure 11D–6), while the breakdown of deep sleep and the introduction of REM sleep are mostly associated with subtypes A2 (Figure 11D–7) or A3 of CAP.

CAP AND NONRESTORATIVE SLEEP

CAP is a marker of sleep instability swinging between poles of greater arousal (phase A) and lesser arousal (phase B). CAP is increased by perturbing conditions such as acoustic stimulation (Figure 11D–8) and correlates with the subjective sensation of nonrestorative sleep. The amount of CAP and the representation of phase A subtypes can be deeply influenced in the different sleep disorders.

Primary insomnia is characterized by an exaggeration of the physiological amounts of CAP, which is also increased

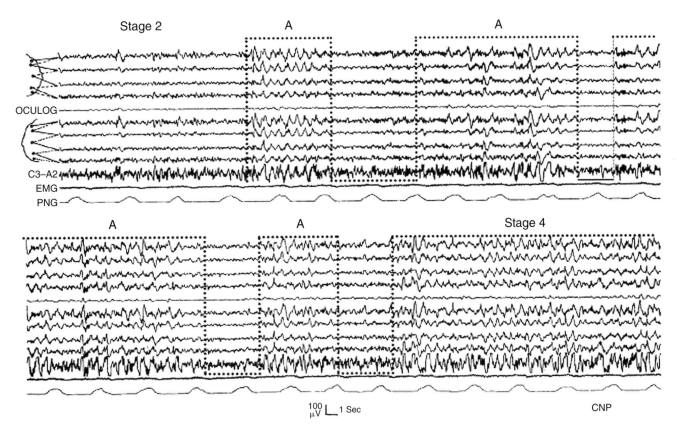

FIGURE 11D–6. *Transition from stage II to stage IV accompanied and smoothed by a CAP sequence composed of phase A1 subtypes (bottom-open dotted boxes). OCULOG, Oculogram; EMG, electromyogram; PNG, pneumogram. EEG derivations as in Figure 11D–1 (top and middle segments).*

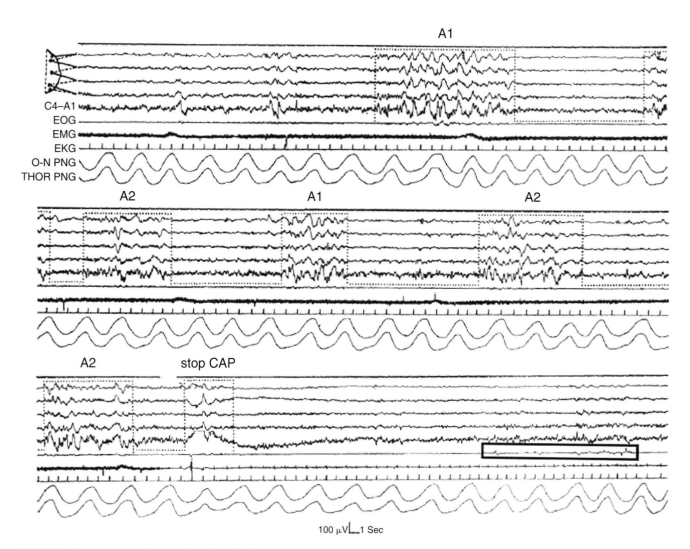

100 μV⌊__1 Sec

FIGURE 11D–7. *Onset of REM sleep heralded by a CAP sequence in stage II. The transition to REM sleep is defined by the abrupt drop of muscle tone, the interruption of the CAP sequence (stop CAP), and the occurrence of a burst of REMs (black box). EOG, Electrooculogram; EMG, electromyogram; EKG, electrocardiogram; O-N PNG, oronasal airflow; THOR-PNG, thoracic pneumogram. EEG channel derivations as in Figure 11D–1 (top segment).*

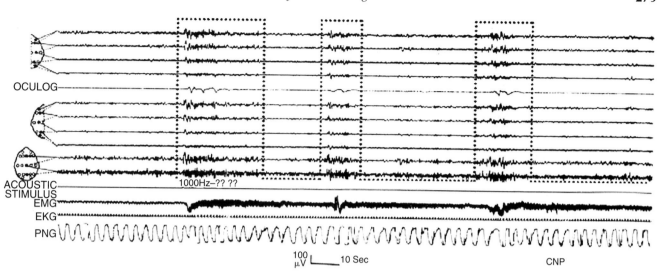

FIGURE 11D–8. *A rapid shift from stage II non-CAP (left side of the trace) to stage II CAP, induced by a single acoustic stimulus. The A phases of the CAP (bottom-open dotted boxes) are associated with a reinforcement of muscle tone.*
EEG channel derivations: channels 1-4 as in Figure 11D–1 (top segment); channels 6-9 as in Figure 11D–1 (middle segment); channels 10-11: Fz-Cz; Cz-Pz. OCULOG, Oculogram; EMG, electromyogram; EKG, electrocardiogram; PNG, pneumogram.

in psychiatric-related insomnia (major depression, dysthymia), in primary generalized epilepsy, in PLM disorders, in sleep apnea syndrome, and when sleep is recovered in the morning hours.

Sleep-promoting medication reduces the excessive amount of CAP in both primary and secondary insomnia.

THE CAP PHASES AND SLEEP DISORDERS

The phase A of CAP is associated with an activation of cardiac and autonomic functions (Figure 11D–9). It reflects a gate through which pathological events are more likely to occur. A gating effect has been established for interictal EEG bursts (Figure 11D–10), epileptic motor events (Figure 11D–11), periodic limb movements (Figure 11D–12), sleep bruxism (Figure 11D–13), and post-apnea respiratory recovery (Figure 11D–14).

Phase B exerts a powerful inhibition on generalized (see Figure 11D–10) and focal lesional (Figure 11D–15) EEG discharges, on myoclonic jerks (see Figure 11D–12), and on sleep bruxism (see Figure 11D–13). Phase B triggers breathing interruption in sleep apnea syndrome (see Figure 11D–14).

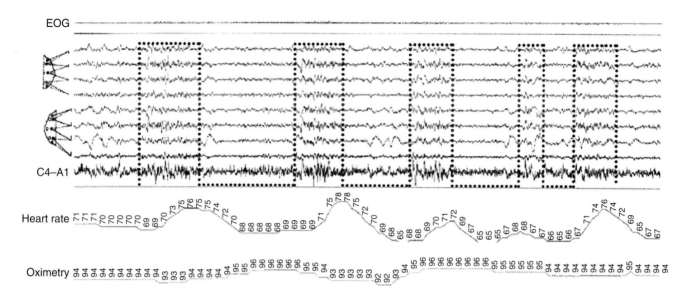

FIGURE 11D–9. *CAP sequence coupled with on-line monitoring of heart rate and oximetry (patient with PLM and mild SDB). Notice the close time-relation between the onset of the A phases (bottom-open dotted boxes) and the acceleration of cardiac activity (in parallel with the delayed saturation fall). EOG, Electrooculogram. Top 4 EEG channels as in Figure 11D–1 (top segment); EEG channels 5-8 as in Figure 11D–1 (middle segment).*

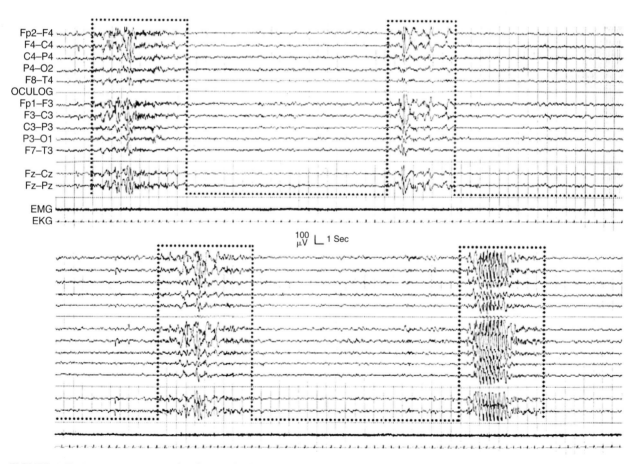

FIGURE 11D–10. *Primary generalized EEG discharges recurring in clusters boxed within the A phases of a CAP sequence. Notice the absence of EEG bursts during phase B. EMG, Electromyogram; EKG, electrocardiogram; OCULOG, oculogram.*

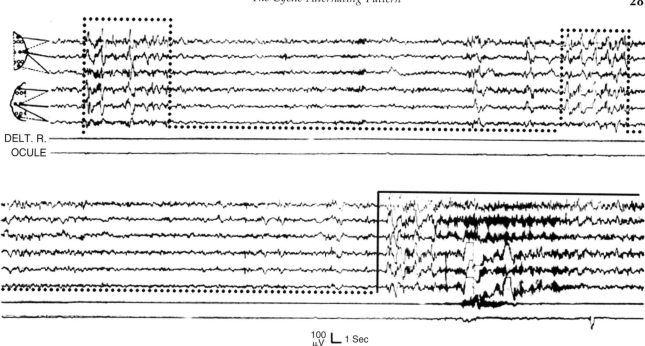

DELT. R.

OCULE

$$100 \ \mu V \ \llcorner \ 1 \ Sec$$

FIGURE 11D–11. *Nocturnal motor seizure* (black continuous outline) *in stage II sleep preceded by a CAP sequence with A phases* (dotted bottom-open boxes) *containing interictal EEG abnormalities.* DELT R, *right deltoid muscle;* OCULO, *oculogram. EEG channels 1-6 from the top: FP_2-C_4, FP_2-T_4, T_4-O_2; FP_1-C_3, FP_1-T_3, T_3-O_1.*

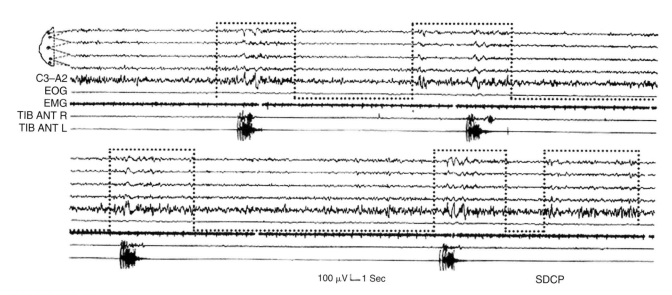

C3–A2
EOG
EMG
TIB ANT R
TIB ANT L

100 μV ⌊—1 Sec   SDCP

FIGURE 11D–12. *A CAP sequence associated with periodic limb jerks which occur in close relation with the A phases of CAP (and never during the B phases). The motor phenomena coincide with or follow the onset of the A phases* (dotted bottom-open boxes). *Notice that the last phase A is not associated with any muscle event.* EOG, *Electrooculogram;* EMG, *electromyogram;* TIB ANT R, *right anterior tibialis muscle;* TIB ANT L, *left anterior tibialis muscle. EEG channel derivations as in Figure 11D–1 (middle segment).*

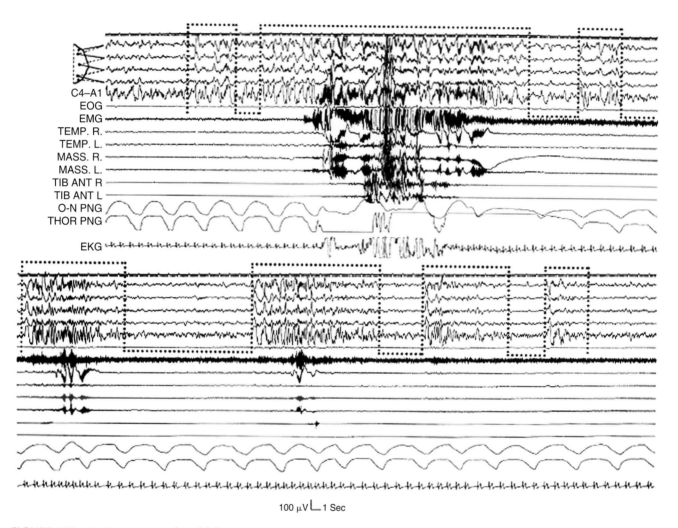

100 μV ⌐ 1 Sec

FIGURE 11D–13. *Bruxism episodes of different intensities associated with the recurring A phases of CAP (dotted bottom-open boxes) in the transition from deep to light NREM sleep. Motor events and cardiorespiratory activation occur after the onset of the A phases dominated by desynchronized EEG patterns (especially A3 subtypes). EOG, Electrooculogram; EMG, electromyogram; TEMP. R, right temporalis muscle; TEMP. L, left temporalis muscle; MASS. R, right masseter muscle; MASS. L, left masseter muscle; TIB ANT R, right anterior tibialis muscle; TIB ANT L, left anterior tibialis muscle; O-N PNG, oronasal airflow; THOR-PNG, thoracic pneumogram; EKG, electrocardiogram. EEG channel derivations as in Figure 11D–1 (top segment).*

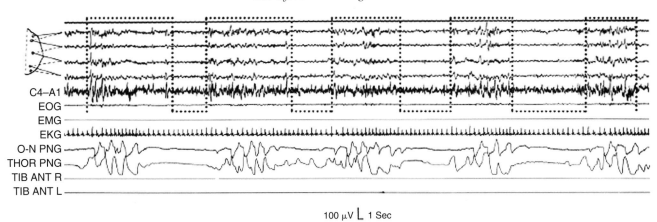

100 µV L 1 Sec

FIGURE 11D–14. *Repetitive sequence of different respiratory events (obstructive, mixed, and central), which always occur during a phase B and are interrupted by a phase A (dotted bottom-open boxes). EOG, electrooculogram; EMG, electromyogram; EKG, electrocardiogram; O-N PNG, oronasal airflow; THOR-PNG, thoracic pneumogram; TIB ANT R, right anterior tibialis muscle; TIB ANT L, left anterior tibialis muscle. EEG channel derivations as in Figure 11D–1 (top segment).*

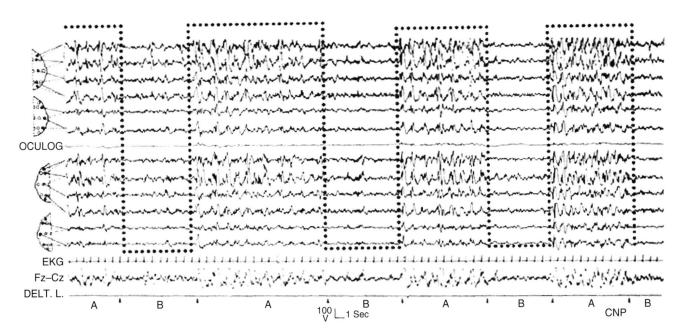

FIGURE 11D–15. *Secondary generalization of interictal EEG discharges (right anterior cerebral focus) modulated by the A phases of CAP (dotted bottom-open boxes). OCULOG, Oculogram; EKG, electrocardiogram; DELT L, left deltoid muscle. EEG channel derivations as in Figure 11D–3. (Channels 1–6 and 8–11 from top); Channels 12, 13 from top: F7-T3; T3-T5.*

BIBLIOGRAPHY

Halasz P, Terzano MG, Parrino L, Bodizs R. The nature of arousal in sleep. *J Sleep Res* 2004;13:1–23.

Hirshkowitz M. Standing on the shoulders of giants: The Standardized Sleep Manual after 30 years. *Sleep Med Rev* 2000;4:169–179.

Parrino L, Smerieri A, Spaggiari MC, Terzano MG. Cyclic alternating pattern (CAP) and epilepsy during sleep: How a physiological rhythm modulates a pathological event. *Clin Neurophysiol* 2000;111(Suppl 2):S39–S46.

Parrino L, Boselli M, Spaggiari MC, Smerieri A, Terzano MG. Cyclic alternating pattern (CAP) in normal sleep: Polysomnographic parameters in different age groups. *Electroenceph Clin Neurophysiol* 1998;107:439–450.

Rechtschaffen A, Kales A, eds. *A Manual of Standardized Terminology, Techniques and Scoring System for Sleep Stages of Human Subjects.* Washington, DC: U.S. Government Printing Office, NIH Publication No. 204, 1968.

Terzano MG, Mancia D, Salati MR, Costani G, Decembrino A, Parrino L. The cyclic alternating pattern as a physiologic component of normal NREM sleep. *Sleep* 1985;8:137–145.

Terzano MG, Parrino L. Clinical applications of cyclic alternating pattern. *Physiol Behav* 1993;54:807–813.

Terzano, MG, Parrino L. Origin and significance of the cyclic alternating pattern (CAP). *Sleep Med Rev* 2000;4:101–123.

Terzano MG, Parrino L, Smerieri A, et al. Atlas, rules and recording techniques for the scoring of cyclic alternating pattern (CAP) in human sleep. *Sleep Med* 2001;2;537–553.

Terzano MG, Parrino L, Smerieri A, et al. Atlas, rules, and recording techniques for the scoring of cyclic alternating pattern (CAP) in human sleep: Consensus report. *Sleep Med* 2002;3:187–199.

Terzano MG, Parrino L, Spaggiari MC, Palomba V, Rossi M, Smerieri A. CAP variables and arousals as sleep electroencephalogram markers for primary insomnia. *Clin Neurophysiol* 2003;114:1715–1723.

Chapter 11E

Peripheral Arterial Tonometry

STEPHEN D. PITTMAN AND ROBERT J. THOMAS

Disclosure Statement: Stephen Pittman has received research support from Itamar Medical Ltd., Respironics Inc., WideMED Ltd., and the Alfred Mann Foundation; served as a remunerated consultant for Itamar Medical Ltd., the developer of the PAT technology; and is currently employed by Respironics, Inc.

Transient arousal from sleep is associated with increased bursts of sympathetic nerve activity (SNA) in normal adults. This leads to increased heart rate and blood pressure as well as peripheral vasoconstriction. Sleep fragmentation resulting from frequent arousals has been implicated in daytime impairment of cognitive and psychomotor performance based on investigation of experimental sleep fragmentation in healthy adults. Thus, quantifying brief arousals may be important for the assessment of sleep quality, independent of alternative sleep quality measures such as sleep latency, sleep efficiency, and wake after sleep onset. This response is nonspecific, not dependent on the cause of arousal, but in the appropriate clinical context (such as obesity, heart failure) or with the appropriate phase-linked associations (such as oxygen desaturations), disease states may be predicted.

THEORETICAL PRINCIPLES

Exposure to cold results in reflex digital vasoconstriction whereas heat exposure produces vasodilatation. The digit vascular bed has a dense network of arteriovenous anastomoses that allow considerable variation in skin blood flow. The finger pulse wave amplitude decreases with brachial artery infusion of norepinephrine (α-receptor agonist) during wakefulness in a dose-dependent manner. The sympathetic discharges associated with recurrent transient arousals from sleep induce recurrent cycles of digital vasoconstriction, providing an alternative method to EEG for arousal detection in those with a functioning sympathetic nervous system. The peripheral arterial tonometry (PAT) signal is attenuated in response to obstructive breathing during sleep. The signal's attenuation at the termination of apnea has been shown to be reduced in a dose-dependent manner using the α-receptor antagonist phentolamine (Figure 11E–1). Thus, the finger pulse wave amplitude reflecting digital vasoconstriction is α-adrenoreceptor mediated. O'Donnell and coworkers evaluated the effects of experimental airflow limitation and arousal on digital vascular tone in human subjects with OSA using PAT signal recordings. Subjects were maintained at a therapeutic positive airway pressure and then nasal positive pressure was reduced over a range of pressures for three to five breaths during NREM sleep as shown in Figure 11E–2. EEG arousal in response to airflow obstruction attenuated the PAT signal more (23.3 percent reduction) than in the absence of arousal (7.7 percent reduction). This suggests acute digital vasoconstriction is accentuated in the presence of EEG arousal.

The signal detected has no overlap with PTT (Chapter 11 C), but the basic target is identical—the identification of bursts of sympathetic activity. Similar information may be obtained from the recording of muscle or skin sympathetic nerve activity, skin blood flow, and heart rate variability. However, sympathetic innervation and discharge patterns have regional differences, and not all activators result in an increased autonomic flow to all targets.

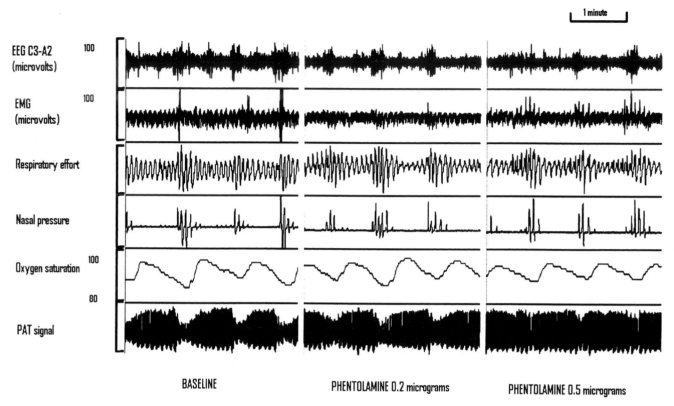

EEG C3-A2 (microvolts)   100

EMG (microvolts)   100

Respiratory effort

Nasal pressure

Oxygen saturation   100 / 80

PAT signal

BASELINE   PHENTOLAMINE 0.2 micrograms   PHENTOLAMINE 0.5 micrograms

1 minute

FIGURE 11E–1. *PAT signal in sleep-disordered breathing. The cyclic attenuation of the PAT signal is seen to occur phase-locked with respiratory recovery* (left panel). *Low-dose phentolamine infusion attenuates* (middle panel), *and higher dose eliminates, digital vasoconstriction. Thus, normal sympathetic function and peripheral innervation is necessary to detect the signal, which is a limitation in patients with severe autonomic neuropathy. (From Zou et al, Sleep 2004;27:487 Fig. 1)*

SUMMARY OF TECHNOLOGY

PAT is a plethysmographic technique that uses a finger-mounted pneumo-optical sensor for the continuous measurement of the digital arterial pulse wave volume. The finger sensor applies a uniform, subdiastolic pressure field to the distal two thirds of the finger and fingertip that (1) clamps the probe to the finger, (2) facilitates the unloading of arterial wall tension, which increases the dynamic range of the PAT signal, and (3) prevents distal venous pooling and distention to avoid the induction of venoarterial-mediated vasoconstriction. Thus, attenuation of the PAT signal reflects digital vasoconstriction, increased SNA, and can serve as a marker for arousal from sleep. It has also been reported that the PAT signal can detect the peripheral vasoconstriction associated with REM sleep.

CLINICAL APPLICATIONS

A number of recent reports have investigated automated analysis of the PAT signal (attenuation and pulse rate),

oxyhemoglobin saturation, and wrist actigraphy for detecting episodes of obstructive sleep disordered breathing. One investigation included standard PSG laboratory studies to define the severity of OSA and concurrent PAT technology studies in the laboratory and home studies on a separate night with only the PAT technology. Based on the likelihood ratios for the home study results, the system yielded a very large increase (LR+ = 8) in the probability of having moderate-severe OSA (RDI = 15 events/hour) and a large reduction (LR– = 0.05, 95% CI: 0.01–0.31) in the probability of having moderate-severe OSA. Investigations by Pillar and coworkers assessed automated PAT signal detection of arousals and then validated their technique against ASDA defined arousals using concurrent laboratory PSG recordings. Using the Watch-PAT device for the detection of OSA, there was a significant correlation (R = 0.87, p < 0.001) between ASDA defined arousals derived from the PSG and autonomic arousals detected with the PAT signal. The sensitivity and specificity of PAT in detecting patients with at least 20 arousals per hour of sleep were 0.80 and 0.79, respectively. However, arousals from sleep demonstrate

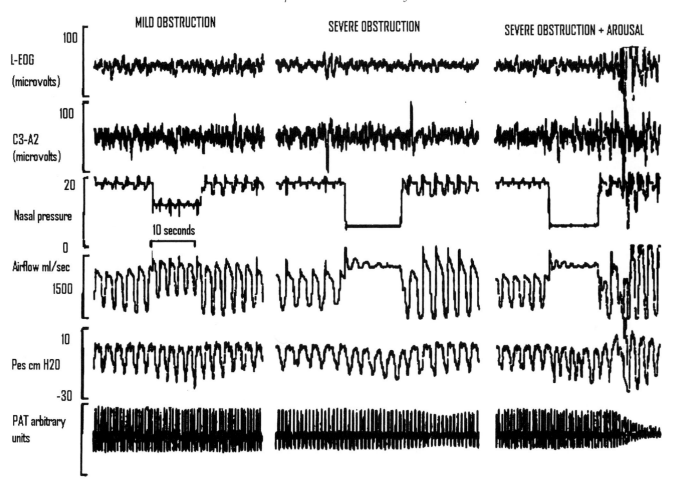

FIGURE 11E–2. *Interaction of obstruction and arousal. Sleep, airflow, nasal positive airway pressure, esophageal pressure (Pes), and the PAT signal are recorded simultaneously. Mild obstruction induced by partial lowering of positive airway pressure does not result in an EEG arousal attenuation of the PAT signal. Dropping the pressure to induce an obstructive apnea results in severe obstruction and mild attenuation of the PAT signal (middle panel), while the occurrence of an arousal results in severe digital vasoconstriction. (From O'Donnell et al, Am J Resp Crit Care Med 2002;166:967 Fig. 1)*

wider patterns than the AASM 3-second arousal, and in fact the PAT technology should be able to detect more subtle but possibly clinically significant arousals. It may be more useful to develop autonomic arousal/activation concepts relatively unconstrained by the AASM arousal definition.

CONCLUSIONS

The PAT signal can detect digital vasoconstriction associated with bursts of sympathetic activity that are characteristic of transient arousals from sleep. The signal provides one measure of autonomic activation. Integration of such signals into the clinical practice of sleep medicine may provide a complementary role in assessing the detection and clinical impact of disturbed sleep.

REFERENCES

1. Somers VK, Dyken ME, Mark AL, Abboud FM. Sympathetic-nerve activity during sleep in normal subjects. *N Engl J Med* 1993;328:303–307.
2. Davies RJ, Belt PJ, Roberts SJ, Ali NJ, Stradling JR. Arterial blood pressure responses to graded transient arousal from sleep in normal humans. *J Appl Physiol* 1993;74:1123–1130.
3. Morgan BJ, Crabtree DC, Puleo DS, Badr MS, Toiber F, Skatrud JB. Neurocirculatory consequences of abrupt change in sleep state in humans. *J Appl Physiol* 1996;80:1627–1636.
4. Stepanski E, Lamphere J, Roehrs T, Zorick F, Roth T. Experimental sleep fragmentation in normal subjects. *Int J Neurosci* 1987;33:207–214.
5. Grote L, Zou D, Kraiczi H, Hedner J. Finger plethysmography—A method for monitoring finger blood flow during

sleep disordered breathing. *Respir Physiol Neurobiol* 2003; 136:141–152.

6. Zou D, Grote L, Eder DN, Peker Y, Hedner J. Obstructive apneic events induce alpha-receptor mediated digital vasoconstriction. *Sleep* 2004;27:485–489.

7. O'Donnell CP, Allan L, Atkinson P, Schwartz AR. The effect of upper airway obstruction and arousal on peripheral arterial tonometry in obstructive sleep apnea. *Am J Respir Crit Care Med* 2002;166:965–971.

8. Schnall RP, Shlitner A, Sheffy J, Kedar R, Lavie P. Periodic, profound peripheral vasoconstriction—A new marker of obstructive sleep apnea. *Sleep* 1999;22:939–946.

9. Bar A, Pillar G, Dvir I, Sheffy J, Schnall RP, Lavie P. Evaluation of a portable device based on peripheral arterial tone for unattended home sleep studies. *Chest* 2003;123:695–703.

10. Lavie P, Schnall RP, Sheffy J, Shlitner A. Peripheral vasoconstriction during REM sleep detected by a new plethysmographic method. *Nat Med* 2000;6:606.

11. Dvir I, Adler Y, Freimark D, Lavie P. Evidence for fractal correlation properties in variations of peripheral arterial tone during REM sleep. *Am J Physiol Heart Circ Physiol* 2002; 283:H434–H439.

12. Ayas NT, Pittman S, MacDonald M, White DP. Assessment of a wrist-worn device in the detection of obstructive sleep apnea. *Sleep Med* 2003;4:435–442.

13. Penzel T, Kesper K, Pinnow I, Becker HF, Vogelmeier C. Peripheral arterial tonometry, oximetry and actigraphy for ambulatory recording of sleep apnea. *Physiol Meas* 2004;25: 1025–1036.

14. Pittman SD, Ayas NT, MacDonald MM, Malhotra A, Fogel RB, White DP. Using a wrist-worn device based on peripheral arterial tonometry to diagnose obstructive sleep apnea: In-laboratory and ambulatory validation. *Sleep* 2004;27: 923–933.

15. Pillar G, Bar A, Betito M et al. An automatic ambulatory device for detection of AASM defined arousals from sleep: The WP100. *Sleep Med* 2003;4:207–212.

16. Pillar G, Bar A, Shlitner A, Schnall R, Shefy J, Lavie P. Autonomic arousal index: An automated detection based on peripheral arterial tonometry. *Sleep* 2002;25:543–549.

17. EEG arousals: Scoring rules and examples: a preliminary report from the Sleep Disorders Atlas Task Force of the American Sleep Disorders Association. *Sleep* 1992;15: 173–184.

12

Therapy and PSG: Continuous Positive Airway Pressure and Bilevel Positive Airway Pressure

ROBERT J. THOMAS

CONTINUOUS POSITIVE AIRWAYS PRESSURE

The ultimate goal of continuous positive airway pressure (CPAP) titration is complete elimination of flow limitation. This may or may not be achieved at an acceptable "cost" (of inducing arousals and central respiratory events, or patient discomfort). The next best goal is good quality sleep, and some residual flow limitation (with occasional arousals). *Anything less than this is unsatisfactory.* An in-line pneumotachograph (inbuilt into the PAP machine or a separate unit in the circuit) or mask pressure monitoring through a differential pressure transducer is required. Thermistors are useless during titration and should not be used except perhaps to monitor mouth breathing.

Some General Guidelines

1. The starting pressure is usually 4 centimeters (cms) of H_2O. Less pressure can cause significant carbon dioxide rebreathing, and the 4-centimeter minimum is a recommendation by the Food and Drug Administration (FDA). Lower pressures may be used if the patient specifically asks (and seems unable to tolerate 4 centimeters) for it, but document this. It may also be dropped if the patient seems to have central apneas at 4 cms H_2O itself, though this usually implies either insufficient pressure ("central" events can be obstructive in pathophysiology), severe sleep-onset respiratory instability (wait a bit, check that the lights-out time is not much earlier than usual bedtime, try a slightly higher pressure if flow limitation is obvious),

or the need to move to bilevel positive airway pressure (BiPAP) fairly quickly.

2. Occasional patients will not be able to enter sleep due to repetitive obstructive apneas or hypopneas. Though the technician often waits for the patient to sleep before raising the pressure, if this phenomenon is recognized, the CPAP should be slowly increased even though the patient may not be "sleeping yet."

3. There is no strict standardized rule for increasing the rate of CPAP pressure. It can be raised every few minutes, or even every few breaths if obstructive apneas, hypopneas, and flow limitation are obvious. The maximum waiting time should be in the range of 3 to 15 minutes (except in slow-wave sleep [SWS] or non–cyclic alternating pattern [non-CAP], see below) if you want to be sure that the pressure is insufficient at that stage of the titration. If the patient wakes up and states that the pressure is too much, you can slow the rate of increase.

4. Most patients, especially older individuals or those on benzodiazepines/sedative drugs, exhibit periods of sleep that are not scored as stage III or IV by conventional criteria, but clearly have excessive slow-wave frequency waves. Respiration is usually quite stable during this period (functionally, think of it as SWS), and if recognized the same precautions as during conventionally scored SWS apply. Those who study the cyclic alternating pattern (CAP) will recognize this type of "stable" NREM sleep as non-CAP. In fact, for the purpose of titration, dividing sleep into CAP, non-CAP, and REM works well and may be

better than Rechtschaffen-Kales (RK) stages II, III, and IV and REM sleep.

The stability of this non-CAP or slow-wave–like (frequency but not amplitude) sleep can cause a false sense of security (of treatment efficacy, CPAP or BPAP); it is also important not to change pressures if this state is recognized (unless obstructions and flow limitation are quite overt). Do not respond to subtle flow limitation in non-CAP. More often, flow looks absolutely normal in non-CAP, and then quite abnormal when CAP or REM occurs.

5. Do not aggressively increase the pressure in SWS/non-CAP unless the obstructions are obvious. Apneas and major hypopneas, clear snoring, or marked flow limitation should not be ignored, while subtle hypopneas and minimal/mild flow limitation can simply be observed until the patient is in stage II/CAP. This is to avoid going beyond the patient's pressure tolerance during SWS/non-CAP (where arousability is reduced) and then facing the problem of excessive pressure-induced respiratory events and arousals when that period of slow-wave/non-CAP sleep is complete. Moreover, 1- to 2-centimeter pressure changes during non-CAP typically result in no/minimal effect on the polysomnographic (PSG) patterns. *Straight obstructive events are maximal in CAP and REM sleep; periodic breathing is maximal in CAP, minimal/absent in non-CAP and REM sleep. Periodic breathing patterns are often more subtle than overt Cheyne-Stokes respiration.*

6. Significant repetitive oxygen desaturations will not generally occur in SWS in the presence of normal cardiac and pulmonary function unless there are respiratory events. Respiration is often quite stable in SWS/non-CAP even in individuals with severe obstructive sleep apnea. Flow can look normal in SWS/non-CAP and revert to marked limitation immediately after termination of non-CAP/SWS. If an auto-titrating machine is being used, pressures in SWS/non-CAP may drop to quite minimal (4 to 6 centimeters) levels.

7. Some variability of respiration during REM sleep is normal, especially in phasic REM. Hypopneas should not be "chased" unless they are associated with arousals or oxygen desaturation. Brief central apneas may occur normally during REM, especially phasic REM. *Flow limitation remains a valid indicator of increased upper airway resistance during REM sleep, but mild intermittent degrees of abnormality that is not associated with arousals or desaturations can be tolerated.* If there are obvious obstructive apneas and hypopneas or progressive flow limitation in REM, increase the pressure.

8. If oxygen desaturation (e.g., 3 percent to 4 percent, or drops to less than 90 percent) occurs and persists during REM sleep in spite of what seems to be reasonable control of obstructive events—the first step would be a small increase in CPAP. If this does not resolve the problem, the options include doing nothing (if the changes are minor), adding oxygen, or switching to BiPAP. When considering oxygen administration, the patient may need to be investigated for the presence of cardiorespiratory disease.

9. Most periodic limb movements in sleep (PLMS) that are seen in individuals with sleep-disordered breathing (SDB) in the absence of restless legs syndrome are usually related to the respiratory events. Persistence of PLMS on what looks like reasonably good control of sleep apnea may mean residual subtle hypopneas, especially if they occur during REM sleep or during the latter half of the night. If this is the case, try a small increase in CPAP (or IPAP of the BiPAP), but not more than 3 to 4 cm H_2O beyond the level needed to abolish flow limitation, or until central apneas appear.

10. If a patient seems to be doing well at a certain pressure (they have done well during prior NREM and REM sleep periods), *but there is persistent flow limitation*, with or without brief and infrequent arousals, gradually increase pressure in 1-centimeter increments (maximum: 4 or until increasing respiratory events are noted) to try and abolish it, unless the patient is in non-CAP/SWS (if so, wait and watch for CAP/more unstable stage II sleep). If arousals increase or hypopneas/central apneas appear, reduce pressure to the previously well-tolerated level. In certain individuals, mild persisting flow limitation is a practical tradeoff to pressure tolerance.

11. Snoring should never be tolerated. However, beware of subtle vibrations picked up on the microphone that may have no physiological significance.

12. Heated humidification should be routine, but an occasional patient may choose not to use it at the onset. Table 12–1 suggests guidelines for a CPAP titration protocol.

BILEVEL POSITIVE AIRWAY PRESSURE

WHAT IT IS: Independently adjusted inspiratory (I) and expiratory (E) pressures. The difference between the two pressures determines the "drive input" of the system—the greater it is, the greater the active contribution to ventilation.

WHAT IT IS NOT: Intrinsically superior to CPAP in the treatment of obstructive SDB, if patients are

Table 12–1. Suggested Guidelines for CPAP Titration

Goal	Action	Indicator	Defaults
1. Abolish obstructive apneas and severe obstructive hypopneas.	Increase CPAP by 1 centimeter every 5 to 10 minutes (or even every few breaths if the evidence for obstruction is clear) to a maximum of 18 centimeters.	Monitor nasal pressure and effort bands for evidence of cyclic decreases and increases, flow limitation with an abrupt return to a sinusoidal waveform, and abrupt termination of events with a large recovery breath.	If events persist: 1. Check for mask leak or open mouth. 2. Full face mask (preferred) or chinstrap (this is not very efficient). 3. Increase humidifier setting, check for nasal congestion (consider decongestant). 4. Consider BiPAP.
2. Eliminate inspiratory flow limitation.	Increase CPAP by 1 centimeter every few (3 to 15) minutes up to 18 centimeters. Tolerance to pressures is a real-time judgment. The "3–15" minutes is just a guideline. When the EEG morphology is CAP/unstable NREM sleep, aggressive increases in pressures are reasonable, when unstable flow limitation is seen.	1. Monitor nasal pressure for progressive flow limitation terminating in arousals. 2. Recognize "stable/progressive" and "unstable/nonprogressive" forms of flow limitation. 3. Recognize periodic breathing—It is often less than Cheyne-Stokes. One clue is a *mirror-image* pattern of recurrent events. The other is *improvement* when the patient goes into REM sleep.	If flattening/flow limitation persists, consider defaults as under #1. *Do not make aggressive pressure changes for mild abnormalities when the EEG morphology is non-CAP.*
3. Eliminate arousal and PLMs (hypothesis: subtle obstructive events drive PLMS).	Increase CPAP by 1 centimeter every 3 to 15 minutes, but not more than 2 to 3 cm H$_2$O beyond level needed to abolish visible flow limitation or until increasing hypopneas or central apneas appear.	Monitor EEG for arousals and anterior tibialis for PLMs.	If arousals and PLMs persist, decrease CPAP to lowest level that accomplishes goal #2 and consider BiPAP.
4. Eliminate saturation decreases to less than 88 percent to 90 percent, if they persist in spite of apparently normal flow.	1. Increase CPAP by 1 centimeter every 5 to 10 minutes, but not more than 4 cm H$_2$O beyond level needed to abolish flow limitation or until increasing hypopneas or central apneas appear. 2. If there is no response, drop back to a pressure that normalizes flow.	Monitor SaO$_2$ for drops below 88 percent to 90 percent.	If SaO$_2$ is less than 88 percent to 90 percent despite increased CPAP: Options: Consider increased CPAP (superior choice). 2. Low-flow O$_2$ administration (1 to 4 L/minute) may be considered but patient may also need to be investigated for presence of cardiorespiratory disorders.

unselected. A significant minority of patients may also not "like" the way BiPAP feels.

SOME COMMON ERRORS IN THE CLINICAL USE OF BIPAP

1. Late recognition of the lack or inadequate efficacy of CPAP.
2. Inadequate Expiratory support (E). This is a serious error (100 percent failure is expected). Besides the fact that apneas cannot be eliminated by an increase in IPAP alone, expiratory airway instability in general is a more recently recognized and clinically important phenomenon.
3. Inadequate (typically less than 3 to 4 centimeters) I-E difference, especially if hypoventilation is the main indication (the closer, the more like CPAP it is).
4. Trying to use a fixed "formula" for titration.
5. Simultaneously increasing I and E, especially if this is done repeatedly.
6. Not recognizing significant degrees of mouth leak.
7. Inadequate humidification with resultant increase in nasal resistance.
8. Worsening of inspiratory airflow due to possible glottic narrowing while using the timed mode.
9. Too high a starting pressure (always taking off from the "end" of CPAP).

THE FOLLOWING PRACTICAL POINTS SHOULD BE CONSIDERED

1. It is best to increase pressure in 1-centimeter increments. With experience, it will be possible to judge when greater increases are required at the individual steps.
2. Increase either the I or the E at any step during learning—with experience, there may be comfort increasing both, but there is then a danger of simply "playing" with the pressures.
3. It can be more difficult to recognize hypopneas and flow limitation while on BiPAP (compared to CPAP), but use all data available (arousals, snoring, effort channels).
4. Do not increase I to more than 18 to 20 centimeters (even if available on some of the newer machines) without consulting the physician.
5. The final IPAP will usually be at least close to (or even higher than) the CPAP required (if known) to eliminate most, if not all, hypopneas and flow limitation.

The ideal end point of titration is to normalize sleep, prevent desaturations and overt airflow obstructions (apneas, hypopneas), and eliminate flow limitation.

6. There is increasing experimental and clinical (human) evidence that expiratory airway narrowing is an important component of upper airway pathophysiology in patients with obstructive SDB. Real-time video recording of the upper airway and pressure profile measurements have often shown narrowing of the airway to be maximal (or very close to that) in end expiration. This can vary from patient to patient. What this means in a practical sense is that if expiratory positive airway pressure (EPAP) is inadequate, it may be manifested as inspiratory flow limitation or otherwise unstable breathing and arousals. If reasonable IPAP increases (I-E difference of 4 to 5 cms) do not seem to be improving things, go up on the EPAP.
7. It is a common error not to choose adequate EPAPs when switching to BiPAP from CPAP. Technicians may fall into a pattern of using "standard" starting BiPAP levels, such as 5/3, 6/3-4. This can be completely inappropriate if the pressure requirements are higher, and this is best judged based on response to previous CPAP. Use guidelines and examples given below.
8. It is advantageous to simultaneously monitor pneumotachograph (independent in-line or PAP machine) flow, and the pressure-time profile (mask pressure). The information obtained is complementary, and the implications of the patterns of the pressure profile are well described in the mechanical ventilation literature (e.g., inadequate triggering, overlap of neural expiration and machine inspiration).
9. It is advisable to accurately identify the inspiratory signal early, such as during biocalibrations (this may not be as easy as it may seem once the study is running). A good intercostal electromyogram (EMG) is useful in this discrimination, but may not be available, especially in overweight individuals. The inspiratory part of the curve is usually of lesser duration. Have this part of the flow profile above the baseline, as it is easier, from a visuospatial basis, to appreciate flow limitation (like a "slice cut from the top of a mountain"). With a good pressure trace, flattening and "wobbling" during inspiratory flow limitation, somewhat similar to that seen during CPAP, should be visible.
10. The issues raised (see CPAP titration above) regarding less and more stable forms of NREM sleep and respiration, based on recognizing CAP and non-CAP, are also valid for BiPAP titration.
11. The upper airway may be more unstable on BiPAP than on CPAP in individual patients. This phenomenon is characterized by the requirement of an EPAP

of very close to or greater than CPAP required to normalize flow, repetitive obstructive apneas in spite of increasing EPAP, and generally increased arousals or patient's perceived discomfort.

12. Recognizing subtle forms of periodic breathing, especially during CPAP titration (and even induced or worsened by it), is a critical part of a superior titration. Reductions in CPAP or a switch to BiPAP are all possible measures, depending on the clinical situation.

Periodic breathing resolves during REM sleep, so a patient who is far worse in stage II (specifically CAP) than in REM sleep may have this pattern. Increasing CPAP does not generally improve periodic breathing unless obstructions are still overt. If the pattern is mild, allowing some more time to settle down and reach a new equilibrium is reasonable. Those with severe CO_2 retention due to obstruction may manifest this pattern once the airway is open as they are now hyperventilating in a relative sense (with a reduction of P_{CO_2}).

Patients with exceptionally dysrhythmic breathing, or severe periodic breathing such as those with heart failure, may be impossible to "control" on a single night. In these patients, repeat titrations are usually required, with each consecutive assessment achieving a superior end point. The other option that is likely to see increasing use is "acclimatization" to CPAP/BiPAP or use of technology such as smart bilevel machines that improve Cheyne-Stokes respiration with use over several weeks.

Sleep and titration are dynamic interactive processes. No number (e.g., "x" minutes to allow a certain pattern or remain on a certain pressure) is absolute, and moment to moment changes may be required, especially as sleep switches from REM to NREM and between non-CAP and CAP. Too much pressure is as disruptive as inadequate pressure.

Table 12–2 outlines certain clinical situations and BiPAP titration end points. Table 12–3 lists some general guidelines for practical clinical use of BiPAP in SDB. Some suggested guidelines for BiPAP titration protocol are listed in Table 12–4.

Gas Modulation

Altering the composition of the gas content within the PAP circuit will likely see increasing use in the treatment

Table 12–2. BiPAP Titration End Points

Clinical Situations	Possible End Points
Central sleep apnea	Provide ventilatory drive, provide ventilatory timing. Prevent CO_2/O_2 cycling, prevent arousals.
Periodic breathing in cardiac failure	Reduce ventilatory oscillations. Reduce CO_2 and O_2 cycling. Improve gas exchange, improve cardiac function. Prevent arousals and its neurohumeral consequences.
Periodic breathing in neurologic or metabolic disease	Reduce ventilatory oscillations, CO_2 and O_2 cycling. Prevent arousals.
Acute ventilatory failure due to neuromuscular disease	Provide ventilatory support. Improve daytime acid-base balance. Reduce sleep fragmentation.
Acute ventilatory failure in chronic respiratory disease	Provide ventilatory support. Sleep fragmentation is a secondary end point.
Chronic ventilatory failure in chronic respiratory disease	Provide ventilatory support. Improve daytime acid-base balance. Reduce sleep fragmentation.
Classic obstructive SDB	Provide adequate "E" to prevent expiratory airway collapse and enough "I" to prevent inspiratory flow limitation. Improve pressure tolerance.
REM-hypoventilation	Provide ventilatory support by manipulating I-E difference—the subject is effectively in relative neuromuscular paralysis.
Induction of non-obstructive SDB	Presumably CPAP unmasks abnormalities in ventilatory control that then requires optimizing drive, timing, and preventing major fluctuations of CO_2 and O_2. Excessive CPAP can induce this pattern.
Pressure intolerance	Lessen the "pressure experience."

Table 12–3. General Guidelines for Practical Clinical Use of BiPAP in SDB

Clinical Situations	Suggested Steps
A. CPAP titration is begun and the patient almost immediately starts having central apneas; flow limitation is minimal.	1. This usually means that the pressure to keep the airway open is not high, and low initial pressures of BiPAP should be applied. Waiting a few minutes is reasonable, to allow time to settle down, as sleep-onset breathing instability is prominent in some patients with obstructive sleep apnea. Occasionally, this waiting period is all that is required to go on with CPAP itself. 2. Once a decision is made to move to BiPAP, a reasonable starting point is 5/3 or 6/4. Increase the IPAP by 1-centimeter increments to 7 or 8, then increase the E to 4 and then 5. The duration between increments should follow flexible guidelines. Allow 5 to 10 minutes at least unless the pressure is obviously inappropriate. Further increments should follow the general titration protocol. This is the only situation to use starting pressures in this low range. 3. Do not adjust pressures if the patient quickly goes into SWS/non-CAP (as can often happen). Wait until this period is complete. An exception can be made if obstructions are really very obvious (such as snoring, repetitive desaturations due to obstructive apneas, and major obstructive hypopneas). It is then more important to provide adequate E. Unfortunately, there is no easy way to give a "rule" in this instance; experience is what helps the most. 4. The ultimate pressure to obtain optimal control may not be very low. It could just mean that the sleep-wake transition period cannot tolerate higher E pressures.
B. The patient starts off well enough on CPAP, but as you try to control flow limitation and more subtle hypopneas, central events or an increasing number of arousals are seen.	1. This is a common situation. Technician responses include either to continue to "chase" the hypopneas with increasing pressure (serious error) or to drop back to the best tolerated pressure (compromise). It is critical to first try to eliminate flow limitation, to be sure that inadequate pressure is not the issue. It may be an issue of judgment to leave small degrees of flow limitation alone, and indeed, in some patients a normal flow profile cannot be obtained by any pressure generated by machines in routine clinical use, even if tolerated. 2. If you choose to switch to BiPAP, IPAP = approximate CPAP, which was the highest tolerated reasonably well, EPAP = lowest CPAP required to prevent all apneas and major hypopneas. Example: CPAP 12, BiPAP 10/6-12/8. The I-E difference will be at least 3-4, usually. Then increase IPAP in 1-centimeter increments. If there is no positive response to 2 to 3 centimeters of increase, the E is probably too low and needs to be increased. Further adjustments will follow the general titration protocol. If a range of higher pressures does not work, choose lower levels. The starting pressure may have been too high. If the CPAP was high in the first place, you may choose to start BiPAP settings that are also high.
C. Straight BiPAP titration (indications may include intolerance to pressure at home, persistent arousals, daytime symptoms, REM-hypoventilation not treated on prior study).	1. Increase CPAP by 1 to 2 centimeters every 5 to 10 minutes up to 14 to 15 centimeters (or to pressure that was most effective and best tolerated on prior titration, if known). This is to get a sense of the individual breathing pattern and the improvement in flow in relation to pressure increments, to obtain a visual impression of abnormal flow patterns at various pressures, and to help choose appropriate initial IPAP and EPAP. 2. Increase IPAP by 1 centimeter every 3 to 15 minutes up to a maximal IPAP of 18 to 20 centimeters. If the I-E difference is greater than 5 to 6 centimeters and the IPAP is greater than 15 centimeters, and hypopneas or inspiratory flow limitation persists, consider increasing EPAP, as expiratory airway instability may be the cause of persistent hypopneas. See B above to help choose initial settings. 3. The physician may request a "Bilevel PAP all night." In that case, the previous CPAP report can serve the same purpose.
D. Patient is doing well in NREM sleep, enters REM, and then develops profound desaturations. You look at the tracing, and there does not seem to be a major increase in obstructive events (if there is, increase CPAP).	1. This is REM-hypoventilation. The first step is still an increase in CPAP, as the flow tracings are not quantitative, hypopneas are a normal part of REM, and obstruction may still be important. If this does not help, the choices are BiPAP (preferred) or the addition of oxygen. Keep IPAP at current levels of CPAP, drop EPAP by 3 to 4 centimeters, but not lower than the CPAP that was "almost enough." The other option is to keep EPAP at the current level of CPAP, and use an IPAP that is 3 to 4 centimeters higher. The problem with the second approach is that excessive E may be used. The end result may be pressures that patients do not tolerate when the REM period is complete. 2. Increase IPAP to control desaturations. If the difference in I-E is more than 5 to 7 centimeters and desaturations persist, maybe more IPAP is required (try going higher), or the EPAP is too low (try raising EPAP next), or additional oxygen is required.

Table 12–3. General Guidelines for Practical Clinical Use of BiPAP in SDB—cont'd

Clinical Situations	Suggested Steps
E. Indication for BiPAP titration in non-obstructive SDB associated with neuromuscular diseases.	1. This may include acute conditions such as myasthenia gravis, snakebite neuroparalysis, and acute demyelinating polyneuropathy. The basic idea is to use minimal EPAP (usually more than 4 or 5 centimeters is not necessary) and an increased I-E differential (6 to 8 centimeters) to provide maximal tolerable ventilatory support. This is often used with no regard to sleep stages (such as in the MICU), but more accurate titration can be done during full PSG, especially as control during REM sleep may be the crucial issue. Blood gas is the typical end point. REM-hypoventilation may be profound, requiring the addition of oxygen. 2. Upper airway collapsibility and obstruction can be significant in such patients. Though generally lower EPAPs are generally adequate, this may not always be the case. 3. There may be different settings for wake and sleep. Use the non-REM settings, or slightly lower if not tolerated, while awake. The more chronic the condition, the more important to titrate with simultaneous sleep recording.
F. Indication is noninvasive ventilation in patients with chronic respiratory failure due to obstructive lung disease, and the obstructive element is mild.	During the acute exacerbations, the principles are similar to those while dealing with acute neuromuscular disorders. Sleep is less critical than improvements in blood gas. A PSG-defined titration will offer superior control, but there are practical limitations to this. There should be no strong history of a significant obstructive element (no snoring, spacious oropharynx, but this is no guarantee). The target is acceptable blood gas values. The goal is not to obtain "normal values" (which will usually imply relative hyperventilation) but to be closer to the patient's stable chronic condition (PCO_2 not less than 45 to 50 mm Hg). REM-hypoventilation may be profound, requiring an increase in I-E difference or the addition of oxygen.
G. Addition of oxygen.	The actual delivered amount to the patient is not predictable due to variable dilution and washout. Saturations (or if necessary, blood gas) are a reasonable surrogate. It is absolutely critical that oxygen be added to patients with chronic hypercapnic respiratory failure and obstructive sleep apnea on CPAP (with persistent hypoxia, such as during REM) with the greatest caution. Loss of the hypoxic drive + altered ventilation-perfusion match + the Haldane effect (the promotion of carbon dioxide dissociation by oxygenation of hemoglobin) can result in worsening gas status and severe hypercapnia. The saturation may look OK, but CO_2 may rise dangerously. A switch to BiPAP is preferred, and the physician should be brought into the decision loop. A blood gas may have to be done on the spot.
H. Addition of a backup rate "timed" mode	This is often a judgment call. There are two types of central disease: hypercapnic (primary reduction of central drive such as severe hypoventilation states) and hypocapnic (CO_2 oscillations around the apneic set-point, such as in congestive heart failure). Persistence of central apneas (or prominent periodic breathing), in spite of seemingly adequate levels of pressure to eliminate obstructive events, and lack of triggering of the BiPAP is the usual indication. This mode cannot compensate for inappropriate or inadequate pressures, or typically control hypocapnia-induced central apneas (may induce glottic closure). The timed beats provide ventilatory support, and damp major fluctuations in O_2 and CO_2, but can also worsen hypocapnia. In this instance, the ventilator essentially tries to take over much of sleep respiration. Typically, periodic respiratory cycling and arousals persist, although major deviations of O_2 and CO_2 (by preventing long central apneas) are minimized.
I. Use of different I/E time ratios and rise times.	Newer machines will have the option of adjusting the inspiratory-expiratory time ratios and rise times in the spontaneous mode (this is already available in the timed, but not spontaneous/timed mode of commercial BiPAP devices). This can significantly improve patient comfort and tolerance, and minimize patient-BiPAP synchrony difficulties. Using these options in real time for titration will be possible only with sufficient understanding of the physiology and pathophysiology of pressure support ventilation waveforms.

Table 12–4. Suggested Guidelines for BiPAP Titration

Goal	Action	Indicator	Defaults
A. Abolish obstructive apneas and severe obstructive hypopneas.	1. Increase pressure in CPAP mode by 1 centimeter every 5 to 10 (or even every few breaths if the evidence for obstruction is clear) minutes to a maximum of 14 to 15 cm H_2O. 2. Add IPAP, and keep a 3- to 4-cm H_2O I-E difference. 3. EPAP greater than this is not practical with many current BiPAP machines (max IPAP 30 cms in some lab machines), and presence of severe obstruction at such pressures usually implies the need to check the defaults.	Monitor nasal pressure and effort bands for evidence of cyclic decreases and increases, flow limitation with an abrupt return to a sinusoidal waveform, and abrupt termination of events with a large recovery breath.	If events persist: 1. Check for mask leak or open mouth. 2. Full face mask (preferred) or chinstrap. 3. Heated humidifier.
B. Eliminate inspiratory flow limitation.	1. Increase IPAP (at any given pressure of EPAP) by 1 centimeter every 3 to 15 minutes. Do not change EPAP simultaneously "routinely." 2. The "3–15" minutes is just a guideline. When the EEG morphology is CAP, aggressive increases in pressures are reasonable, when unstable flow limitation is seen. 3. *Inadequate EPAP can cause inspiratory flow limitation. You will likely need to consider EPAP adjustments throughout the study.*	1. Monitor nasal pressure for progressive flow limitation terminating in arousals. 2. Recognize "stable/progressive" and "unstable/nonprogressive" forms of flow limitation. 3. Recognize periodic breathing. It is often less than Cheyne-Stokes. One clue is a mirror-image pattern of recurrent events. The other is improvement when the patient goes into REM sleep.	1. If flattening/flow limitation persists, consider defaults as under #A. 2. *If obstructive apneas appear in the absence of leak, EPAP must be increased. No amount of IPAP can compensate for inadequate EPAP.* 3. *Do not make pressure changes for mild abnormality when the EEG morphology is non-CAP.*
C. Eliminate arousal and PLMs (hypothesis: subtle obstructive events are driving PLMs)	Increase IPAP 1 centimeter every 3 to 15 minutes but not more than 2 to 3 cms H_2O beyond level needed to abolish visible flow limitation or until increasing hypopneas or central apneas appear.	Monitor EEG for arousals and anterior tibialis for PLMs	If arousals and PLMs persist, decrease IPAP to lowest level that accomplishes goal #B. IPAP is usually greater than EPAP by 3 to 4 centimeters at all times.
D. Eliminate SaO_2 less than 88 percent to 90 percent, if they persist in spite of apparently normal flow.	Increase IPAP 1 centimeter every 5 to 10 minutes but not more than 3 to 4 cm H_2O beyond that to abolish flow limitation or until increasing hypopneas or central apneas appear.	Monitor SaO_2 for drops below 88 percent to 90 percent.	If SaO_2 is less than 88 percent to 90 percent despite increased IPAP, and obstruction does not seem to be persistent, add O_2 at 1 to 4 L/minute.

of non-obstructive SDB, such as periodic breathing, idiopathic central sleep apneas, and those with mixed patterns. These patients are hard to treat by positive airway pressure alone. Hypoxia and hypocarbia are destabilizing to respiratory control, and the latter is perhaps the most critical factor in the pathogenesis of non-obstructive disease outside sleep or REM-specific hypoventilation. There is no formal guideline for the use of O_2 in the sleep laboratory.

There is convincing evidence from over 50 years of research that much of periodic breathing and central SDB, irrespective of the associated etiology, requires a degree of hypocapnia. Oxygen can blunt periodic cycling induced by hypocapnia, but can rarely, if ever, eliminate it. Minimizing or reversing hypocapnia is central to any strategy to treat mixed or central disease. These strategies include the following:

1. Careful use of a backup rate to prevent wide swings in O_2 and CO_2 that can perpetuate a hypoventilation-hyperventilation cycle.

2. Additional oxygen (2 to 4 L/minute) to reduce hypoxia-mediated periodic breathing and respiratory control instability. Hypoxia amplifies hypocapnia-induced periodic breathing.

3. Preventing excessive CO_2 blow-off may be theoretically achieved by adding CO_2 to the PAP circuit or increasing effective dead space. The former strategy will require flow-independent concentration regulation; the latter is a practical challenge as small leaks will eliminate the effect of additional dead space. Use of non-vented masks and 150 to 200 cc of additional dead space is well tolerated and efficacious in the sleep lab for the treatment of central/mixed disease when used with PAP. Translating that efficacy to use at home is much more difficult. End-tidal and/or transcutaneous CO_2 monitoring are necessary components of strategies to safely change CO_2 kinetics.

Figures 12–1 through 12–22 are taken from several overnight PSG segments to bring out the problems during CPAP-BiPAP titration.

Text continued on p. 323

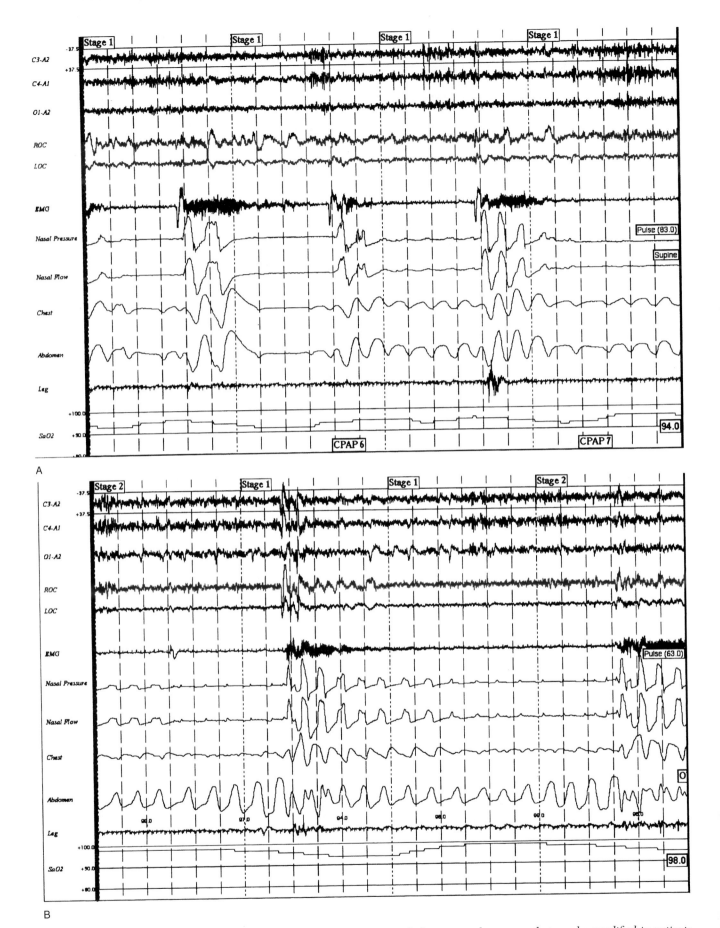

FIGURE 12–1. *CPAP titration.* **A:** *Onset of titration, demonstrating typical sleep-onset phenomena that can be amplified in patients with SDB—periodic breathing, central events, flow limitation, arousals. Desaturations would be distinctly uncommon in healthy individuals. Nasal pressure is mask pressure. 120-second epoch.* **B:** *Severe obstructive disease on 8 centimeters CPAP. Note the prolonged event evolution sequence of nearly a minute. 120-second epoch.*

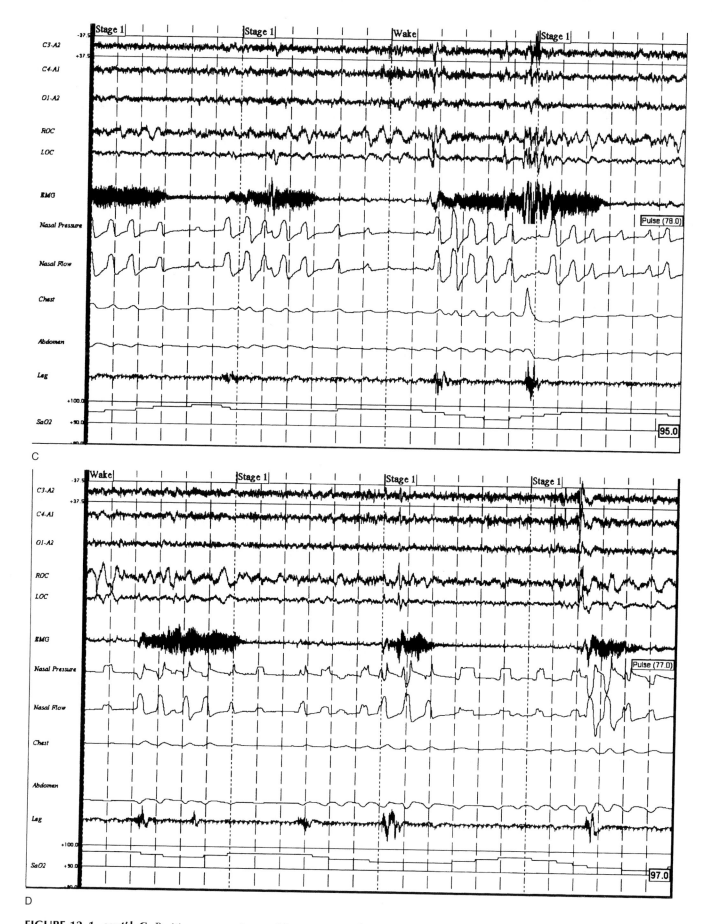

FIGURE 12–1, cont'd C: *Positive pressure is now 10 centimeters. The respiratory events do not look as purely obstructive as before, and this pattern can be seen if there is pressure intolerance. However, this may have been a sleep-wake transition period. 120-second epoch.* **D:** *Positive pressure is 12 centimeters, but intermittent mask leak is disrupting efficacy. Though noted by the technician from the digital readouts, it is also suggested by the opposite movement of the pressure and flow signals associated with the arousals—As flow increases, the mask pressure drops. 120-second epoch.*

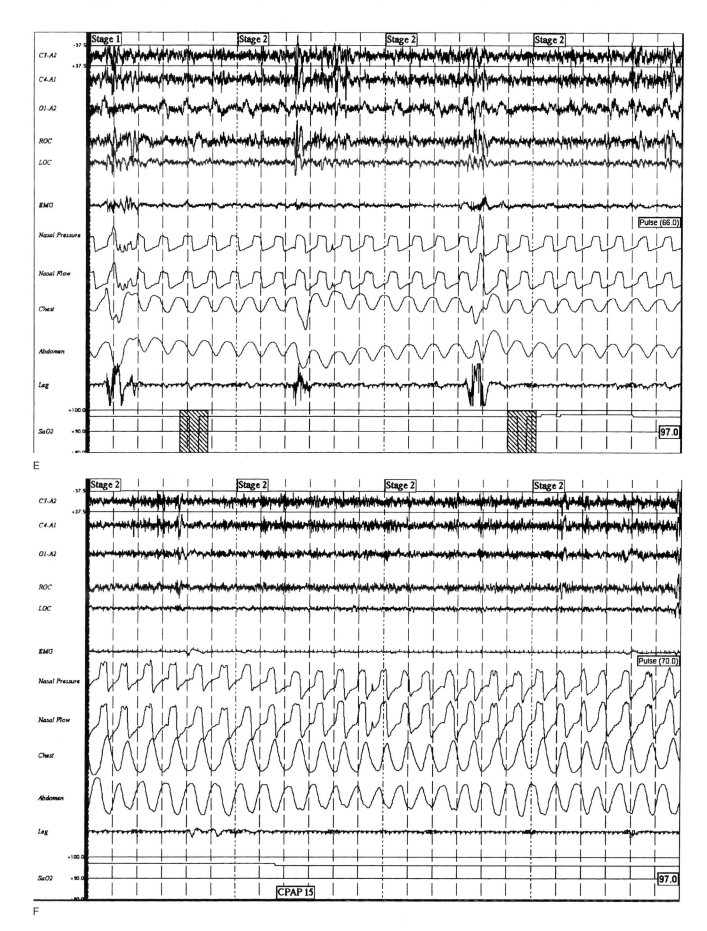

FIGURE 12–1, cont'd *E: Correction of mask leak results in improved control, but inspiratory flow limitation continues, and PLMS are associated with respiratory arousals. As a simple practical rule, as long as flow is abnormal, PLMS should not be considered as an independent cause of arousals. 120-second epoch. F: Flow is nearly normal, and this was the final prescribed pressure as further increases did not result in a clear improvement. Minimal to mild intermittent flow limitation is seen, but 15 percent to 20 percent of breaths in healthy individuals can show some nonprogressive flow limitation. 120-second epoch.*

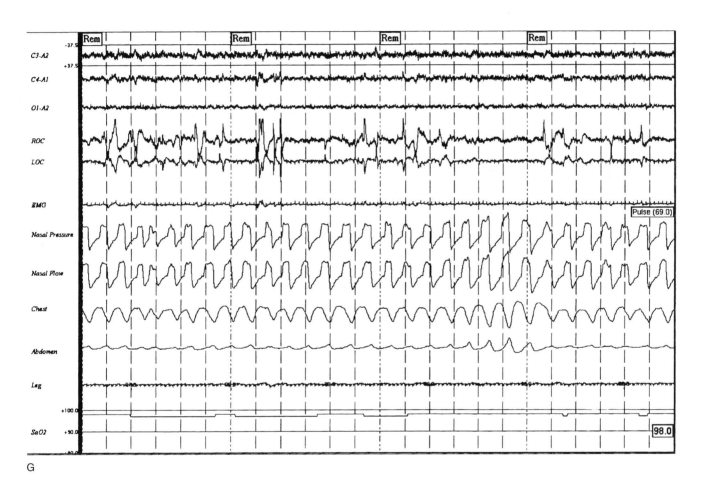

G

FIGURE 12–1, cont'd G: *Adequate control during REM sleep with 15 cm H$_2$O CPAP. It is often not possible or even necessary to try and eliminate ALL evidence of flow limitation during this stage. Lack of arousals or desaturation and a nonprogressive sequence help determine what can be tolerated, without exposing the patient to excessive pressures. 120-second epoch.*

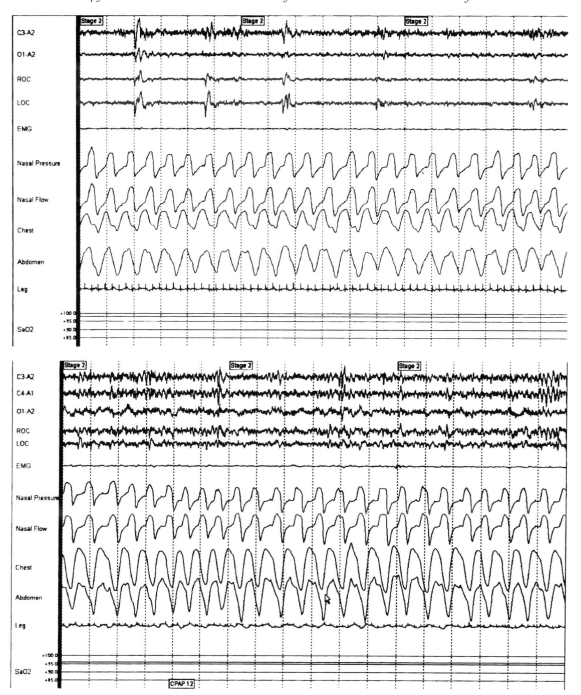

FIGURE 12–2. *CPAP titration. Two examples of perfect responses in NREM sleep— normal flow, no arousals or desaturations. Although this is the ideal end point, in practice this is hard to obtain. There is no evidence yet that this degree of control is necessary to obtain clinical benefit. An important area of research is the dosing aspects of positive airway pressure - is it necessary to eliminate all evidence of flow-limitation? 90-second epochs.*

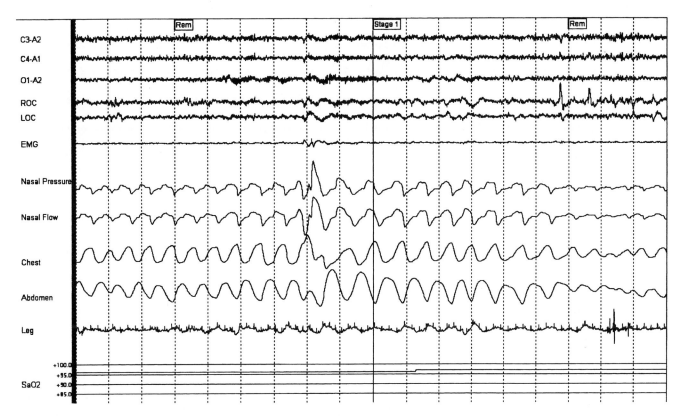

FIGURE 12–3. *CPAP titration. Inadequate pressure during REM sleep. Flow limitation was physiologically significant, as it caused an arousal, even if there was no desaturation. 90-second epoch.*

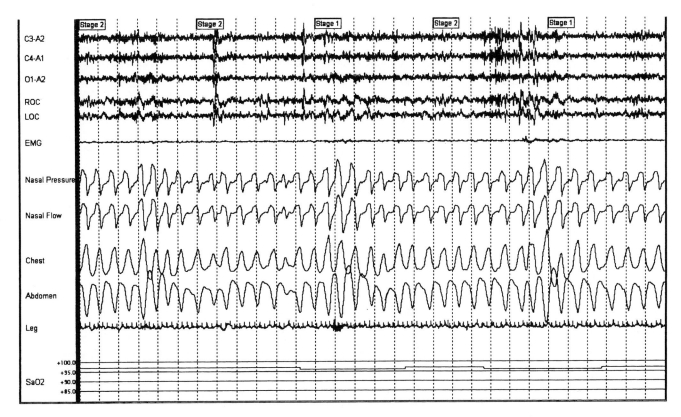

FIGURE 12–4. *CPAP titration. Excessive pressure (12 cms H$_2$O) inducing periodic breathing in NREM sleep. An increase in pressure worsened the pattern, resulting in frank central apnea, while a reduction to 10 centimeters normalized flow and sleep. Assessing the response to small increments and decrements in pressure is usually adequate to address this issue. 150-second epoch.*

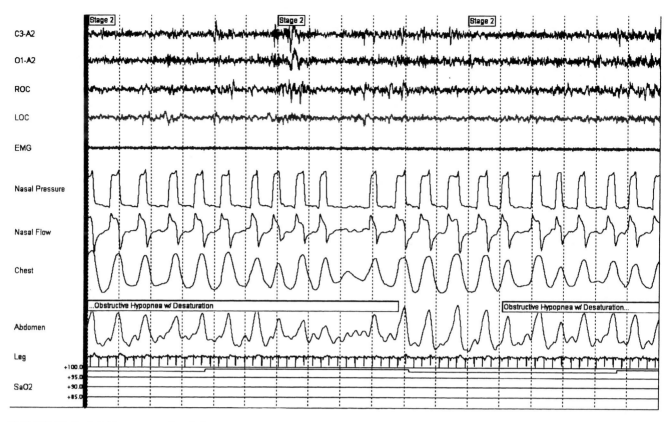

FIGURE 12–5. *BiPAP titration. Brief obstructive apnea. An increase in EPAP is necessary. 90-second epoch.*

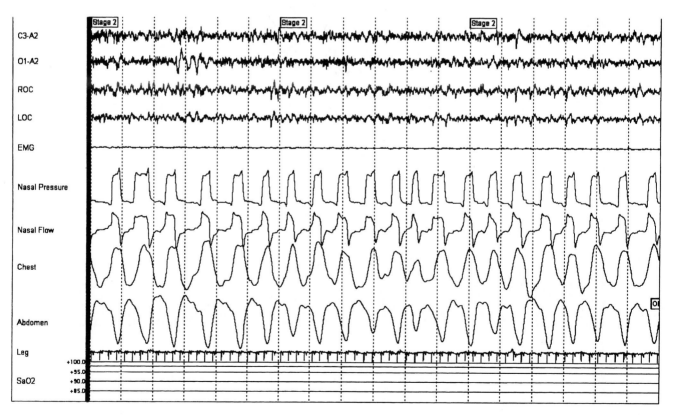

FIGURE 12–6. *BiPAP titration. Good control in NREM sleep—reasonably normal flow (no progressive flow limitation), no arousals or desaturations. 90-second epoch.*

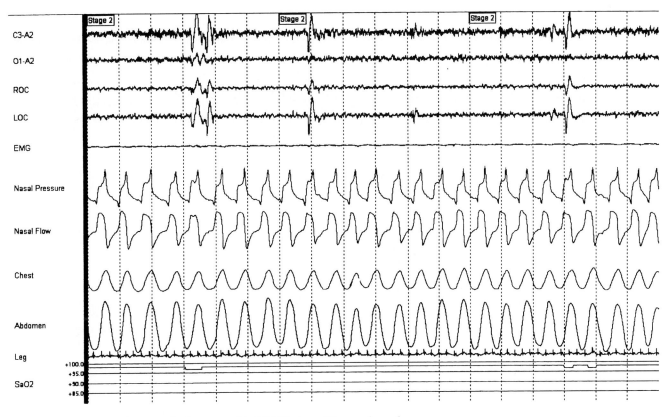

FIGURE 12–7. *BiPAP titration. Perfect control in NREM sleep. 90-second epoch.*

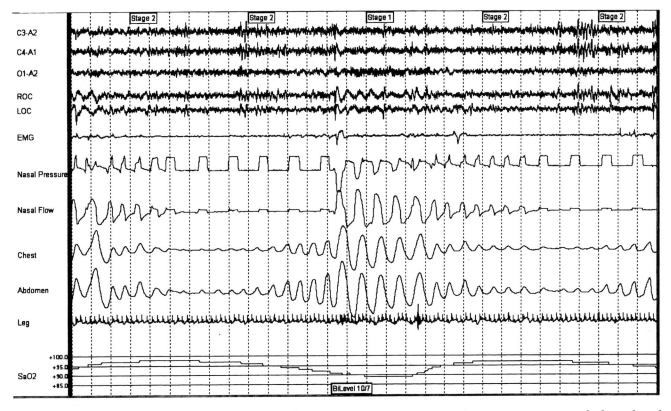

FIGURE 12–8. *BiPAP titration. Periodic breathing/respiratory instability induced by BiPAP of 10/7 centimeters. Patient had complained of difficulty exhaling at 14 centimeters. The final effective treatment was C-Flex at 14 centimeters, setting 3. This form of treatment (proportional PAP) tracks flow and provides enough support during expiration, with increased ease of exhalation. Bilevel ventilation may have induced hypocapnia. 150-second epoch.*

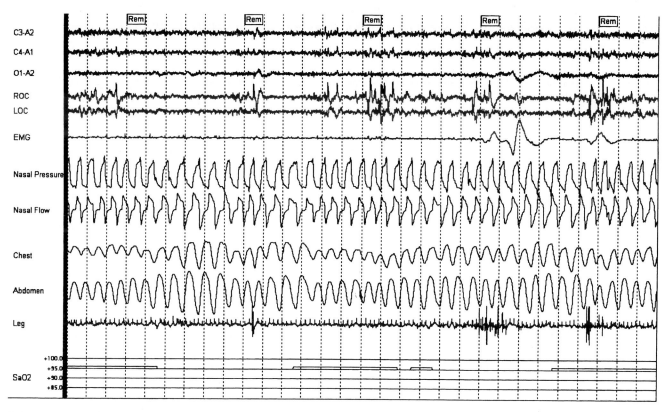

FIGURE 12–9. *BiPAP titration. Adequate control in REM sleep at 17/8 cm H₂O in a patient with severe REM hypoventilation (desaturations to 60 percent). 150-second epoch.*

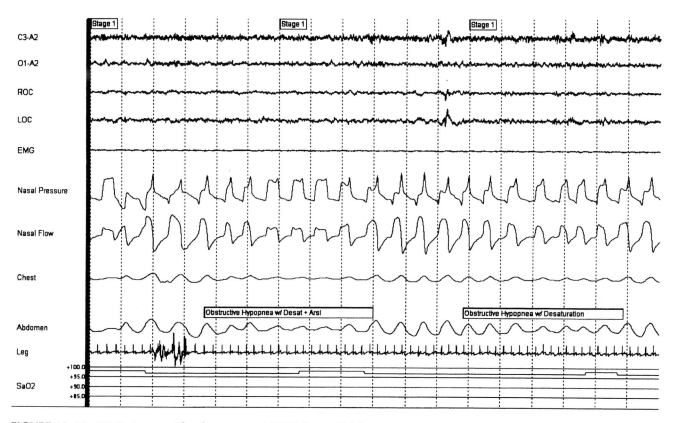

FIGURE 12–10. *BiPAP titration. Flow limitation in NREM sleep. Mild desaturations at 12/8 cm H₂O. Final optimal pressure was 14/8 cm H₂O. 90-second epoch.*

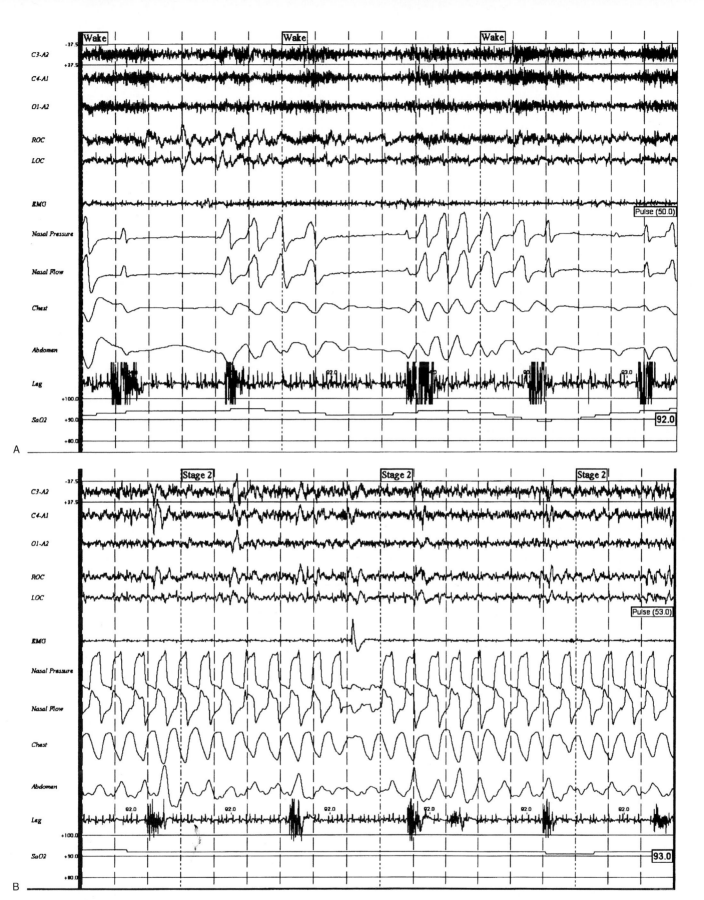

FIGURE 12–11. *Failed auto-titration.* **A:** *A 56-year-old man with severe SDB (four-channel study; respiratory disturbance index (RDI): 62; oxygen desaturation index (ODI) (4 percent): 51; lowest saturation: 72 percent) was started on home treatment with an auto-titrating device, with poor results. He was re-titrated in the sleep laboratory, and the reason for poor response was immediately evident as soon as the study was begun—central SDB unmasked or induced by CPAP. Fixed CPAP did not control the respiratory disorder; BiPAP did (following snapshots). 90-second epoch.* **B:** *BiPAP 13/8 cm H$_2$O, spontaneous mode. EPAP is inadequate, resulting in brief obstructive apneas during NREM sleep. PLMS continue but are of uncertain significance at this stage. Sleep and breathing are markedly improved relative to CPAP treatment. 90-second epoch.*

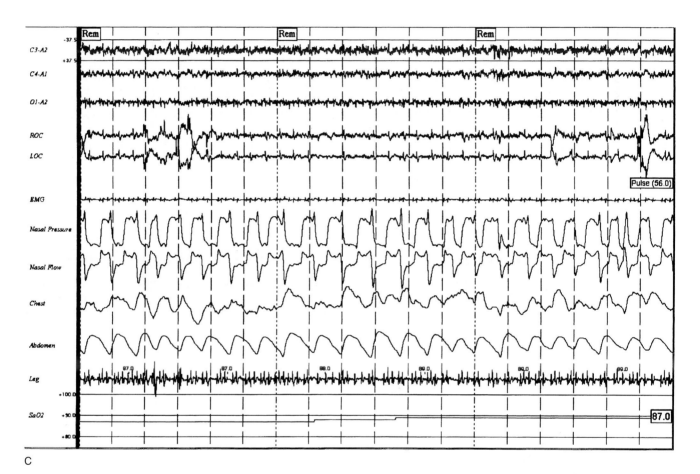

C

FIGURE 12–11, cont'd C: *BiPAP 15/10 cm H$_2$O, spontaneous mode. Inspiratory flow limitation and desaturations in REM sleep, but sleep and overall breathing are stable. Final setting was 18/10 cm H$_2$O, which eliminated flow limitation and maintained oxygen saturations in REM sleep greater than 90 percent. Auto-CPAP devices are not to be used in the setting of non-obstructive SDB. Thus, correct phenotyping of the disorder during the diagnostic study is important. One clinical clue for non-obstructive disease is a clear improvement of severe disease during REM sleep. 90-second epoch.*

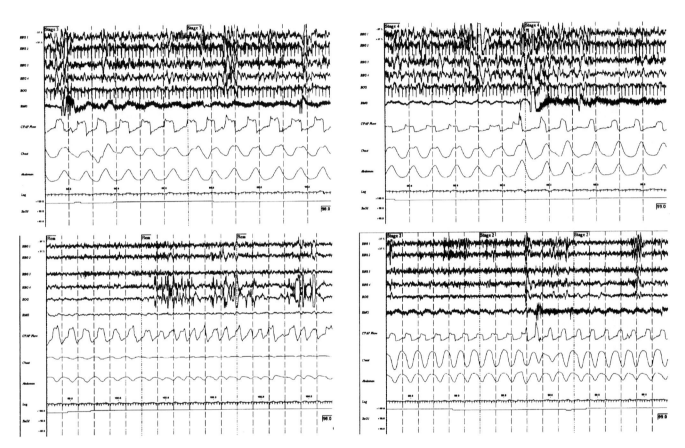

FIGURE 12–12. *Clinically successful auto-titration. A 33-year-old woman could not tolerate fixed CPAP at 9 centimeters, which was adequate to control sleep apnea. An auto-titrating device was well tolerated, and the patient is satisfied with the response. A full night PSG was performed on the home device, and pressures ranged from 5 to 10 centimeters. However, the machine responded sluggishly to several episodes of clearly abnormal flow, as demonstrated. Auto-CPAP machines differ in response characteristics, and still have a way to go before they fulfill their abundant promise.*

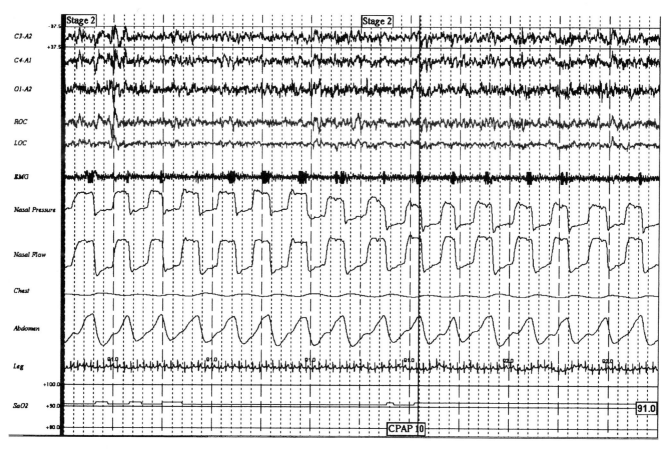

FIGURE 12–13. *Inadequate CPAP. Snoring and inspiratory flow limitation. 60-second epoch.*

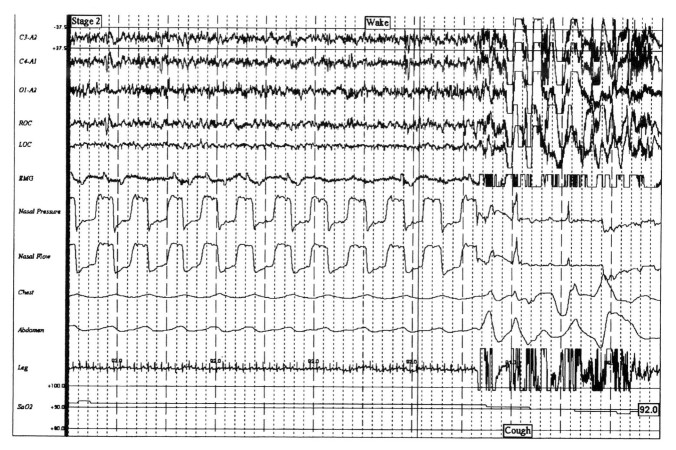

FIGURE 12–14. *Inadequate CPAP. Inspiratory flow limitation that resulted in an arousal. 60-second epoch.*

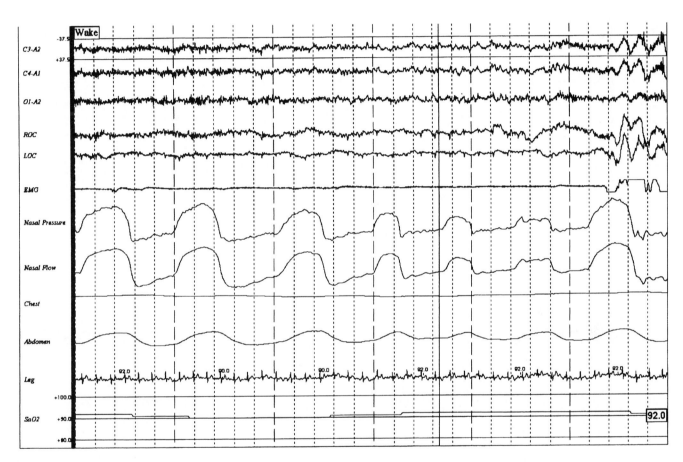

FIGURE 12–15. *Sleep-onset during CPAP titration. There is flow-limitation at sleep onset and an arousal occurs. Upper airway resistance predictably increases at sleep onset. If the pressure is not increased, it may not allow the patient to easily establish continuous sleep, as recurrent arousals will promote a prolonged sleep-wake transition phase. 30-second epoch.*

312

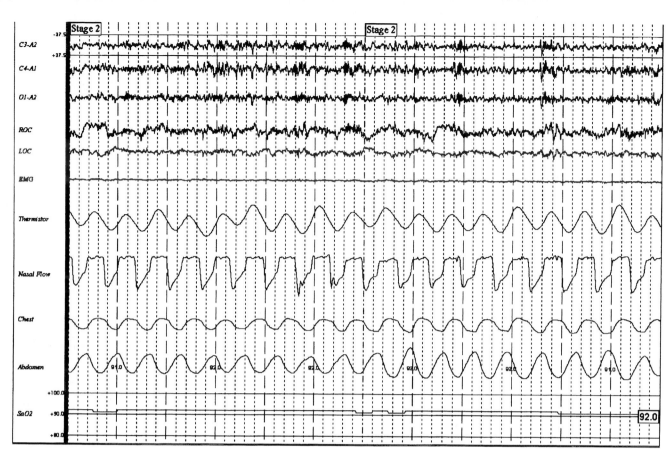

FIGURE 12–16. *Plateau flow limitation in a patient on benzodiazepines. This class of drugs (and others such as 5HT2-antagonists, Tiagabine) increase the percent of non-CAP type of NREM sleep. Respiration is quite stable in this state, even if obstructed. SWS exhibits similar behavior. Increased spindles are consistent with a benzodiazepine effect. During positive pressure titration in this patient, prolonged periods of stable sleep and flow can be expected even at subtherapeutic settings. 60-second epoch.*

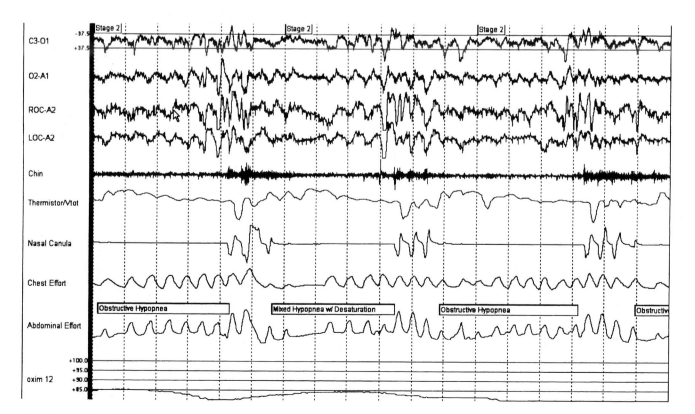

FIGURE 12–17. *NREM-dominant obstructive SDB—diagnostic snapshot. Severe obstructions, but the cycles are relatively short and symmetric. The effort band shows a suggestion of periodic breathing, but the flow signals are consistent with severe obstruction. 90-second epoch.*

313

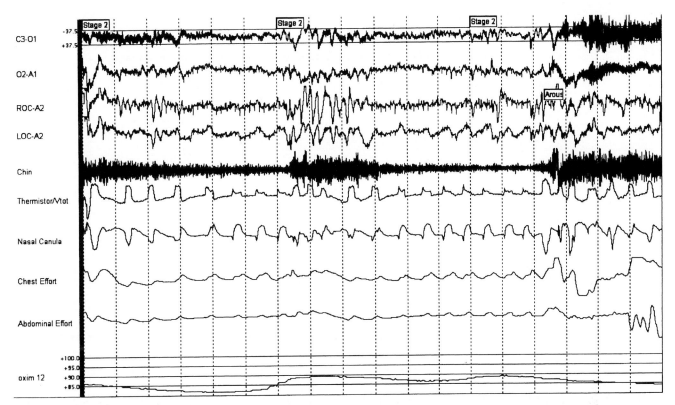

FIGURE 12–18. *NREM-dominant obstructive SDB—unstable NREM sleep. The same patient as in Figure 12–17, during positive pressure titration. Poor control in CAP-type NREM sleep. The pressure in this instance was BiPAP 15/11 cm H_2O, and the pattern was quite similar for CPAP between 12 and 15 centimeters. Higher pressures resulted in a small improvement in flow limitation, but worsened periodic breathing. Thus, there was no optimal pressure setting for CAP-NREM sleep. Low concentration CO_2 (0.5 percent to 0.75 percent) immediately normalized this pattern, consistent with hypocapnia driving the ventilatory instability. 90-second epoch.*

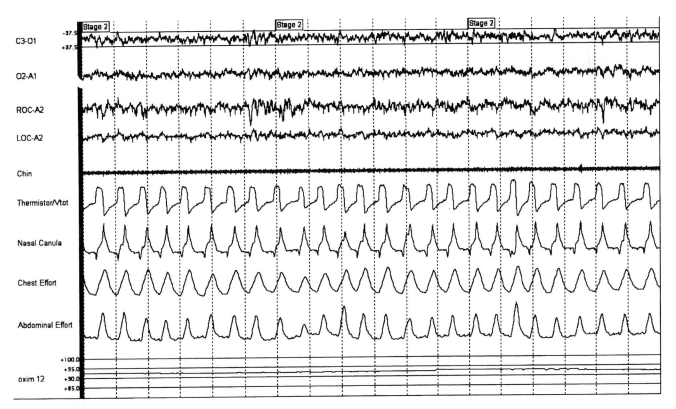

FIGURE 12–19. *NREM-dominant obstructive SDB—stable NREM sleep. The same patient as in Figure 12–17 during positive pressure titration. No respiratory events. Sleep and breathing are usually stable in slow-wave/non-CAP NREM sleep, and the percent of the titration night that such a pattern is seen is really "lost" titration time, even though it is a rebound phenomenon that required positive airway pressure to allow its occurence. 90-second epoch.*

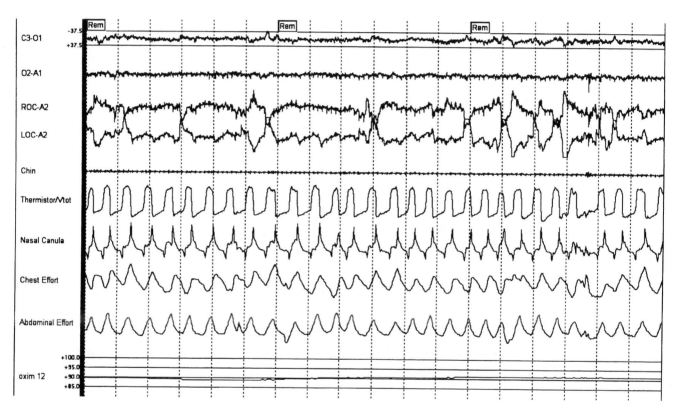

FIGURE 12–20. *A segment of REM sleep in a patient with NREM-dominant obstructive SDB. The same patient as in Figure 12–17, during positive pressure titration. Very good control at settings that were unable to treat disease during CAP-type NREM sleep. The stability of respiration during REM sleep suggests the presence of underlying periodic breathing-type physiology. 90-second snapshot.*

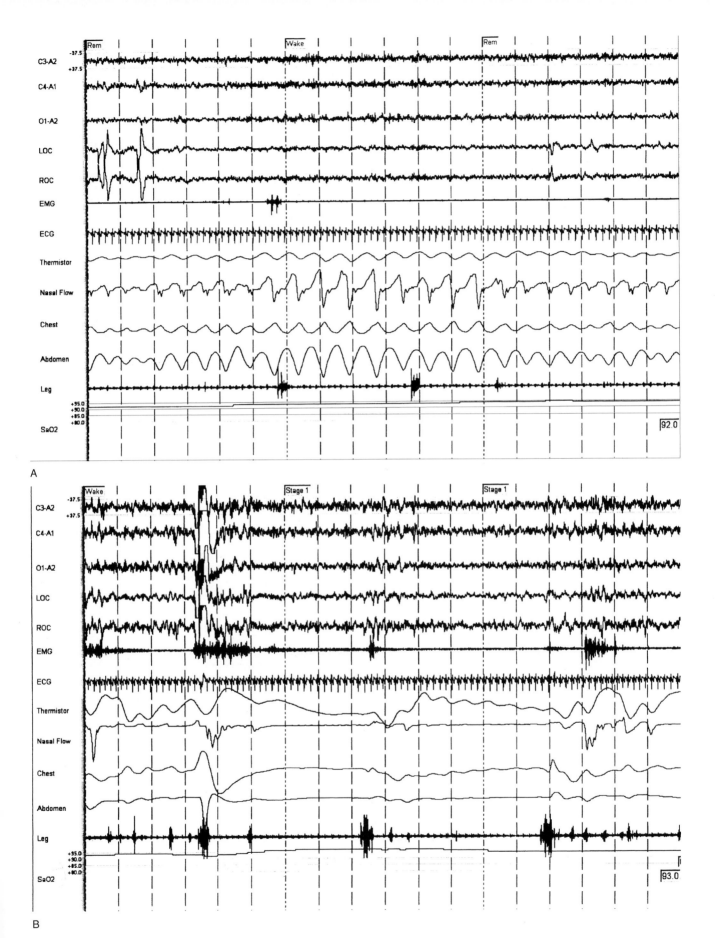

FIGURE 12–21. *Bilevel PAP + timed mode.* **A:** *A 77-year-old man with daytime sleepiness and snoring. Diagnostic snapshot in REM sleep showing minimal SDB.* **B:** *Same patient as in* **A**, *NREM sleep. Predominantly central apnea. Non-obstructive disease, including periodic breathing and high-altitude SDB, is often remarkably less severe in REM sleep.*

316

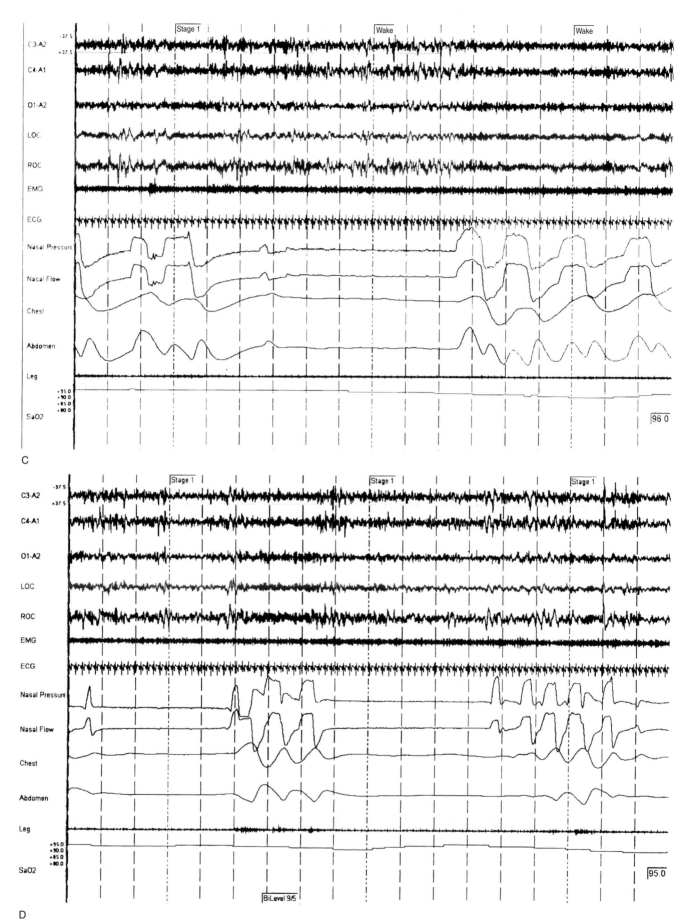

C

D

FIGURE 12–21, cont'd C: *CPAP titration results in repetitive central apneas, as shown.* **D:** *A switch to BiPAP in the spontaneous mode was no better and possibly worsens the central disease, presumably by inducing or worsening hypocapnia. Note that hypoxia is relatively mild.*

317

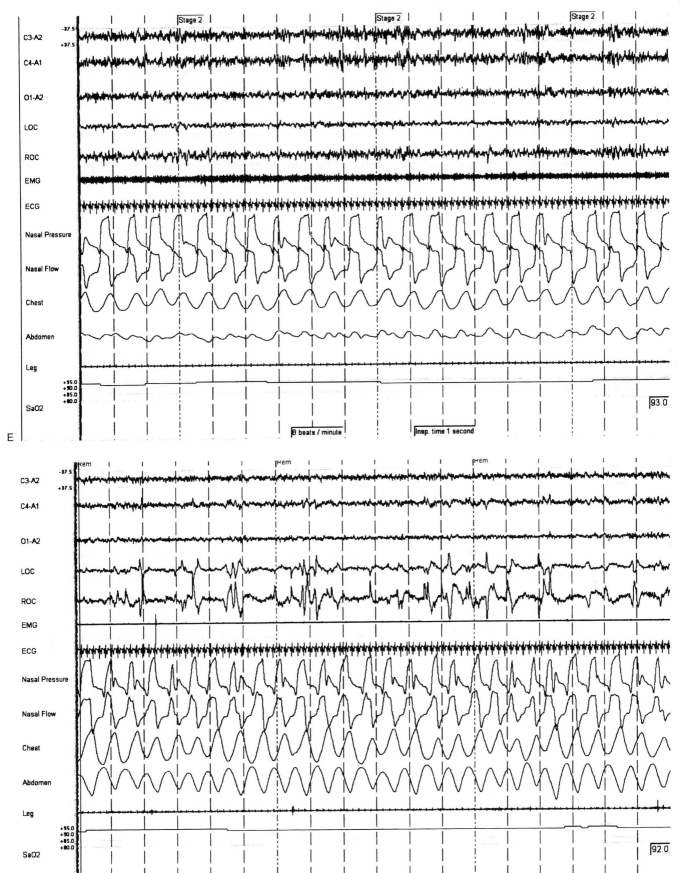

FIGURE 12–21, cont'd E: *Immediate stabilization of sleep and breathing following addition of a* <u>backup rate of 8 breaths per minute</u>, *and this response was maintained for the night. Although adding a backup rate in individual patients can also worsen disease by inducing even more hypocapnia, in some patients the timed breaths reduce the overall fluctuations in O_2 and CO_2 enough to stabilize breathing. The only way to assess the individual response is to "try it."* **F:** *Same patient as in* **E**, *REM sleep, BiPAP 9/5 cm H_2O, 8 beats/minute backup rate. Stability was expected anyway, based on the diagnostic component of the PSG, and this response in REM sleep has no correlation with the NREM sleep response.*

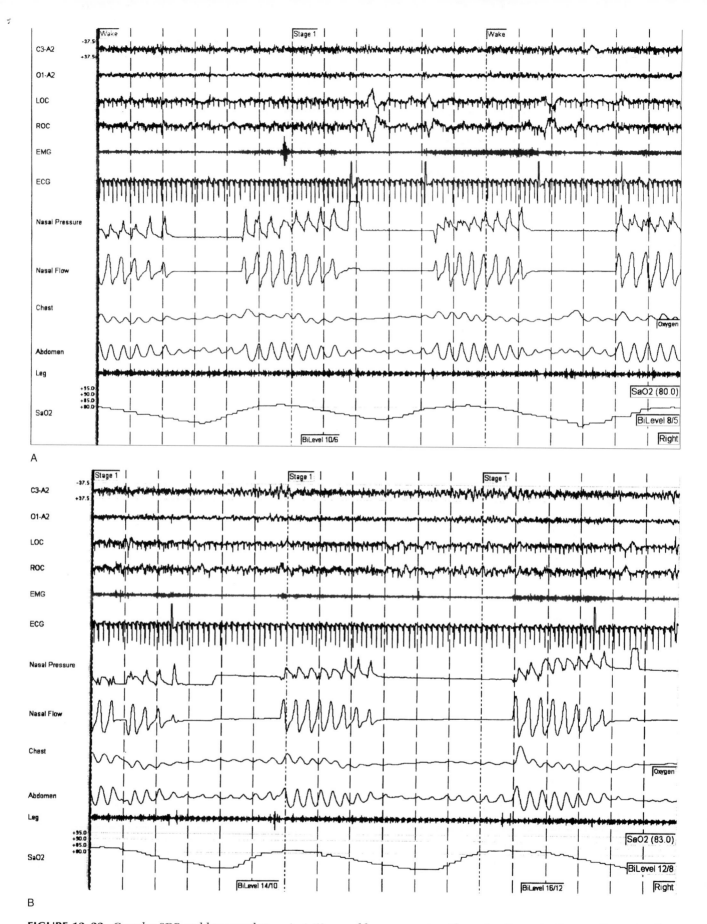

FIGURE 12–22. *Complex SDB and hypoventilation.* **A:** *A 56-year-old man presents with a prior diagnosis of severe obstructive sleep apnea, failure of tolerance/efficacy of CPAP, pulmonary hypertension, moderate obesity (BMI: 32), and class III exertional dyspnea. Echocardiogram does not show LV dysfunction. Pulmonary function tests show mild restriction. Re-titration is initiated with BiPAP. Obstruction, symmetric desaturations, and periodic breathing are noted. $PaCO_2$ is 66 mm Hg, PaO_2 50 mm Hg, on room air.* **B:** *Severe mixed events, with a Cheyne-Stokes pattern, desaturations and obstruction that are more or less unchanged at BiPAP settings ranging from 12/8 to 16/12 cms H_2O in the spontaneous mode.*

319

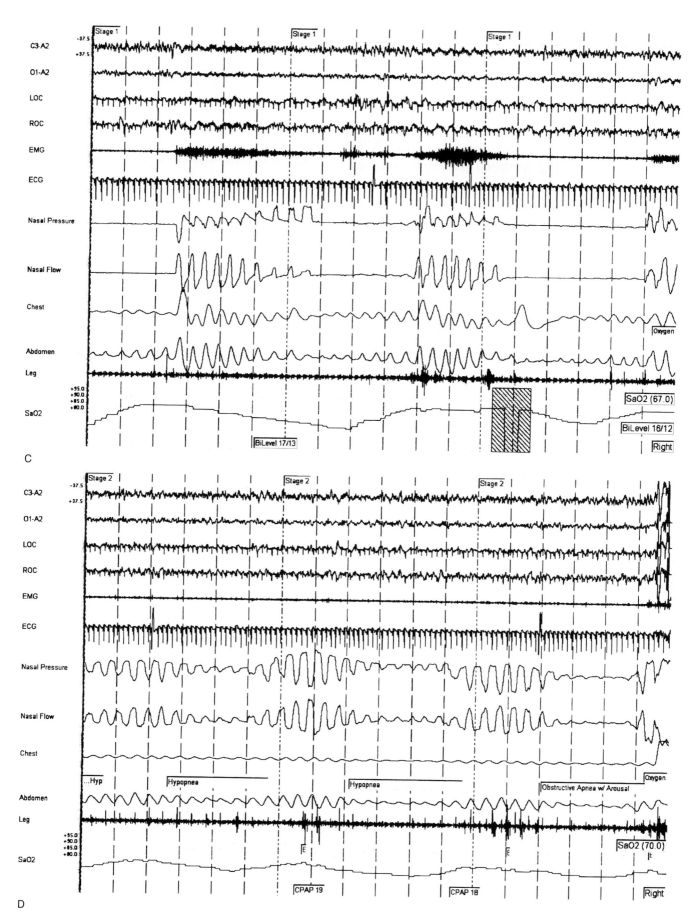

FIGURE 12–22, cont'd C: *An attempt is made to overcome obstruction by increasing the EPAP to 12 and 13 centimeters, with no benefit.* **D:** *CPAP is briefly evaluated to assess the amount of obstruction. Periodic breathing with symmetric waxing and waning effort, oxygen desaturations, and airflow are all noted.*

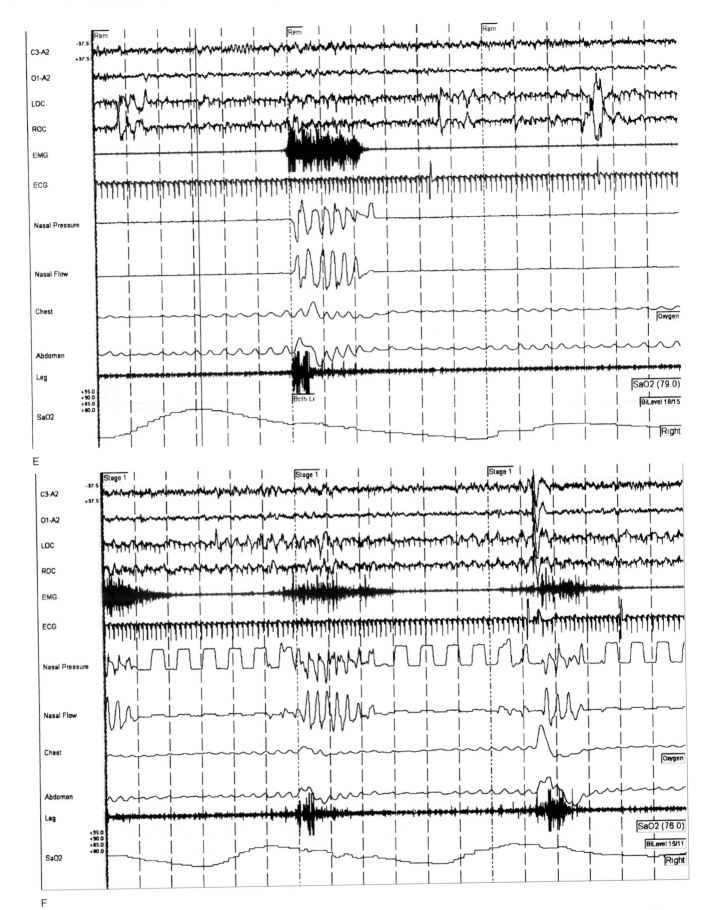

FIGURE 12–22, cont'd E: *BiPAP is 18/15 cms H₂O, spontaneous mode. Severe oxygen desaturation and obstructions are noted during REM sleep. Respiratory effort seems poor, even with uncalibrated effort signals. Flow is either obstructed or too small to trigger the BiPAP machine.* **F:** *A backup rate of 16 per minute is added (spontaneous/timed), and the pressure dropped to 15/11 centimeter as there is a concern that the high EPAP may be contributing to an excessive load on the respiratory muscles. Cyclic desaturations and arousals continue. The machine-supported timed breaths result in the near-square-wave pressure profile. Spontaneous effort is faster but unable to trigger breaths.*

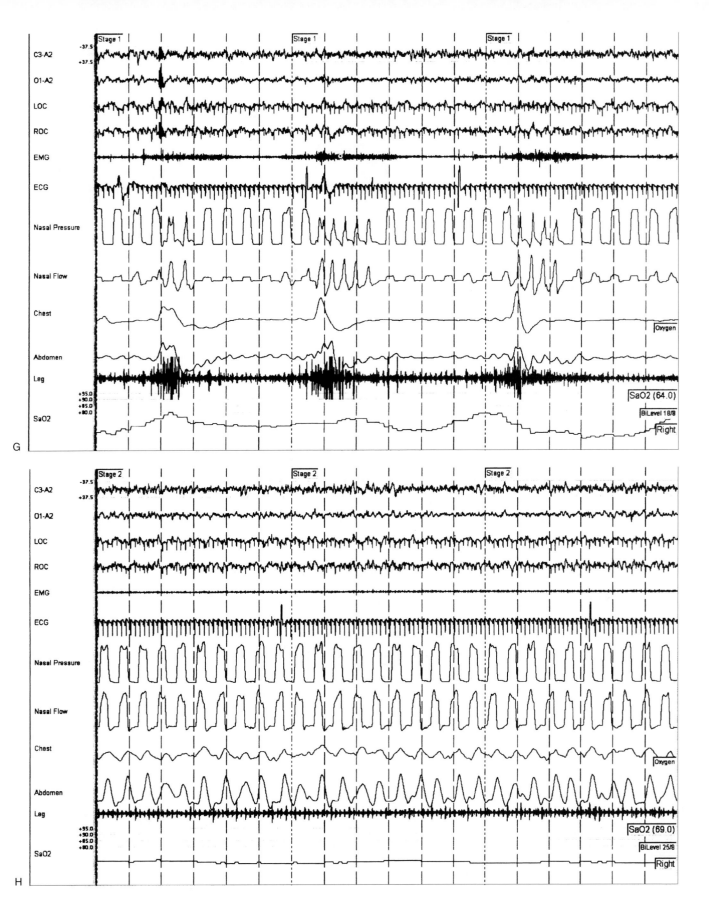

FIGURE 12–22, cont'd G: *An attempt is made to increase ventilatory support by increasing the I-E difference by a change from 15/11 to 18/8 cm H$_2$O. Backup rate is increased to 20 per minute. The actual tidal volume is not known during this titration, as the flow signal is not quantitative.* **H:** *Adequate control of obstruction in stable NREM sleep but strong suggestion of hypoventilation (persistent desaturation). Intracardiac shunting (e.g., across a patent foramen ovale) or V/Q (ventilation-perfusion) mismatches can contribute but are typically less likely in patients seen in sleep laboratories. Disproportionate desaturations are a surrogate marker of hypoventilation in this instance. Sleep type is non-CAP, which demonstrates stability similar to classic delta sleep. BiPAP is 25/8 cms without a backup rate (which was temporarily discontinued to assess need during this type of sleep).*

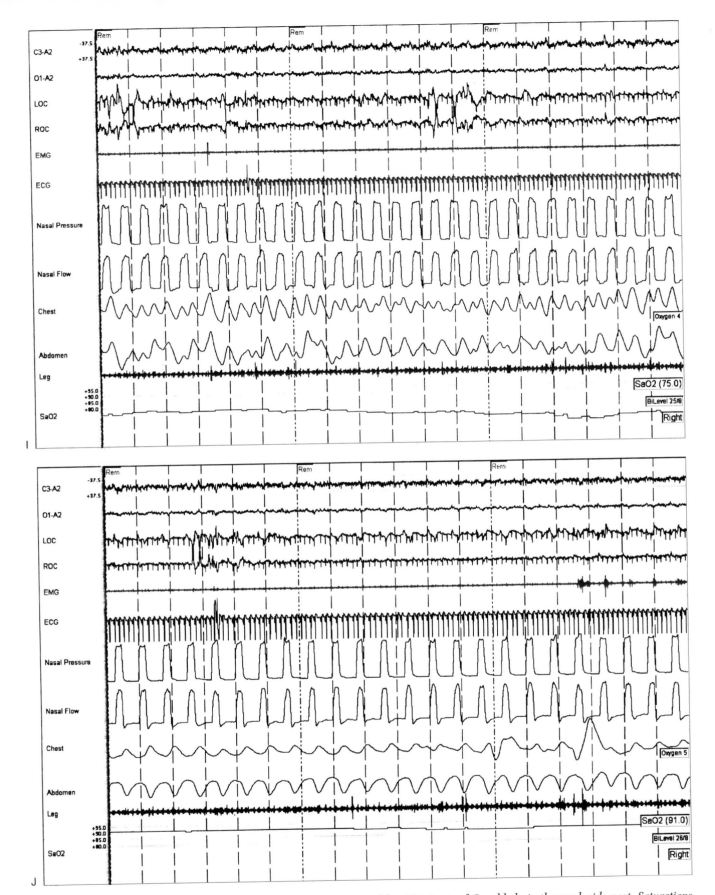

FIGURE 12–22, cont'd I: *In REM sleep, desaturations are improved by 4 L/minute of O_2 added via the mask side-port. Saturations remain unsatisfactory, despite an I-E difference of 17 cm H_2O (BiPAP is 25/8 centimeters). Respiratory rate is 20 per minute, which seems to be largely patient initiated. Backup rate is decreased to 16 per minute.* **J:** *An increase in supplemental oxygen to 6 L/minute results in satisfactory oxygen saturations. Improved saturations have slowed the respiratory rate to about 16 per minute, and breaths are spontaneously triggered. The patient has refused (or is unable to) sleep supine during this study—a potential limitation. Transcutaneous CO_2 monitoring will be an ideal additional variable if available. The percent of O_2 in the inhaled gas is not consistent and predictable, given variable dilution effects.*

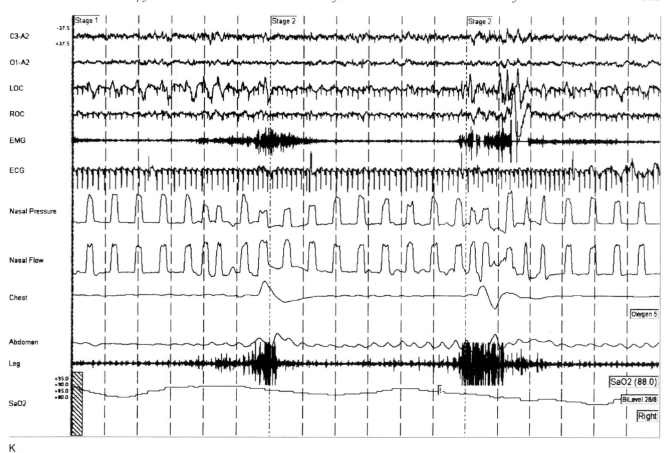

FIGURE 12–22, cont'd *K:* *It is now close to the end of the study. Periodic breathing continues at settings (26/8, 16 breaths per minute, 6 liters of additional oxygen) that were effective in REM sleep. Several breaths are likely machine initiated, given the rate discrepancy between effort and flow channels. Desaturations are less severe than during the early part of the night. Perfect control is not usually obtainable on a single night in such a patient, and a re-titration after a few weeks or months of regular use will allow further fine-tuning. Home oxymetry may be useful to track progress in this instance. On follow-up, this setting has resulted in a remarkable subjective clinical improvement. Room air wake PaO$_2$ is 58 mm Hg, and PaCO$_2$ is 55 mm Hg, consistent with an overall improvement in ventilatory drive.*

BIBLIOGRAPHY

Pepperell JC, Maskell NA, Jones DR, Langford-Wiley BA, Crosthwaite N, Stradling JR, Davies RJ. A randomized controlled trial of adaptive ventilation for Cheyne-Stokes breathing in heart failure. *Am J Respir Crit Care Med* 2003; 168:1109–1114.

Khayat RN, Xie A, Patel AK, Kaminski A, Skatrud JB. Cardio-respiratory effects of added dead space in patients with heart failure and central sleep apnea. *Chest* 2003;123:1551–1560.

Sanders MH, Kern N. Obstructive sleep apnea treated by independently adjusted inspiratory and expiratory positive airway pressures via nasal mask. Physiologic and clinical implications. *Chest* 1990;98:317–324.

Guilleminault C, Kreutzer M, Chang JL. Pregnancy, sleep disordered breathing and treatment with nasal continuous positive airway pressure. *Sleep Med* 2004;5:43–51.

Dempsey JA, Smith CA, Przybylowski T, Chenuel B, Xie A, Nakayama H, Skatrud JB. The ventilatory responsiveness to CO$_2$ below eupnoea as a determinant of ventilatory stability in sleep. *J Physiol* 2004;560:1–11.

d'Ortho MP. Auto-titrating continuous positive airway pressure for treating adult patients with sleep apnea syndrome. *Curr Opin Pulm Med* 2004;10:495–499.

Thomas RJ. Cyclic alternating pattern and positive airway pressure titration. *Sleep Med* 2002;3:315–322.

Naughton MT. Sleep disorders in patients with congestive heart failure. *Curr Opin Pulm Med* 2003;9:453–458.

Roux FJ, Hilbert J. Continuous positive airway pressure: new generations. *Clin Chest Med* 2003;24:315–342.

Yan AT, Bradley TD, Liu PP. The role of continuous positive airway pressure in the treatment of congestive heart failure. *Chest* 2001;120:1675–1685.

Farre R, Montserrat JM, Rigau J, Trepat X, Pinto P, Navajas D. Response of automatic continuous positive airway pressure devices to different sleep breathing patterns: a bench study. *Am J Respir Crit Care Med* 2002;166:469–473.

Pevernagie DA, Proot PM, Hertegonne KB, Neyens MC, Hoornaert KP, Pauwels RA. Efficacy of flow- vs impedance-guided autoadjustable continuous positive airway pressure: a randomized cross-over trial. *Chest* 2004;126:25–30.

Parreira VF, Delguste P, Jounieaux V, Aubert G, Dury M, Rodenstein DO. Glottic aperture and effective minute venti-lation during nasal two-level positive pressure ventilation in spontaneous mode. *Am J Respir Crit Care Med* 1996;154:1857–1863.

Jounieaux V, Aubert G, Dury M, Delguste P, Rodenstein DO. Effects of nasal positive-pressure hyperventilation on the glottis in normal sleeping subjects. *J Appl Physiol* 1995;79:186–193.

13

Pediatric Polysomnography

Timothy F. Hoban

NORMAL PSG FINDINGS AND SAMPLE MONTAGES FOR CHILDREN

Pediatric Polysomnography: General Considerations

Although polysomnography (PSG) represents the most reliable means for the investigation of pediatric sleep, the methods and facilities used for the study of adult patients do not always meet the needs of young children. There are several methods by which both children's families and the sleep lab may maximize patient comfort and the likelihood of successful pediatric studies.

Sleep laboratories that study children regularly usually find it helpful to prepare a child-friendly environment. An appropriately decorated pediatric room with an additional bed for a parent is optimal, but often feasible only for labs studying large numbers of children. The lab should provide age-appropriate distractions during setup, such as nonstimulating and nonfrightening videos. Stuffed animals, toys, and stickers are useful for both distraction and reward. Snacks such as crackers, milk, or juice should also be available. Proper preparation of the laboratory technical staff is essential. The study should be performed by staff who are comfortable with and oriented toward children. Setup for younger children may sometimes require additional staff. Finally, the lab should schedule pediatric studies to coincide as closely as possible with the child's typical sleep schedule, particularly for younger children with early bedtimes. Advance preparation of families for the study is also quite important. Children should be told what to expect during the study at a level appropriate for age, and an advance tour of the sleep lab will help acclimate youngsters to the equipment that will be used. Any potentially uncomfortable aspects of the study such as esophageal pressure monitoring (Pes) should be discussed with parents in advance.

NORMAL SLEEP AND BASELINE RECORDING MONTAGE FOR CHILDREN
(Figure 13–1)

These 30-second epochs demonstrate a standard recording montage for children. Electroencephalography (EEG) monitoring typically includes at least one central channel (C3-A2 and/or C4-A1) in addition to the occipital leads to provide increased sensitivity for the vertex sharp waves, K complexes, and sleep spindles used in scoring. Bilateral electrooculography (EOG) leads permit detection of the slow eye movements of light sleep and the rapid movements of REM sleep. Surface electromyography (EMG) is typically recorded over the mentalis or submentalis muscles, allowing the detection of movement that may accompany arousals. Additional EMG leads over the right and left anterior tibialis muscles permit detection of periodic limb movements in sleep (PLMS). Nasal-oral airflow monitoring, oximetry, and assessment of thoracoabdominal effort via strain gauges are performed in the same manner used for adults. Figure 13–1**A** demonstrates normal stage III sleep in a 4-year-old boy, characterized by high-amplitude slow-wave forms on EEG, striking regularity of respiratory rate and effort, and preserved muscle tone on chin EMG.

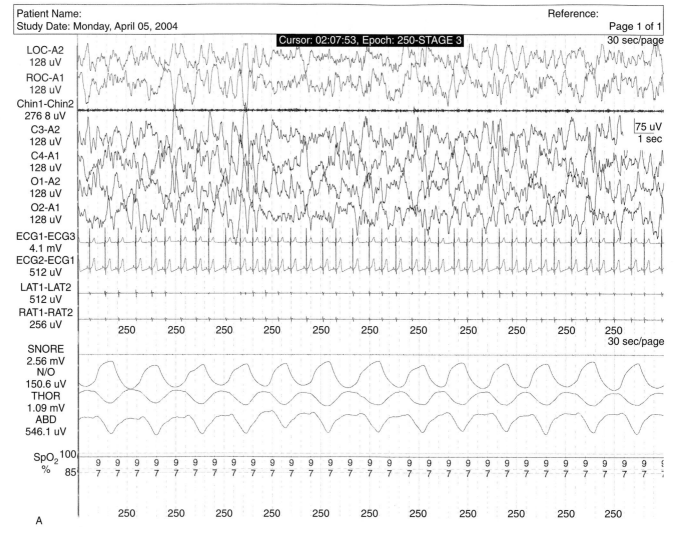

FIGURE 13–1. **A:** *Baseline recording montage and normal stage III sleep.*

Figure 13–1**B** demonstrates normal REM sleep in the same patient. In addition to rapid eye movements, the epoch is characterized by mixed EEG frequencies, by absent EMG tone, and by variable respiratory rate and effort.

USE OF THE HYPNOGRAM IN PEDIATRIC STUDIES (Figure 13–2)

The software used for the interpretation of digital PSGs usually allows data to be viewed graphically in the form of a hypnogram displaying the changes in certain data parameters during the night. The hypnogram at minimum includes sleep stage, body position, and SaO_2 but may also chart the frequency of apnea, periodic limb movements,

or other events. Review of the hypnogram permits rapid assessment of sleep architecture and the influence of sleep state or position upon the frequency of desaturation or apnea. This hypnogram illustrates sleep cycling in an 8-year-old girl with the Chiari II malformation. In spite of normal sleep cycling and only minor disruption of sleep continuity, the hypnogram clearly illustrates a consistent pattern of REM-related hypoxemia during sleep due to central and obstructive apneas.

CUSTOM MONTAGES IN CHILDREN

Standard recording montages for children are often customized depending on the variety of sleep disorder being investigated. End-tidal or transcutaneous carbon dioxide

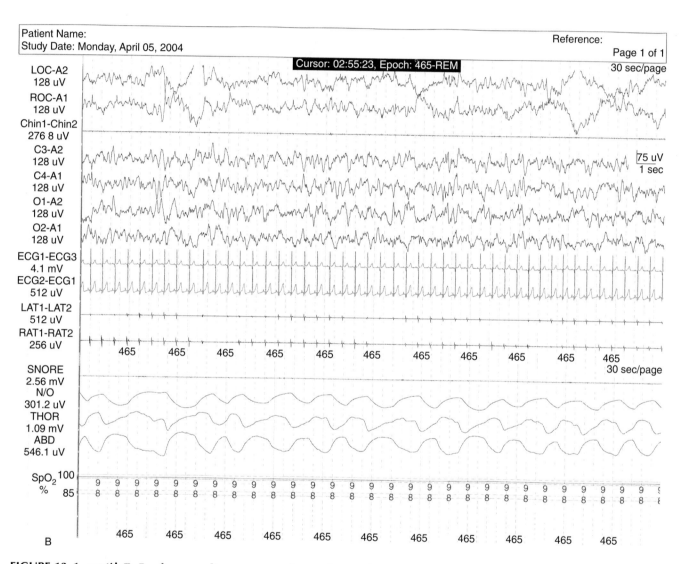

FIGURE 13–1, cont'd B: *Baseline recording montage and normal REM sleep.*

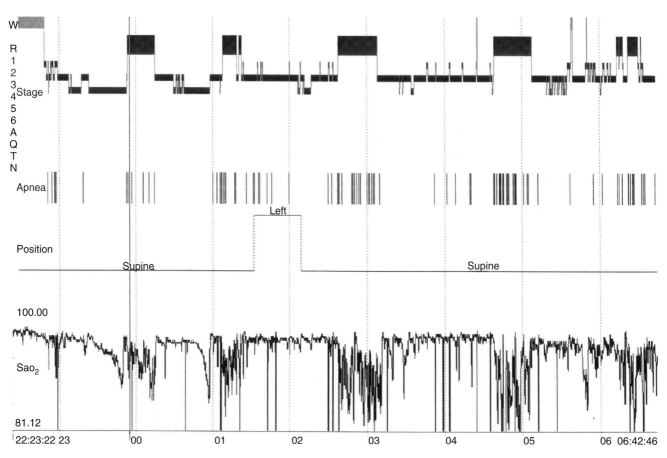

FIGURE 13–2. *Use of the hypnogram in pediatric studies.*

monitoring is usually performed when there is clinical suspicion of nocturnal hypercapnia, such as may occur in youngsters with neuromuscular disorders, morbid obesity, or congenital central alveolar hypoventilation (Ondine's curse). Figure 13–3 is a 30-second epoch of stage III sleep from a 4-year-old girl with Aicardi syndrome. This tracing demonstrates normal waveforms for capnography (CAPN), with maximal values detected at the end of expiration. The ETCO2 signal demonstrates both graphically and numerically a rolling average derived from the capnogram. Incidentally demonstrated is low baseline oxygen saturation in the absence of respiratory events.

Esophageal Pressure Monitoring and Nasal Pressure Transducers

Respiratory monitoring during pediatric PSG has traditionally measured oral-nasal airflow using thermistors or thermocouples, which provide a semiquantitative estimate of airflow. This has been supplanted in recent years by nasal pressure recording, which is thought to be more sensitive to small decrements and restriction of airflow. Lack of published pediatric experience and accepted normative data limit use of this technique at present. Esophageal pressure monitoring (Pes) is a technique in which a small, water-filled esophageal catheter attached to a transducer provides direct measurement of esophageal pressure fluctuations. In children with the upper airway resistance syndrome (UARS), where increased respiratory effort leading to arousal may occur in the absence of discrete apneas and hypopneas, Pes may reveal excessive pressure fluctuations due to partial airway obstruction. Figure 13–4 is a 60-second epoch that demonstrates partial airway obstruction in a 17-year-old girl with sickle cell disease and UARS. Despite normal oximetry and only minimal snoring, the nasal pressure tracing demonstrates a "plateau" at the top of the waveform indicative of flow limitation. Peak-to-nadir Pes fluctuations nearing 30 centimeters of water

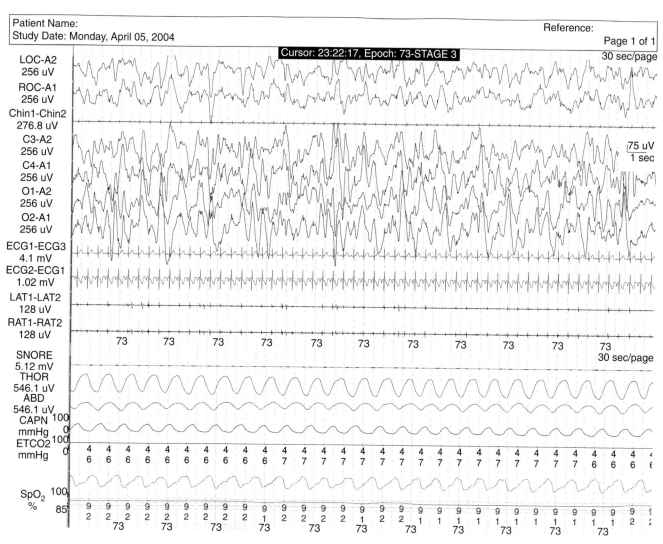

FIGURE 13–3. *Normal capnogram.*

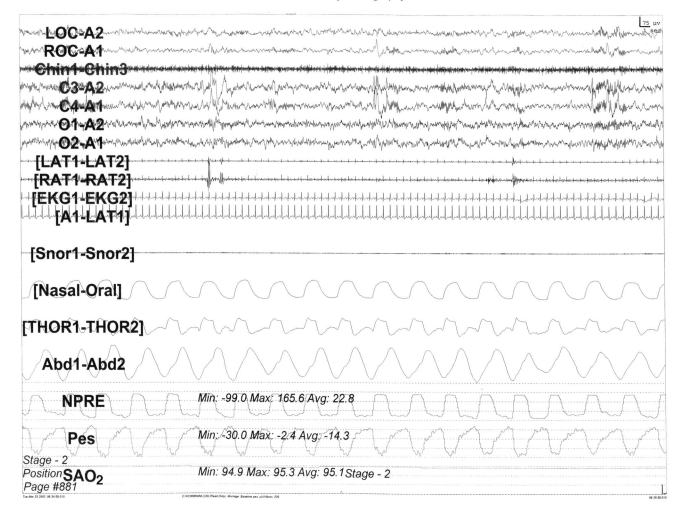

FIGURE 13–4. *Custom montages for children: esophageal pressure monitoring (Pes) and nasal pressure transducers.*

(normal <= 10) confirm the presence of significant partial obstruction and increased work of breathing.

16-Channel Electroencephalogram

Among the advantages of digital PSG is the ability to accommodate full 16-channel EEG in addition to the baseline recording montage when sleep-related seizures are suspected in a child. Figure 13–5 is a 30-second epoch that demonstrates multifocal epileptiform discharges during light non-REM sleep in a 5-year-old boy with Prader-Willi syndrome who presented with a history of a 20-second sleep-related seizure characterized by nonfocal upper body shaking followed by extension of both arms over the head. This tracing demonstrates frequent spike discharges emanating from the right central-temporal region (near the C4 and T6 electrodes) and less frequently from an independent focus near the P4 electrode.

NORMAL SLEEP IN INFANTS

The EEG characteristics of normal sleep in infants are immature and poorly differentiated as compared to the sleep of normal children and adults. As a result, the classification of sleep stages for infants reflects these differences and distinguishes three states: *active sleep, quiet sleep,* and *indeterminate sleep.*

Active Sleep

Infants typically enter sleep with a period of active sleep, which is the infant equivalent of REM sleep and comprises almost half of total sleep time in term infants. As demonstrated in this 30-second epoch for a 3-month-old infant (Figure 13–6), the EEG background is characterized by mixed frequencies of somewhat higher amplitude than those seen in older children. The rapid eye movements

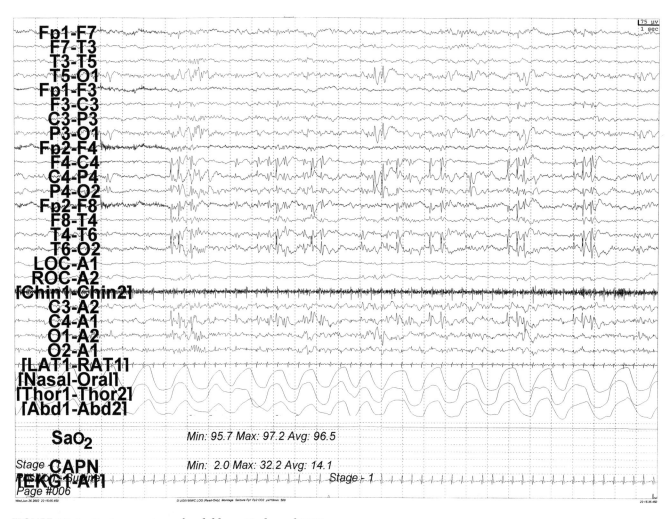

FIGURE 13–5. *Custom montages for children: 16-channel EEG.*

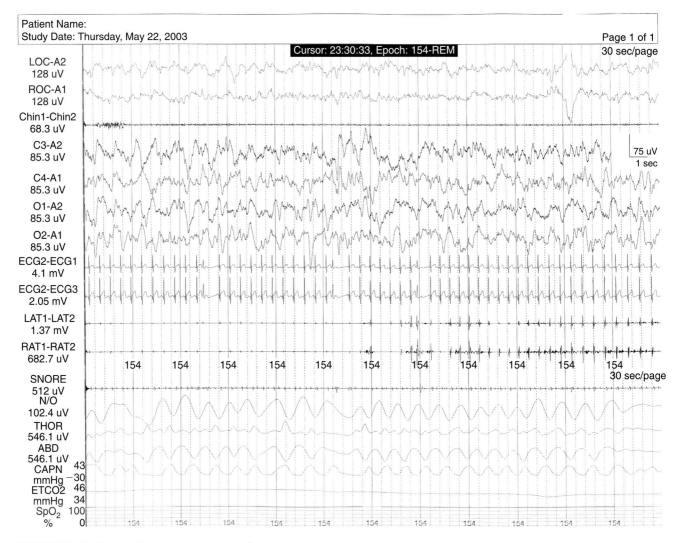

FIGURE 13–6. *Normal sleep in infants: active sleep.*

demonstrated in this segment are not always apparent in infants, whereas the reduced EMG activity, increased heart rate variability, and irregular respiration demonstrated represent somewhat more consistent findings.

Specific scoring criteria for infant sleep have been described by Anders *et al.* In addition to the characteristic physiologic activity described above, active sleep is also characterized by phasic bursts of motor activity, which may include facial movement (smiles, frowns, sucking), gross and fine body movements, and even brief vocalization.

Quiet Sleep

Quiet sleep is demonstrated in this 30 second epoch for the same 3-month-old patient (Figure 13–7). The heart rate is reduced and EMG activity increased compared to

active sleep. EEG reveals intermixed delta and theta activity with an asymmetric and an immature sleep spindle in the C3 lead during the last 5 seconds of the epoch. Respirations are deep, regular, and unlabored throughout the segment.

Other manifestations of quiet sleep described by Anders *et al* include behavioral quiescence, paucity of movement, and high EMG tone. Epochs not clearly correlating to active or quiet sleep may be scored as *indeterminate sleep*.

Periodic Breathing

Periodic breathing (Figure 13–8) in infants is characterized by alternating periods of regular respiration separated by 5- to 10-second central pauses. This pattern may arise during either active or quiet sleep and is most commonly

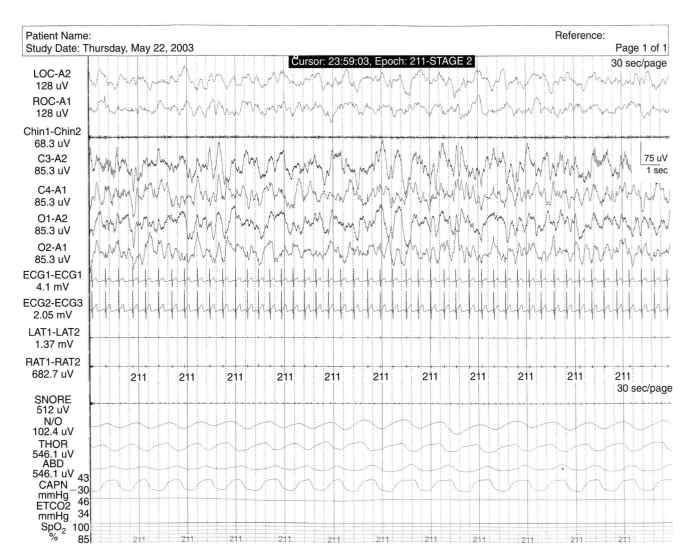

FIGURE 13–7. *Normal sleep in infants: quiet sleep.*

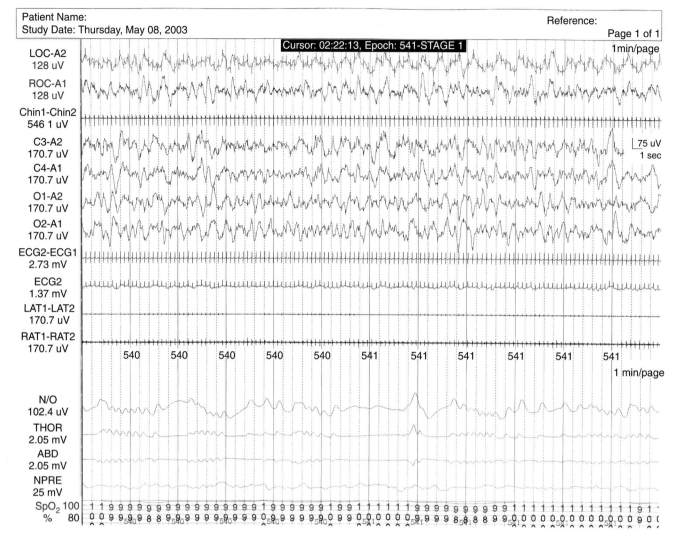

FIGURE 13–8. *Normal sleep in infants: periodic breathing.*

exhibited by premature infants, although it is seen occasionally in term infants as well. A periodic pattern of respiratory effort and airflow is demonstrated on this 1-minute epoch of sleep for a 2-month-old infant. No desaturation or sleep disruption is seen in association with the respiratory variation demonstrated.

ABNORMAL PSG FINDINGS IN CHILDREN

Sleep-Disordered Breathing

Obstructive Apnea

Figure 13–9 shows a 60-second segment recorded from a 2-year-old girl with micrognathia due to Pierre-Robin syndrome. The onset of the 15-second apnea is accompanied by a slight reduction of heart rate that persists until the end of the apnea and is followed by brief tachycardia. Despite the short duration of the event, oxygen saturation reaches a nadir of 80.6 percent.

Brief Obstructive Apnea

This 30-second epoch (Figure 13–10) was recorded from the same 2-year-old patient with Pierre-Robin syndrome. Although the duration of obstructed flow is less than the 10 seconds required for scoring an apnea for adults, it exceeds the duration of two respiratory cycle lengths generally used for scoring apneas in children. Although the apnea does not cause any oxygen desaturations, it is accompanied by paradoxical (out of phase) chest

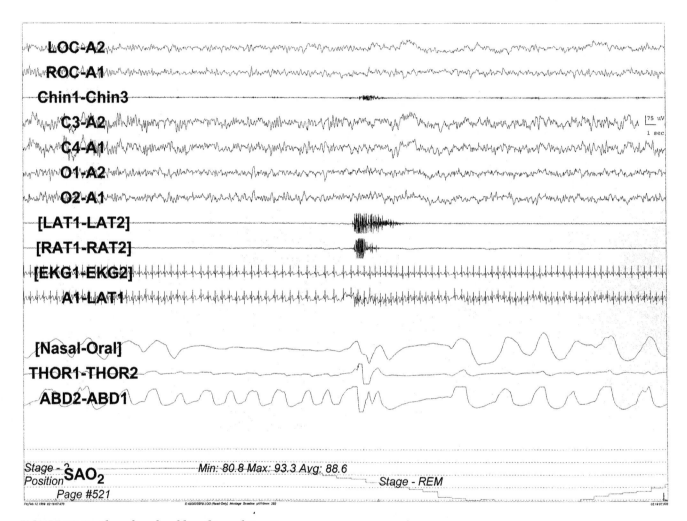

FIGURE 13–9. *Sleep-disordered breathing: obstructive apnea.*

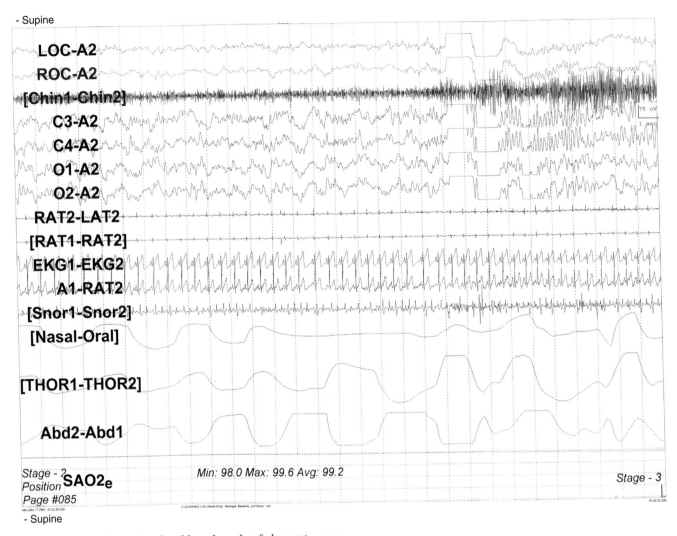

FIGURE 13–10. *Sleep-disordered breathing: brief obstructive apnea.*

wall movements and causes prominent arousal from sleep.

Complex Obstruction

This 60-second segment (Figure 13–11) was recorded from a teenager with spina bifida and hydrocephalus due to the Chiari II malformation who presented with profound nocturnal oxygen desaturations and obstructive symptoms while being observed in the intensive care unit following revision of a ventriculoperitoneal shunt. In addition to prolonged apnea lasting 50 seconds, the epoch demonstrates only slow and irregular respiratory effort at a rate of only 6 to 8 breaths per minute.

Hypopnea

Hypopneas are events characterized by reduced airflow or effort sufficient to cause either arousal or desaturations.

Unfortunately, there is considerable variability among sleep laboratories regarding the duration or severity required to score hypopneas and no universally accepted definition exists. At the University of Michigan, hypopnea may be scored for any reduction of airflow or effort that exceeds 10 seconds and results in arousal or a 4 percent desaturation. The middle third of this 30-second epoch (Figure 13–12) recorded from a teenager with sickle cell disease reveals a hypopnea characterized by moderate reduction of airflow in the nasal-oral channel and crescendo snoring near the end of the event. Although no oxygen desaturation occurs, the hypopnea results in a brief arousal from sleep and is accompanied by CO_2 levels of 57.7 mm Hg on the capnogram near the end of the event. Esophageal pressure fluctuations exceeding 30 centimeters of water (normal = 10) underscore the severity of obstruction present.

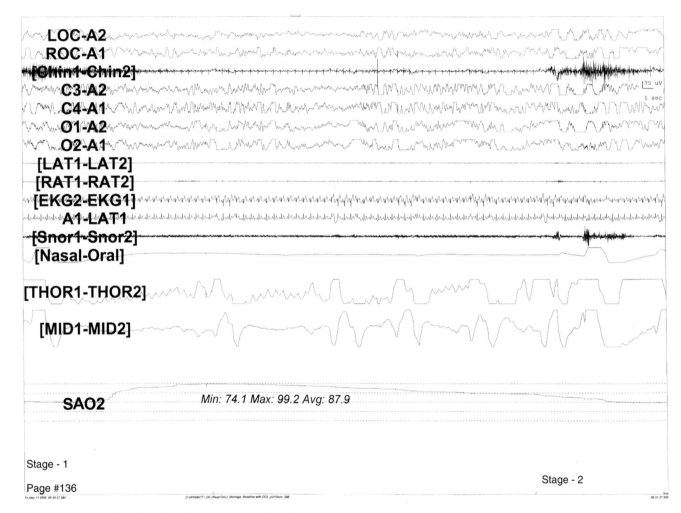

FIGURE 13–11. *Sleep-disordered breathing: complex obstruction.*

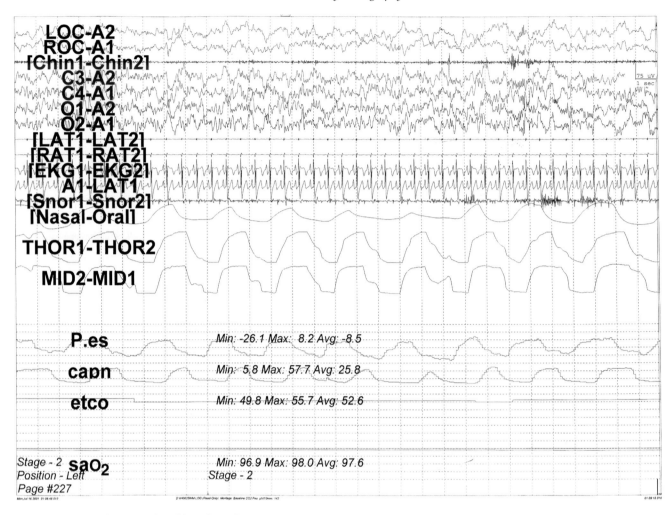

FIGURE 13–12. *Sleep-disordered breathing: hypopnea.*

Central Apnea

Central apneas represent pauses in respiration caused by absent or delayed respiratory effort rather than upper airway obstruction. As is the case for other varieties of apnea, a duration of 10 seconds is required to score a central apnea for adults, whereas some labs require a duration of only two respiratory cycle lengths for children. This 60-second segment (Figure 13–13) was recorded from a 12-year-old boy with longstanding insomnia and suspected Asperger syndrome (a variety of high-functioning autism). The study revealed an apnea-hypopnea index of 10.2 events per hour, consisting primarily of brief central apneas with only minimal desaturations. The central apnea demonstrated in this epoch follows a deep sigh and is characterized by absent airflow as determined by the nasal-oral and nasal pressure leads. The minor oscillations apparent on the capnogram

are synchronous with the electrocardiogram, representing minute airflow from cardioballistic forces rather than functional respiration.

Prolonged Central Apnea

This 60-second epoch (Figure 13–14) from a 3-year-old boy with developmental delay and seizures demonstrates a prolonged central apnea arising from REM sleep and causing arterial oxygen desaturation to 78.4 percent.

Mixed Apnea and Periodic Respiration

Mixed apneas begin with a centrally mediated pause in respiration followed by resumption of respiratory effort impeded by an obstructed upper airway. The first 2-minute epoch (Figure 13–15) from a 13-year-old boy with Alexander disease, a progressive cerebral degeneration, demonstrated an unusual cyclical pattern of mixed apneas with

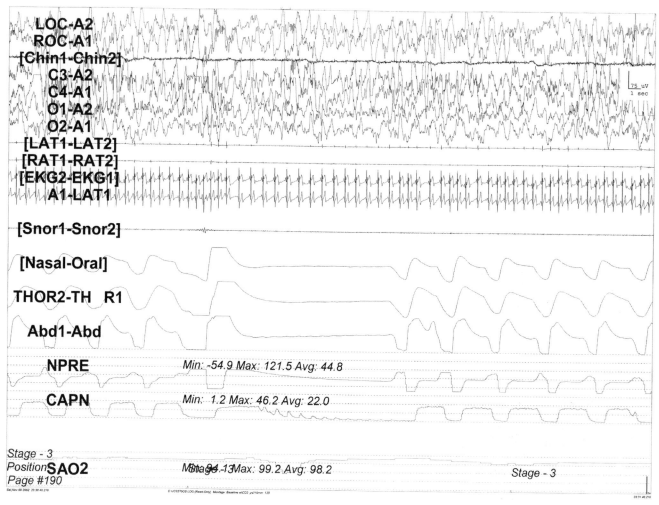

LOC-A2
ROC-A1
[Chin1-Chin2]
C3-A2
C4-A1
O1-A2
O2-A1
[LAT1-LAT2]
[RAT1-RAT2]
[EKG2-EKG1]
A1-LAT1

[Snor1-Snor2]

[Nasal-Oral]

THOR2-TH R1

Abd1-Abd

NPRE   Min: -54.9 Max: 121.5 Avg: 44.8

CAPN   Min: 1.2 Max: 46.2 Avg: 22.0

Stage - 3
Position SAO2   Stage - 13 Max: 99.2 Avg: 98.2   Stage - 3
Page #190

75 uV
1 sec

FIGURE 13–13. *Sleep-disordered breathing: central apnea.*

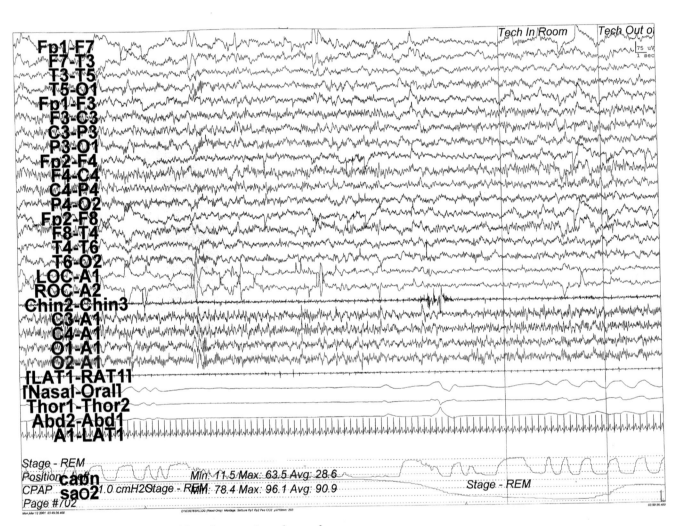

FIGURE 13–14. *Sleep-disordered breathing: prolonged central apnea.*

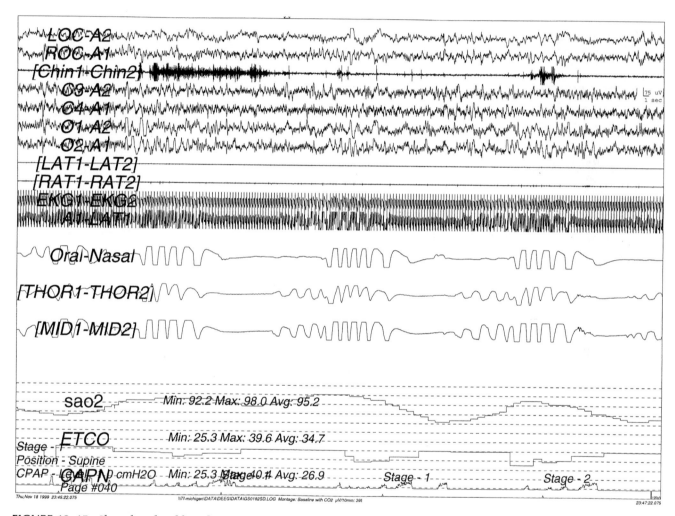

FIGURE 13–15. *Sleep-disordered breathing: mixed apnea.*

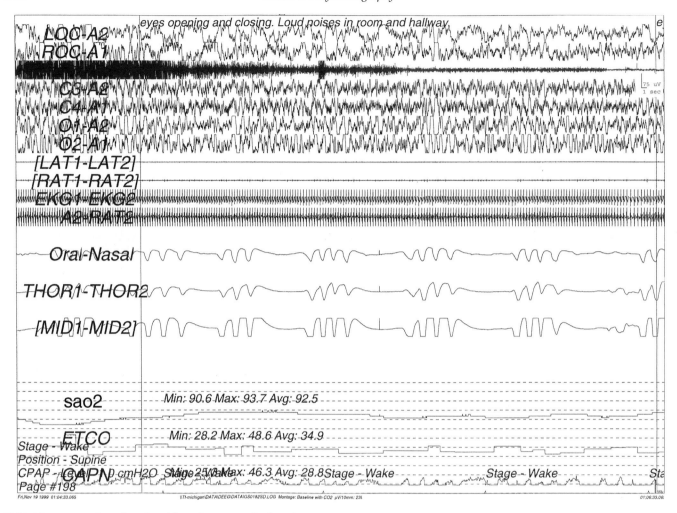

FIGURE 13–16. *Sleep-disordered breathing: periodic breathing.*

minimal oxygen desaturation. The second epoch (Figure 13–16), from the same study, demonstrates prominent periodic respiration during wakefulness, which is extremely uncommon in healthy older children.

Obesity-Hypoventilation Syndrome

Hypoventilation is defined as impairment of pulmonary ventilation sufficient to produce hypoxemia and/or hypercapnia. The etiology of hypoventilation in morbidly obese youngsters may be multifactorial as a result of both chronic upper airway obstruction as well as physical restriction of chest wall and diaphragmatic movement due to obesity. This 30-second epoch (Figure 13–17) of slow-wave sleep is recorded from an 8-year-old with morbid obesity and aniridia whose weight was 85 kilograms near the time of the study. Although the respiratory disturbance index during the study was only 5.6 apneas and hypopneas per hour, the PSG revealed long periods of sustained hypox-

emia and hypercapnia such as that demonstrated in this segment. The concurrent snoring exhibited during this epoch and frequently during the remainder of the study suggests an obstructive component for this patient's hypoventilation.

Non-obstructive Hypoventilation

Hypoventilation may also occur purely on a non-obstructive basis in the case of children with cervical spinal cord lesions, muscular dystrophy, and many neuromuscular disorders. This 60-second epoch (Figure 13–18) begins in REM sleep with a long period of hypoxemia as low as 82 percent and hypercapnia exceeding 72 mm Hg. No snoring or other evidence of upper airway obstruction is evident. Hypoventilation ends abruptly with arousal from sleep and brisk improvement of oxygen saturation and reduction of the elevated end-tidal CO_2 levels on the capnogram.

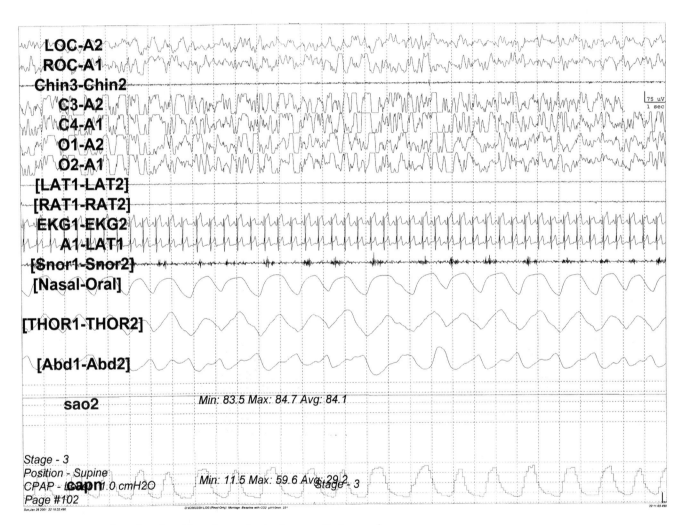

FIGURE 13–17. *Sleep-disordered breathing: obesity-hypoventilation syndrome.*

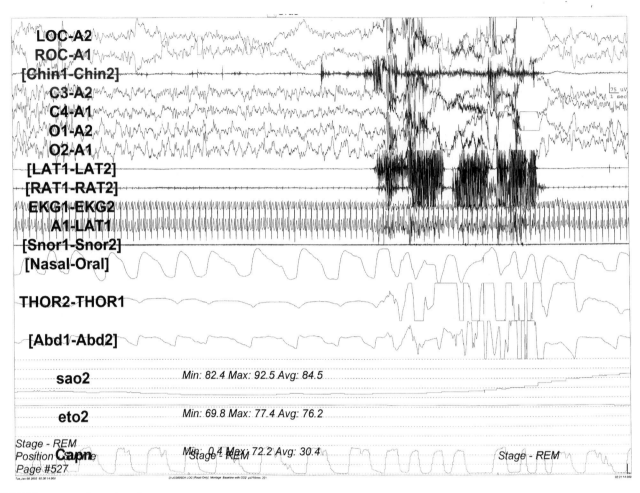

FIGURE 13–18. *Sleep-disordered breathing: non-obstructive hypoventilation.*

Bradypnea

This 60-second PSG epoch (Figure 13–19) from an 8-year-old girl with spina bifida and Chiari II malformation demonstrates a decreased respiratory rate of only 7 breaths per minute during REM sleep. Although significant gas exchange abnormalities are not demonstrated during this epoch, the study as a whole exhibited frequent REM-related hypoventilation and central apneas with oxygen saturations as low as 69 percent and hypercapnia as high as 65 mm Hg. The patient underwent suboccipital decompression of her Chiari II malformation shortly following this study. Follow-up PSG performed 5 months postoperatively revealed no bradypnea, moderately improved hypoventilation (oximetry nadir of 84 percent), and a reduction of the respiratory disturbance index from 12.2 to 6.8 events per hour.

Upper Airway Resistance Syndrome

UARS, in which increased respiratory effort due to partial airway obstruction disrupts sleep in the absence of gas exchange abnormalities, may cause symptoms virtually indistinguishable from those of traditional OSA. This 60-second segment (Figure 13–20) was recorded from a 12-year-old boy who presented with complaints of excessive somnolence, prominent nighttime snoring, and a significant decline in academic performance. Although the PSG exhibited only one obstructive apnea and seven hypopneas during 6 hours of recorded sleep, long periods of excessive esophageal pressure fluctuations were apparent, often exceeding 40 cm of water (normal = 10).

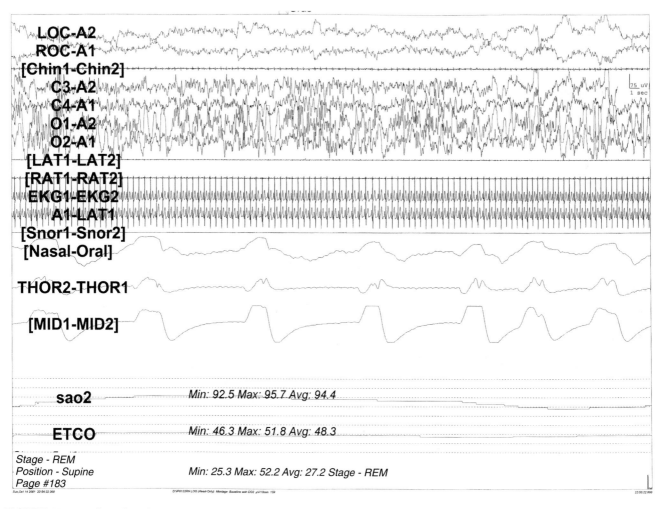

FIGURE 13–19. *Sleep-disordered breathing: bradypnea.*

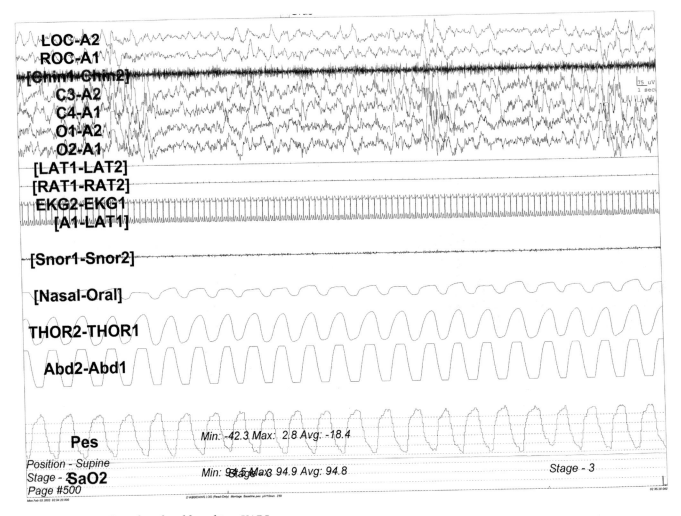

FIGURE 13–20. *Sleep-disordered breathing: UARS.*

Pes Crescendo

This 30-second epoch (Figure 13–21), recorded from the same 12-year-old patient, exhibits Pes crescendo, a characteristic PSG finding in UARS. During the crescendo, gradually increasing esophageal pressure fluctuations reflect increasing respiratory effort in the face of partial airway obstruction, culminating in arousal from sleep. As is demonstrated in this segment, the event is not accompanied by detectable alteration of airflow or oxygen saturation.

Periodic Limb Movements in Sleep

This 240-second epoch (Figure 13–22) demonstrates PLMS in a 12-year-old boy with obstructive sleep apnea. PLMS are characterized by periodic elevations of EMG tone lasting between 0.5 and 5 seconds in duration

and occurring at intervals ranging between 4 and 90 seconds. Arousals may also occur in association with PLMS.

Parasomnias

Non-REM Arousal Disorders

Non-REM arousal parasomnias such as night terrors, sleep walking, and confusional arousals occur commonly in children and are polysomnographically characterized by abrupt partial arousal from slow-wave sleep. This 60-second segment (Figure 13–23) was recorded in a 16-year-old girl with clinical complaints of insomnia and restless leg syndrome. The confusional arousal demonstrated arises abruptly from slow wave and is characterized by talking and arm flinging without return to full wakefulness.

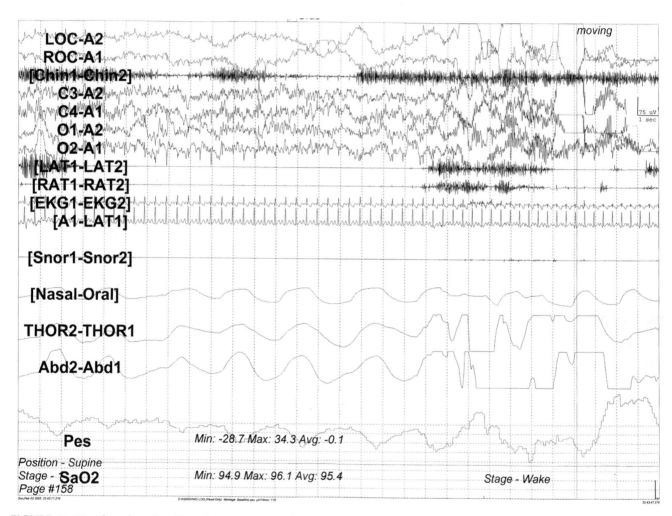

FIGURE 13–21. *Sleep-disordered breathing: Pes crescendo.*

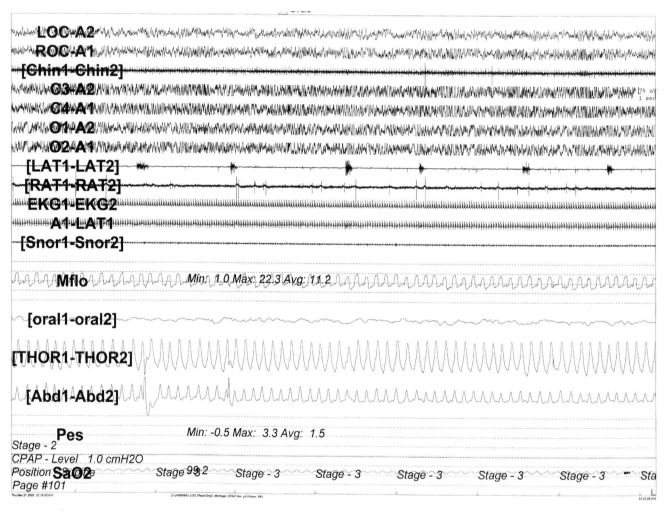

FIGURE 13–22. *PLMS.*

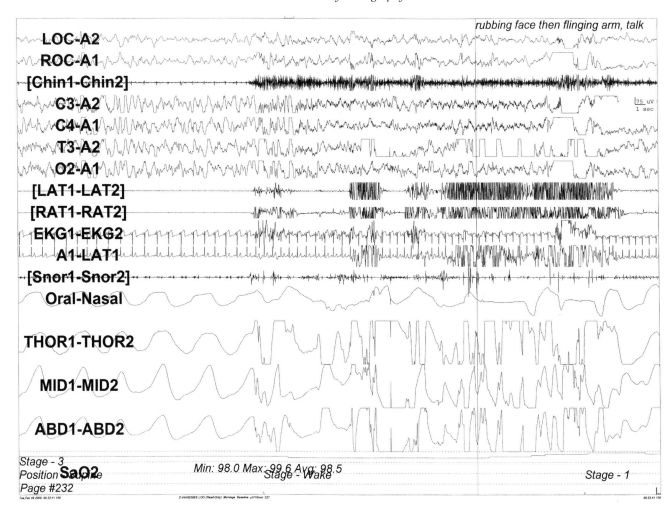

FIGURE 13–23. *Parasomnias: non-REM arousal disorders.*

Bruxism

Bruxism is thought to affect between 4 percent and 6 percent of children but has not been well studied in the pediatric population. This 30-second epoch (Figure 13–24) was recorded in an 11-year-old boy being evaluated for suspected sleep apnea. The episodic tooth grinding recorded causes prominent rhythmic EMG artifact at a rate of 1 to 1.5 hertz in the chin and EEG leads.

Electroencephalography Abnormalities during Polysomnography

Interictal Spikes

Because epilepsy affects approximately 1 percent of children and since sleep often activates epileptiform discharges on EEG, interictal spikes (20 to 70 milliseconds) or sharp waves (70 to 200 milliseconds) are sometimes encountered during PSG. This 30-second epoch (Figure

13–25) was recorded in a 12-year-old girl with tuberous sclerosis and complex partial seizures whose routine EEG had been normal. Spike discharges are seen most frequently in the C3-A2 and O1 leads and independently in the O2-A1 and LOC-A2 leads. The multifocal activity seen in this recording was most prominent in light non-REM sleep with almost complete suppression during REM sleep.

Electrographic Seizure

This 30-second epoch (Figure 13–26) was recorded in a 4-year-old girl being treated with phenytoin for several prior seizures of left parasagittal onset as documented by prior EEG studies. Although she had been clinically seizure-free on treatment for several months before PSG was performed for investigation of suspected OSA, the PSG recorded a 3-minute seizure in which the only clinical manifestation was a brief period of eye

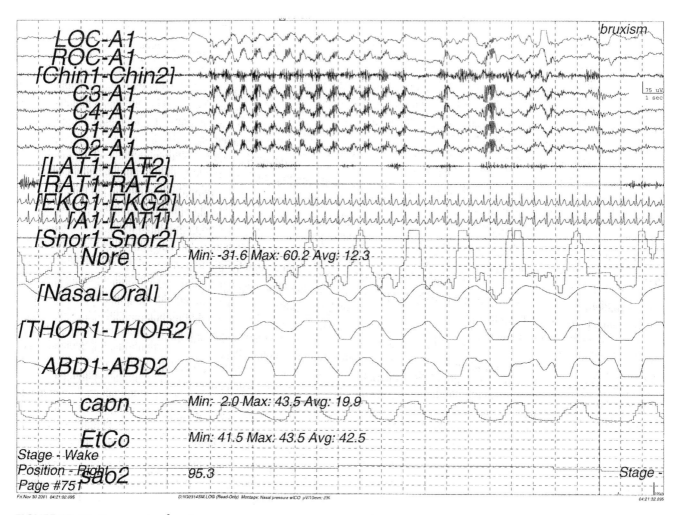

FIGURE 13–24. *Parasomnias: bruxism.*

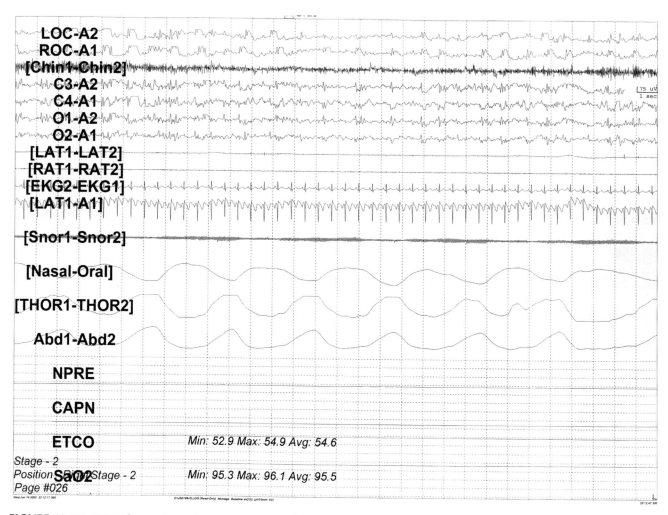

FIGURE 13–25. *EEG abnormalities during PSG: interictal spikes.*

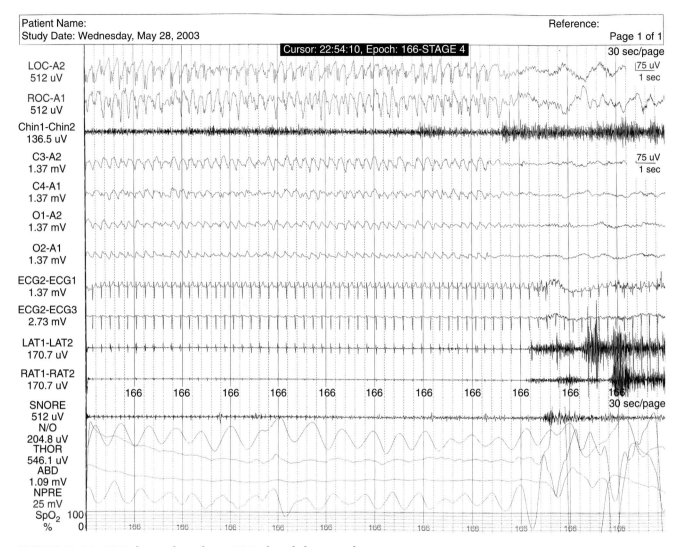

FIGURE 13–26. *EEG abnormalities during PSG: clinical-electrographic seizure.*

opening. The seizure commenced with the gradual development of the rhythmic delta slowing demonstrated on the limited EEG montage used for the study. The higher amplitudes apparent in the C3-A2 channel are consistent with the localization demonstrated on previous full EEG studies. Interestingly, clearly recognizable spike-wave discharges were apparent only late in the seizure and were prominent only in the eye leads, as seen in this epoch. The last 3 seconds of the epoch demonstrate abrupt termination of the seizure accompanied by arousal.

Cardiac Abnormalities during Polysomnography

Ventricular Ectopy

This 30-second segment (Figure 13–27) demonstrates frequent ventricular ectopy in a 2-year-old boy with upper airway resistance syndrome and no other known risk factors for cardiac disease. Although ventricular ectopy and dysrhythmias have been reported in adults with sleep-related breathing disorders, this association has not been well studied in children.

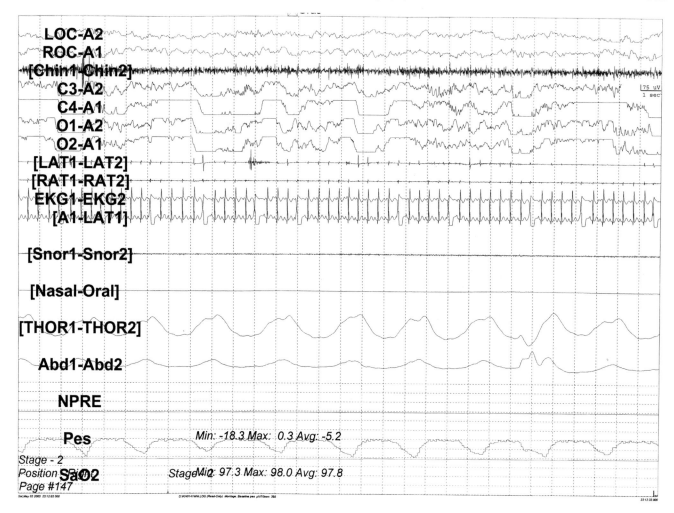

FIGURE 13–27. *Cardiac abnormalities during PSG: ventricular ectopy.*

BIBLIOGRAPHY

Anders T, Emdee A, et al. *A Manual of Standardized Terminology, Techniques, and Criteria for Scoring of States of Sleep and Wakefulness in Newborn Infants.* Los Angeles: UCLA Brain Information Service, NINDS Neurological Information Network, 1971.

Beran RG, Plunkett MJ, et al. Interface of epilepsy and sleep disorders. *Seizure* 1999;8(2):97–102.

Carroll JL, Loughlin GM. Diagnostic criteria for obstructive sleep apnea syndrome in children. *Pediatr Pulmonol* 1992;14:71–74.

Carroll JL, Loughlin GM. Obstruct sleep apnea syndrome in infants and children: Diagnosis and management. In Ferber R, Kryger M, eds. *Principles and Practice of Sleep Medicine in the Child.* Philadelphia: WB Saunders, 1995.

Crabtree VM, Ivanenko A, et al. Periodic limb movement disorder of sleep in children. *J Sleep Res* 2003;12(1):73–81.

Guilleminault C, Pelayo R, et al. Recognition of sleep-disordered breathing in children. *Pediatrics* 1996;98(5):871–882.

Kohrman MH, Carney PR. Sleep-related disorders in neurologic disease during childhood. *Pediatr Neurol* 2000;23(2):107–113.

Laberge L, Tremblay RE, et al. Development of parasomnias from childhood to early adolescence. *Pediatrics* 2000; 106(1 Pt 1):67–74.

Marcus C L, Hamer A, et al. Natural history of primary snoring in children.[see comment]. *Pediatr Pulmonol* 1998;26(1):6–11.

Marcus CL, Keens TG, et al. Obstructive sleep apnea in children with Down syndrome. *Pediatrics* 1991;88(1):132–139.

Marcus CL, Omlin KJ, et al. Normal polysomnographic values for children and adolescents. *Am Rev Respir Dis* 1992; 146(5 Pt 1):1235–1239.

Ng DK, Kwok KL, et al. Habitual snoring and sleep bruxism in a paediatric outpatient population in Hong Kong. *Singapore Med J* 2002;43(11):554–546.

Picchietti DL, Walters AS. Moderate to severe periodic limb movement disorder in childhood and adolescence. *Sleep* 1999;22(3):297–300.

Rosen C L, D'Andrea L, et al. Adult criteria for obstructive sleep apnea do not identify children with serious obstruction. [see comment]. *Am Rev Respir Dis* 1992;146(5 Pt 1):1231–1234.

Ward SL, Marcus CL. Obstructive sleep apnea in infants and young children. *J Clin Neurophysiol* 1996;13(3):198–207.

Index